HEALTHCARE FUNDING AND CHRISTIAN ETHICS

Healthcare has an impact on everyone, and healthcare funding decisions shape how and what healthcare is provided. In this book, Stephen Duckett outlines a Christian, biblically grounded, ethical basis for how decisions about healthcare funding and priority setting ought to be made. Taking a cue from the parable of the Good Samaritan (Luke 10:25–37), Duckett articulates three ethical principles drawn from the story: compassion as a motivator; inclusivity, or social justice as to benefits; and responsible stewardship of the resources required to achieve the goals of treatment and prevention. These are principles, he argues, that should underpin a Christian ethic of healthcare funding. Duckett's book is a must for healthcare professionals and theologians struggling with moral questions about rationing in healthcare. It is also relevant to economists interested in the strengths and weaknesses of the application of their discipline to health policy.

STEPHEN DUCKETT is affiliated with the Religion and Social Policy Network, University of Divinity, and is an honorary professor in the School of Population and Global Health, University of Melbourne. An Australian health economist, with a career that spans academic and senior management and policy roles in healthcare in Australia and Canada, he is a Fellow of the Academy of the Social Sciences in Australia and of the Australian Academy of Health and Medical Sciences.

NEW STUDIES IN CHRISTIAN ETHICS

Christian ethics has increasingly assumed a central place within academic theology. At the same time the growing power and ambiguity of modern science and the rising dissatisfaction within the social sciences about claims to value neutrality have prompted renewed interest in ethics within the secular academic world. There is, therefore, a need for studies in Christian ethics which, as well as being concerned with the relevance of Christian ethics to the present-day secular debate, are well informed about parallel discussions in recent philosophy, science, or social science. New Studies in Christian Ethics aims to provide books that do this at the highest intellectual level and demonstrate that Christian ethics can make a distinctive contribution to this debate – either in moral substance or in terms of underlying moral justifications titles published in the series

1. *Rights and Christian Ethics*, Kieran Cronin
2. *Biblical Interpretation and Christian Ethics*, Ian McDonald
3. *Power and Christian Ethics*, James Mackey
4. *Plurality and Christian Ethics*, Ian S. Markham
5. *Moral Action and Christian Ethics*, Jean Porter
6. *Responsibility and Christian Ethics*, William Schweiker
7. *Justice and Christian Ethics*, E. Clinton Gardner
8. *Feminism and Christian Ethics*, Susan Parsons
9. *Sex, Gender and Christian Ethics*, Lisa Sowle Cahill
10. *The Environment and Christian Ethics*, Michael Northcott
11. *Concepts of Person and Christian Ethics*, Stanley Rudman
12. *Priorities and Christian Ethics*, Garth Hallett
13. *Community, Liberalism and Christian Ethics*, David Fergusson

(continued after the index)

HEALTHCARE FUNDING AND CHRISTIAN ETHICS

STEPHEN DUCKETT
University of Divinity
and
University of Melbourne

CAMBRIDGE
UNIVERSITY PRESS

CAMBRIDGE
UNIVERSITY PRESS

Shaftesbury Road, Cambridge CB2 8EA, United Kingdom

One Liberty Plaza, 20th Floor, New York, NY 10006, USA

477 Williamstown Road, Port Melbourne, VIC 3207, Australia

314–321, 3rd Floor, Plot 3, Splendor Forum, Jasola District Centre, New Delhi – 110025, India

103 Penang Road, #05–06/07, Visioncrest Commercial, Singapore 238467

Cambridge University Press is part of Cambridge University Press & Assessment, a department of the University of Cambridge.

We share the University's mission to contribute to society through the pursuit of education, learning, and research at the highest international levels of excellence.

www.cambridge.org
Information on this title: www.cambridge.org/9781009260664

DOI: 10.1017/9781009260640

First published 2023

A catalogue record for this publication is available from the British Library.

Library of Congress Cataloging-in-Publication Data
NAMES: Duckett, S. J., author.
TITLE: Healthcare funding and Christian ethics / Stephen Duckett, School of Population and Global Health, University of Melbourne.
DESCRIPTION: Cambridge, United Kingdom ; New York, NY, USA : Cambridge University Press, 2022. | Series: New studies in Christian ethics | Includes bibliographical references and index.
IDENTIFIERS: LCCN 2022023432 | ISBN 9781009260664 (hardback) | ISBN 9781009260640 (ebook)
SUBJECTS: LCSH: Medical ethics – Religious aspects – Christianity. | Medical economics – Religious aspects – Christianity.
CLASSIFICATION: LCC R725.56 .D83 2022 | DDC 174.2–dc23/eng/20220826
LC record available at https://lccn.loc.gov/2022023432

ISBN 978-1-009-26066-4 Hardback

Contents

Tables

General Editor's Preface

Stephen Duckett is a world-class healthcare economist who has been a lay reader within the Anglican Church of Australia for many years and, nearing retirement, enrolled for a doctorate in theology awarded by the Archbishop of Canterbury's unique Lambeth Research Degree Program. It has been a joy to work closely with him on this programme and to watch him bringing his two academic worlds together in this stellar contribution to New Studies in Christian Ethics. It joins and adds to the two much-praised contributions to the series of Albino Barrera – *Economic Compulsion and Christian Ethics* (2005) and *Market Complicity and Christian Ethics* (2011). Remarkably, it also adds something new to that most intractable of problems in healthcare ethics – how to justify prioritising (or, more bluntly, rationing) funding for one form of medical intervention over another.

His ambition is no less than to build upon and extend the current dominant paradigm of healthcare funding, arguing that economic evaluation needs to sit in tension with the theologically grounded principles of compassion, social justice, and stewardship. He achieves this magnificently with an extended demonstration that, properly understood, healthcare funding should not simply be about hard choices in healthcare – although he recognises and addresses those – but ought 'to change the way health economics lives in the real world of patients, practitioners and politicians, transforming health economics from a detached calculating machine to a discipline which engages with identifiable, rather than simply statistical lives' by including compassion, social justice, and stewardship within its discipline.

I cannot think of any other book within Christian ethics that addresses this key and timely topic within healthcare ethics with similar authority and comprehensiveness. Both his doctoral examiners and his Cambridge University Press anonymous reviewers unanimously confirmed that this work is authoritative, scholarly (in both economics and theology), original, and accessible (even to non-economists). In short, this is a monograph that admirably matches the exacting academic standards required by Lambeth Palace, Cambridge University Press, and the interdisciplinary expectations of New Studies in Christian Ethics, namely:

(1) To promote monographs in Christian ethics which engage centrally with the present secular moral debate at the highest possible intellectual level.
(2) To encourage contributors to demonstrate that Christian ethics can make a distinctive contribution to this debate – either in moral substance or in terms of underlying moral justifications.

ROBIN GILL

Acknowledgements

This book had a distal origin: I was interested in exploring theodicy and enrolled in a research degree to provide some structure around my reading and thinking about that topic. That slowly morphed into issues of funding palliative care before broadening to the theology of healthcare funding generally. The latter topic was more suited to my Monday to Friday 'day job' as a health economist, but the quest was really about a discomfort with how the field of health economics had evolved, and what was prioritised and what was not.

I was guided in this journey by my thesis supervisor, the Rev'd Canon Emeritus Professor Robin Gill, who was identified by the Lambeth programme as having the right background and skills to supervise my research. I am incredibly grateful for that introduction. Robin encouraged, prodded, challenged, and stimulated me to focus my research on what became a PhD thesis with the degree awarded by the Archbishop of Canterbury, and subsequently this book. I am extremely grateful for Robin's support along the way.

The Dalton McCaughey Library was an invaluable resource for references to browse and borrow.

I prevailed on some friends and colleagues to read and comment on drafts of the thesis or the book: Robert Dixon, Stephanie Dowrick, Maureen Gleeson (RSM), John Goss, and Helen Lapsley. Their comments helped to clarify my thoughts or writing (or both) and thus strengthened this final product, and I thank them for the time they committed to commenting. I also benefited from comments of the thesis examiners and the anonymous referees from Cambridge University Press. The good feedback I received from two presentations to the Religion and Social Policy Network of the University of Divinity, and to the seminar days of the Lambeth Research Degrees in Theology programme, was also very helpful.

Terri Jackson also read the whole thesis, chapter by chapter, made detailed grammatical suggestions, challenged lack of intellectual clarity, and raised issues of logic and ambiguity. Ours is a great partnership and I am very grateful for her support during this period. I would also like to thank our daughter Sarah for tolerating my discussing these issues with her in our interactions.

Author's Note

Unless otherwise stated, all biblical excerpts are from the New Revised Standard Version. Language and spelling in quotations have been retained throughout.

CHAPTER 1

Ethics and Health Economics

Health economics deals with critical questions of life and death, or as Victor Fuchs (1998) phrased it, *Who Shall Live?* Health economics, as with the broader discipline of economics within which it sits, addresses questions of priority and choice. The alchemy of health economics is that it transforms policy decisions from questions of politics and values to technocratic ones, where arcane formulae yield answers with impressive precision about, for example, which drug should be funded from the public purse and for whom. This magic is, of course, a trick: the values do not magically disappear; they are simply obscured from view (Harvard, Werker, and Silva 2020; Romer 2020). In this book, I bring values back into the foreground, identifying three value-based and theologically informed principles that should shape healthcare funding decisions: compassion, social justice, and stewardship.

'When Christians reflect seriously about how to live, they inevitably appeal to Scripture' (Spohn 2005, 93). This book is about *Christian* ethics, in that sense, appealing to Scripture. It draws particularly on a key teaching of Jesus, the parable of the Good Samaritan. It is also about how to live, as it focuses on how people and communities ought to make moral choices and judge their actions, those of others, and the states of affairs in the world (Gustafson 1986).

Specifically, I explore the ethical basis for policy choices and make an argument about what Christian ethical principles should inform healthcare funding decisions – even in multi-faith or secular contexts – and how to apply those principles in practice. It sits at the intersection of ethics, health policy, and economics, developing ethical principles to inform healthcare funding and payment policies.

In this introductory chapter, I address the question: why a theology of healthcare funding? Why is the interrelationship of healthcare funding and Christian ethics important? I will start by discussing health economics generally, what it misses, and what a theology of healthcare funding can contribute. The second part of the chapter will develop a theology of healthcare funding that will be expanded throughout the book.

The Utilitarian Frame of Conventional Economics

Adam Smith, considered one of the founders of economics, famously argued that business owners are led by workings of an invisible hand to actions that are in the public interest (Smith 1775/1979, 456). Although this invisible hand is usually interpreted as market magic, Smith might also have had in mind the action of divine providence (Oslington 2012). Indeed, Waterman argues that one can read Smith's *Wealth of Nations* as a work of (natural) theology where 'God/Nature does not merely wind up "the great machine" and leave it ticking .... She continues to act in various ways, but always wisely and well, so as to make creative use of human folly and wickedness in ways that bring good out of evil' (Waterman 2002, 919; 2004, 105).

Smith posited that the workings of the economy did not rely on altruism or other motivations of those involved, but rather the market and its potential provided the incentive for commerce and interchange: 'It is not from the benevolence of the butcher, the brewer, or the baker, that we expect our dinner, but from their regard to their own interest. We address ourselves, not to their humanity but to their self-love, and never talk to them of our own necessities but of their advantages' (Smith 1775/1979, 26–27).

Smith is talking here about motivations for engaging in the market (Sen 1993); this is not his only view of the totality of a human, nor even *Homo economicus*. Indeed, Smith – especially in later editions of his *Theory of Moral Sentiments* – saw people as moral beings, who make values-based judgements about how they interact with other people (Chen 2017). He argues that they worry both about the consequences of their actions and how they interact with those with whom they trade.

In Smith's view, traders were concerned with whether their actions were morally appropriate, that is, whether their actions were undertaken with a 'sense of propriety quite distinct from the perception of utility' (Smith 1759/1979, 188), perhaps influenced by the 'culture of politeness' expected in contemporary society (Chen 2017, 51). At the time Smith was writing the world of business and the market was seen to be bound by moral codes, for example, the Westminster Larger Catechism (Howe 2013). All traders – and indeed everyone – should, according to Smith, be expected to act with propriety, and some, worthy of praise, would go beyond that minimum standard, to act with 'virtue' (Waszek 1984). Smith is not positing a value-free world of naked self-interest, but rather a world where economic decisions are taken within a social and moral context.

It was the same Adam Smith who wrote both the *Wealth of Nations* and the *Theory of Moral Sentiments*; these works are not in conflict (Newbert 2018), but rather *Theory* provides a framework for *Wealth* and creates a context within which the narrower, exchange-oriented market ought to work. A framework focusing on utility and one on propriety are not in conflict; both can be part of the same world (Otteson 2015). However, voracious greed is not part of that world: Smith put the benefits (or utility) derived from market interactions into perspective, with people responding to a moral compass, a 'man within', to guide towards what is honourable and noble (Chen 2017). He 'decried selfishness often and at length' (Wight 2005, 46), and core to Smith's view was that 'man does not live by self-interest alone' (Bhagwati 2011, 163).

For Smith, human interactions are critically important: 'the chief part of human happiness arises from the consciousness of being beloved' (Smith 1759/1979, 41). Modern economists might term this as suggesting an 'extra-welfarist' approach where the objective of policy is more than simply adding up the utility gains of individuals (Culyer 1989; Richardson and McKie 2005; but see Birch and Donaldson 2003): that there is something extra involved in human interaction, of which 'being beloved' is but one example.

Although theology and economics – the latter initially 'political economy' – happily coexisted for their first century or so together, 'in the twentieth century they went their separate ways and are no longer on speaking terms' (Waterman 2004, 1). Even as late as the first decades of the twentieth century, economics still had a profound social and moral flavour, as leading economists linked the field to the contemporary 'social gospel' movement (Bateman 1998; Bateman and Kapstein 1999).

Alas, this ethical and principled basis of economics has been all but forgotten, especially in the last fifty years, as economics suffered 'physics envy' (Mirowski 1992; Bateman 1998), attempting to emulate the physical sciences (Lang 2008) and postulate laws that predict behaviours (Mirowski 1991, 1992). As Nobel laureate Amartya Sen has noted: 'the nature of modern economics has been substantially impoverished by the distance that has grown between economics and ethics' (Sen 1987, 7), with the discipline essentially forgetting what the late former Commonwealth Chief Rabbi Jonathan Sacks phrased so succinctly: 'markets need morals' (Sacks 2020, 94).

Nelson is probably close to Smith in rejecting 'commodity exchange as economic and asocial'. She argues that we can repair the split of economics and morality 'if we start instead by considering any exchange as a creative event, a world-creating activity that carries ethical meaning as much as it carries any other significance' (Nelson 2003, 139).

I am remiss in my personal life in not acknowledging the humanity of every person who assists me in a retail or hospitality exchange, denying the ethical meaning of that 'creative event', and certainly the reduction of human involvement through the automation of commodity exchanges (self-service) has ethical challenges (Bulmer, Elms, and Moore 2018; Andrews 2020). Nelson challenges all of us, and especially economists, to again write the human and ethical into our considerations.

This split – between the ethical domain and the economics project – has been exacerbated by the increased use of mathematical abstraction, as the utilitarian 'moral calculus' of Bentham (Brunius 1958; Baujard 2009) is replaced in economics journals by a calculus that cannot incorporate morals into the functional form, and this despite initial quantification efforts serving a moral purpose (Bateman 2001). The increasing abstraction and contemporary 'research methods of economists lead them away from social and spiritual concerns' (Havrilesky 1993, 33).

The science of economics has increasingly employed abstract mathematical precision, underpinned by assumptions about human behaviour, assumptions increasingly challenged by emerging understandings from behavioural economics (Angner 2016; Dhami 2016; Boyd 2020).

Economics originated as a science of individual choice, but economics techniques have been adapted to inform discussion of government and societal priorities. This move from individual choices based on individual values and utility assessments to societal application comes with risks, which is where a theology of healthcare funding can contribute.

In practice, the dominant calculus of health economics is utilitarian – how to get the greatest good for the greatest number, taking into account both the costs and the benefits of a health intervention broadly defined. As a person trained in neoclassical economics, I am steeped in this neoliberal economic orthodoxy – that a society's welfare is optimised when resource allocation decisions in healthcare and other sectors use a utilitarian frame, and trade-offs are informed by consideration of the total welfare gain from social investments. The neoliberal orthodoxy recognises a reality that policy decisions must be made, and it is better if those decisions are more (economically) rational than less. There are a number of challenges to this orthodoxy, including the political question of who gets what (Lasswell 1936).

Economics as the Science of Scarcity

Lionel Robbins, a famous British economist of the middle decades of the last century, described economics as a science of scarcity. Although initially contested (Backhouse and Medema 2009), Robbins' description has slowly come to be accepted as definitive. In *An Essay on the Nature and Significance of Economic Science*, which has been described as 'one of the most influential books on economic science that has been written in the 20th century' (Falgueras-Sorauren 2009), Robbins described the economic endeavour thus: 'Economics is the science which studies human behaviour as a relationship between ends and scarce means which have alternative uses' (Robbins 1932, 15).

Central to Robbins' definition is the recognition of scarcity, and that, when resources in the economy are fully employed, this forces choice. The definition incorporates the concept of opportunity cost: that if resources are used for one purpose, they are not available for use for another purpose.

Much of Robbins' explication of his definition related to individual behaviour, but he also recognised that the scarcity problem was one faced by governments in their allocation decisions. Governments face the same problems of scarcity as individuals: 'the same limitations of means in relation to ends as behaviour within the (exchange) economy' (Robbins 1932, 19). Although for Robbins choice is best seen in the way that *individuals* exercise choice, it can also apply to broader exercises of choice such as by government and there is therefore no reason that governments should make their decisions on some different bases. This in turn led to the idea that one could aggregate individual preferences or utilities into an overall 'social welfare' function, which social policies should optimise (Harsanyi 1955).

For Robbins, 'economics is entirely neutral between ends' (Robbins 1932, 23); that is, economic science does not value London as a destination differently from Melbourne, or health outcomes differently from education outcomes. Essentially, the economics project is to create a way of understanding why individuals make particular choices, and from there, to postulate that an individual's welfare is maximised if choices are exercised in line with their rational ordering of options. The rational ordering makes fungible what might previously have been seen as impossible to compare, such as a new drug compared to a preventive intervention, to achieve the best health gains for the community.

At least according to Robbins, economics is not about the ends, nor about the environment in which choice is made, but rather is about the relationship between means to achieve a given end, that is the end is exogenous and economics assumes the end and determines the optimal means to that end (Robbins 1932, 37). If an individual has decided that Melbourne is the preferred destination, or government has decided to pursue health gains over education as part of budget priority setting, economics is about the relative merits of various means to achieve these ends.

However, what is an 'end' is not as clear cut as Robbins might assume: is an end 'reduction in hip pain' and the economic project is what are the best ways of achieving that, or is the end able to be phrased more broadly, 'improving health outcomes' or 'improving social welfare from public funding'? Economics now legitimately contributes to these broader questions which Robbins might have defined as choices among ends (e.g. investing in cancer treatment versus arthritis, or health versus housing).

Although Robbins cautions against aggregating individual preferences into a social calculus, economics is now recognised as being able to contribute to the rational ordering of society's preferences, rather than being limited to being a science of individual behaviour. Economics is now used to inform decision-makers about the consequences of choices about different means of achieving ends such as maximising health outcomes.

According to Robbins' logic, economics will not help in deciding among broad policy goals, as these are value choices. Rather economics, as a science of scarcity, helps decision-makers understand the consequences of these choices, and specifically, helps decision-makers choose among means to the desired ends. Values are assumed only to impinge on the choice of ends, outside the economist's domain, and the path to the ends is untrammelled by any consideration of values.

Robbins argues that economics, which deals with 'ascertainable facts', and ethics, which deals with 'valuations and obligations', are 'not on the same plane of discourse' (Robbins 1932, 132). For Robbins, economics is a neutral science, specifically neutral between ends; its focus is on evaluation and choices between means.

However, this approach is contested (Falgueras-Sorauren 2009; Sen 2017), including by another economics great, John Maynard Keynes (Davis 1991; Atkinson 2009a, 2009b), who wrote in 1938:

> I want to emphasise strongly the point about economics being a moral science. I mentioned before that it deals with introspection and with values. I might have added that it deals with motives, expectations, psychological uncertainties. One has to be constantly on guard against treating the material as constant and homogeneous in the same way that the material of the other sciences, in spite of its complexity, is constant and homogeneous. It is as though the fall of the apple to the ground depended on the

> apple's motives, on whether it is worth while falling to the ground, and whether the ground wanted the apple to fall, and on mistaken calculations on the part of the apple as to how far it was from the centre of the earth. (Keynes 1978, 300)

So, for Keynes, it is the subject matter of economics, dealing with human behaviour, that makes it, and its considerations, fall into the moral realm.

It is increasingly recognised that economic evaluation and priority setting is 'a quintessentially ethical endeavour' (McKie and Richardson 2003, 2417). Economists have come to recognise that aggregating individual preferences and valuations involves assumptions about the relative value that society might place on an additional year of life in pain or not for a 3-year-old, a 35-year-old, and a 95-year-old, and so the application of economics to social policy now inherently involves value choices. Every economic evaluation makes some assumptions about these valuations, some more explicitly than others. There are also technical issues associated with summing individual utilities, and the underlying assumptions of utilitarianism in terms of how and whether individual utilities can be combined is contested (Sen 1979, 2000, 2017). But despite these critiques, the utilitarian flavour of economics continues to dominate, and no effective alternative has achieved wide acceptance.

The utilitarian frame, which is at the basis of the economist's advice, is consequentialist: it assumes a rational ordering of the consequences of means or strategies to achieve an end, with those consequences typically measured in terms of the costs to achieve those outcomes. It tells us nothing about the process of getting to that end, nor who falls by the wayside on that journey (Van Staveren 2007). Distributional consequences are ignored, absurdly so as Williams argues:

> In this light, utilitarianism does emerge as absurdly primitive, and it is much too late in the day to be told that questions of equitable or inequitable distribution do not matter because utilitarianism has no satisfactory way of making them matter. On the criterion of maximising average utility, there is nothing to choose between any two states of society which involve the same number of people sharing the same aggregate amount of utility, even if in one of them it is relatively evenly distributed while on the other a very small number have a very great deal of it; and it is just silly to say that in fact there is nothing to choose here. (Williams 1973, 142–143)

The optimal distribution of resources occurs if 'no one can be made better off without at least one other person being made worse off' (Culyer 2005, 250), a condition known as Pareto optimality. Utilitarians would address the criticism of distributional consequences by arguing that those who gain *could* compensate those who lose in a trade-off so that Pareto optimality might potentially occur, a so-called Kaldor–Hicks improvement. In fact, under the Kaldor–Hicks criterion, the compensation does not actually have to occur, but a hypothetical compensation is enough so that Pareto optimality is possible: the group that gains could potentially compensate the group that loses sufficiently for it to be acceptable. However, this assumes no malevolence by the winners (Boulding 1969) and in fact such a compensation is one of the unicorns of economics, much talked about but never seen.

The utilitarian calculus sums the utility of individual gains from transactions and assumes that the individual is an autonomous economic unit. In fact, each person is a person in community; the person gains benefit from exchanges, but the person also gains benefit from seeing others benefit, whether or not they are part of that exchange. As Camosy (2012, 234) has argued 'one's own interest cannot easily be separated from what is in others' interest – and *vice versa*'; Hollenbach (2002, 1) goes further to argue that 'the good of the individual and the common good are inseparable'.

Homo economicus, the economist's creation of an egoist, rational, utility-maximising individual unit with no social interaction with others, is a fiction and always has been (Doucouliagos 1994; Thaler 2000; Ailon 2020). It is a theoretical abstraction where community becomes 'so little emphasised that it shrivels up and all persons become individuals in exchange relationships' (Meeks 1989, 112).

Humans have always existed in social units – both small and large – with commitments to those social units affecting their ordering of preferences (Sen 1977). An individual in a family unit may see their own utility and that of their family unit as indistinguishable in many aspects: the common good of the unit and the good of the individual are one and the same. As noted earlier, Adam Smith identified the motivation of participating in a market as being self-interest, but he also knew that the individual is broader than self-interest and has a broader life outside a market.

Economics neglects this point: that individuals participate in markets, but they also participate in and create communities which are not commodifiable (Sandel 2012), and societies not dominated by transactional, dyadic exchanges but which are communities of trust (Hollis 1998). Communities create different exchanges, not simply mutual reciprocity, one person exchanging with another and each gaining utility, but also engage in 'univocal reciprocity' involving more than three persons where the participants 'do not benefit each other directly but only indirectly' (Ekeh 1974, 48).

The utilitarian calculus copes poorly once the intrinsic connection between self-love – maximising one's own utility independently of all others – and neighbour love is recognised (Camosy 2012, 234). It may be possible to shoehorn the utility from seeing others benefit into the equation, but it will always be an uncomfortable fit. The utilitarian calculus is important to assess the (economic) value of an intervention, but this calculus must be considered within a broader moral and community framework, where interventions are designed not only to affect individual behaviour but also the way that communities work together (Shiell and Hawe 1996).

Economics' assumption that humans are simply individual units, deemphasising community, and its ubiquitous use in policymaking, comes at a cost as *Homo economicus* crowds out other manifestations of what it is to be human. Economics in this sense changes the world it is studying and makes it even more important that the underlying values of economics are made transparent (Boulding 1969).

The Alternative Frame: Economics as a Moral Science

Society is complex. Decision-makers are not generally faced with deciding about how to achieve one goal only, but also more often the choice is how much we emphasise this goal as against another one, or how much does achievement of this goal compromise achievement of an alternative goal.

Although Tinbergen has shown that decision-makers need to have a separate instrument or policy for each goal (Tinbergen 1952, 27), decision-makers rarely have that luxury. A decision to subsidise a particular drug, for example, has both a cost – including an opportunity cost that some other policy cannot be pursued – and a distribution of benefits. Funding the drug is therefore both a 'health' decision and a social justice one. Because the drug must be paid for somehow, it has economic implications too.

Despite Robbins' claim, economics involves implicit assumptions that are value-laden:

- If a cost-effectiveness study does not explicitly highlight the distribution of costs and benefits, it is implicitly conveying the message that the distribution is not a relevant issue.
- If the design of a population-funding formula fails to include a factor relating to unemployment because it cannot be measured at the relevant geographical level, that is sending a message that the costs of better measurement are not worth the improved equity of the formula.

- If nursing home funding allows money ostensibly allocated for care to be leached out as extra returns to owners, then quality is assumed to be not a concern of the payer.
- A system design that places a higher monetary reward on cosmetic surgery to reshape body parts solely to improve appearance compared to the monetary reward for caring for older patients and people with mental illness sends a signal about the value to be placed on care for the marginalised.
- If provider payment policy incorporates compulsory co-payments, which result in consumer bankruptcies or significant missed care, then equity has been prioritised below provider incomes or long-term system efficiency.

There are moral and value choices inherent in each of these examples, with the hidden assumption rarely unveiled to test whether the economists (or policy advisers) who make the choices are in fact reflecting society's rational ordering, or whether they are simply reflecting their own unquestioned biases.

Because public policy decisions inherently involve value choices (Muers 2020), in its contribution to public policy, economics becomes a 'moral science' (Boulding 1969; Alvey 1999, 2000; Atkinson 2009a). This is all the more true for health policy and health economics, where the decisions involve quintessentially moral decisions about life and death choices. Health economics inevitably involves moral choices about how much priority should be accorded to the other, how much should healthcare be funded from the public purse, and indeed what should be the ethos or underpinning of healthcare policy delivery.

However, these moral choices mostly remain implicit (Harvard, Werker, and Silva 2020), with health economists exercising power by shaping what is included in the policy calculus and the way trade-offs are presented, or in Lukes' terms, what is on the agenda of policy and what is not (Lukes 1974, 2009). Shaping the choice set can occur by ignoring some possibilities, potentially because of measurement or modelling issues, and what is presented in the results. However, a decision – explicit or implicit – not to address an issue is as critical as a decision to address an issue (Bachrach and Baratz 1963) and equally involves assumptions about what is important and what is not.

Robbins may be right though. Economics is not well equipped to determine issues such as what should be society's priorities, what is the value to be placed on unfettered choice, and the value to be placed on ensuring no one is left behind. Typically, the response is that economics highlights the implication of choices. Unfortunately, all too often this highlighting of the implications of recommendations and assumptions does not occur, and, similarly, potential adverse or unintended consequences are de-emphasised (Merton 1936).

The field of health economics has a very broad remit (Culyer and Newhouse 2000), but health economics textbooks generally move quickly into the standard microeconomics of supply and demand curves in the first or second chapter. Market and quasi-market framing are core, with the underlying individualistic assumption that individuals seek to maximise their utility through their market participation. The value questions are rarely highlighted.

Health economists' analyses and model choices sit within a context. In democracies, health policy decisions, with healthcare funding at the core of these, are inevitably shaped by the values of society and its decision-makers. Health economics is mostly silent on these values and their implications. But just as health economics is about clarifying for decision-makers the costs and benefits of choices, it should also acknowledge to decision-makers that health economics is a moral science, that values are core to what it does, and that the health economics calculus is one which involves moral choices, moral underpinnings, and outcomes with moral consequences.

Public health advocates, including health economists, have long recognised the importance of social determinants of health – for example, racism, ageism, poverty, unemployment, and homelessness (Evans, Barer, and Marmor 1994; Marmot 2005a, 2005b, 2020; Commission on Social Determinants of Health 2008; Braveman, Egerter, and Williams 2011; Marmot and Bell 2019; Mikton et al. 2021); commercial determinants of health – sugary drinks, coal, alcohol, and tobacco (Kickbusch, Allen, and Franz 2016; McKee and Stuckler 2018; Maani et al. 2020; Davies and Pearson-Stuttard 2021, Chapter 5) – are also critical. Davies and Pearson-Stuttard (2021, 7) have suggested the term 'drivers' rather than determinants, as the latter term suggests they are immutable, unchangeable, and outside our control. More recently, Berwick (2020) has identified the 'moral determinants of health', calling for a 'morally guided campaign' to build social solidarity, and address social determinants. Whether explicit or not, these determinants provide the context for research designs; choices to take these factors into account or ignore them are moral or value choices. Health economists need to ensure that their work clarifies the place of these contextual determinants, and to do so in such a way that their impact is clear in their conclusions and recommendations.

The Place of a Christian Ethic of Healthcare Funding

Health economics contributes primarily to improved decision-making on the assumption that the overall goals are somehow determined exogenously and within an overall agreed values framework. Most health economics texts and health technology assessments gloss over the implicit values within the models used, and certainly do not address where these implicit values come from. It is this which is missing from most approaches to the application of health economics to policy.

The failure to discuss and highlight the underlying values does not mean that the values are no longer there, just that they are obscured and, implicitly, not able to be challenged. The moral dimension is erased from consideration, consigned to be neither seen nor heard in health economics discourse, and an illegitimate topic of conversation among polite health economists. But this failure contributes to the hegemony that de-emphasises at best and ignores at worst distributions, and the 'collateral damage' of poorly designed funding rules and policies.

By implicitly constraining health economics debate within narrow utilitarian boundaries, health economists miss better engagement with the public about priorities and values, and potentially misrepresent the public's position on key factors informing choice. Ignoring the ethical dimension of their models' approaches and results means that health economists may be inadvertently led to recommendations that are antithetical to society's 'rational ordering of priorities', which is not where Robbins encouraged us to be.

Every health economist starts by thinking about what questions they are to address. Will they focus on pharmaco-economics, insurance design, or valuing health states? Whatever area of health economics, there are choices to be made about techniques. The field of economic evaluation is but one example where there is an ongoing contest about how to measure health states, how to value an additional year of life lived in a particular health state, and how to bring costs and benefits that accrue in the future together.

Choices about each of these involve a moral dimension, implicitly or explicitly. In some cases, there may be a Christian ethical dimension that comes into play. Theology does not provide a checklist about these moral dimensions, but it can provide a framework or scaffolding around the health economics project. A Christian ethic of healthcare funding can be used to fill in these lacunae of the health economics project and utilitarian economics generally, to consider properly the underlying values that should inform the choices of models and approaches.

Although many high-income countries pay obeisance to a Judeo-Christian ethical basis, Christianity is no longer the dominant force in any country, with the possible exception of the United States where a narrow range of public policy issues are the battleground for Christian fundamentalists (Collins 2019, 2), nor is it any longer a moral glue that holds societies together (Gill 2004, Chapter 6), but it remains a source of 'the creation of meaning and identity' in these countries and so public theology should be part of the public square (Habermas 2008, 131). Although theological discourse may be seen as a 'complicating factor' when it enters the public square (Hicks 2000, 94), Christian ethics has a legitimate role to play in informing debates and decisions in secular societies for two main reasons: one to do with the public square and the other to do with the role of Christians in providing healthcare.

Christians are called to participate in the wider world. We are to live and speak the values taught by Jesus two millennia ago, 'to act as a prophetic presence' in the world (Greek Orthodox Archdiocese of America 2020). The Christian contribution should not simply be a voice that relies on talking to other Christians, but it should be able to inform contemporary secular debates from a Christian perspective, whether in explicitly theological language or not. Indeed, the secular consensus in Western societies means that theological arguments in the public square may have greater traction if they are couched in secular terms (Rawls 1997; Habermas 2006), although exclusion of theological language 'unnecessarily impoverishes the resources for discourse in the public sphere' (Hicks 2000, 100). Public theology is thus often 'bilingual', speaking in both secular and sacred languages (Graham 2013). One can 'speak Christian' in many different ways, provided what is said is 'faithful to the language of Scripture' (Hauerwas 2011, 88). Christians should speak in 'one's own voice' (Volf 2011, 130–133), reflecting a serious interaction between ideas of 'good' and 'God' (Keeling 1998, 140) and potentially 'injecting "theological fragments" into public debate' (Forrester 1997, 200).

The 'connections and relation between secular and religious views of the world are more fluid than we sometimes suppose' (Selby 2014, 131), and so injecting a Christian perspective into policy debates may simply aim to reinforce aspects of the secular discussion. There will be areas of distinct difference, but there are also areas of common ground. As Camosy (2012) has shown, there are very many similarities in the conclusions reached by aggressively secular philosopher Peter Singer and Christian ethics. The differences are easy to identify: Singer and the Roman Catholic Church – the focus of Camosy's exploration – differ significantly on the policy about abortion, but according to Camosy, this disagreement is essentially about a quite narrow area, albeit a fundamental one, namely the moral status of the foetus and whether the foetus' potential should count when determining such status (Camosy 2012, 13). There are also very public differences between Singer and the church on issues such as euthanasia but again, Camosy (2012, Chapter 2) identifies areas of overlap such as in the use of brain death as an appropriate criterion.

But in the areas most relevant to exploring a Christian ethic of healthcare funding, the overlaps between Singer's views and those of Catholic social teaching are very great indeed with only minor differences on issues relating to the duties to the poor (Camosy 2012, Chapter 4) and ethical theory (Camosy 2012, Chapter 5).

The moral reasoning of Christian and secular ethicists and philosophers differs not in the groundwork that may be common, but in the fact that Christians accept and use an additional source of revelation (Gill 2004, 4; Novak 2019, Chapter 1) building on 'our own interaction with Scripture' (Gill 2004, 8) and Christian tradition. MacNamara (1998) makes the helpful distinction between differences in content, of which there are few, compared to differences in context. Deliberative democracy requires common ground, a recognition of common humanity, and the reasonableness of reciprocity (Hollenbach 2002, 144–145). This can be undermined by fissures in society, more driven, especially in the United States, by increasingly fractious and rigid political positionings than a Christian-secular divide.

Christians have no legitimacy to claim that they are the sole guardians of moral correctness, nor, in a secular society, that their views should be given greater weight than any others'. But Christians are called to share a revelation and are often more likely to call out questions of values and to do so in language that crosses political divides, and so emphasises common ground. Calling attention to underlying values may therefore be more likely to lead to an agreed consensus against which to judge policies. The Christian voice will often prioritise different things from the dominant discourse and draw attention to uncomfortable realities in the world we live in. This 'deliberate talk' may move society more in the direction of a Christian ethic (Hicks 2000, 246). But this prophetic voice, calling out injustices, is only part of the contributions Christians can make to public policy.

High-income democratic societies are no longer monocultural and certainly no longer share a common memory, but there is a common morality. In 'safe' discourse, this common morality is one of 'modest virtues' (Wolfe 1998, 126) about how we interact with each other every day, showing individual acts of kindness, and being honest. This 'morality writ small', to use Wolfe's language (Wolfe 1998, Chapter VII), is part of the glue that holds us together – it is part of recognising we are all human whatever our race, culture, or creed. Christians, of course, live by these same modest virtues, but the Christian contribution goes beyond that to larger calls of social justice and equity.

From its beginning Christianity has been an uncomfortable religion, not simply one of private morality, but one that seeks to change society. Not all Christians welcome that tradition with some 'complacent brands of Christianity which are quite comfortable with the *status quo* ... [standing] out as alien to its central thrust' (Esler 1998a, 7). A Christian contribution involves holding a mirror to society and pointing out the uncomfortable blemishes we would prefer not to see. Christians are called 'to the prophetic task of helping the world understand what it really is' (Benne 2011, 330). Christians are not called to exist in a safe, protected bubble, living in joyful hope of a transformed world to be ushered in sometime in the future reign of God. Rather, Christians are called to work to transform today's world so it has more of the attributes that Jesus pointed to in his teaching and in his life of 'selfless holiness' (Williams 2012, 13).

Jesus' own message was informed by and directed towards the very real social conditions of his day – conditions of poverty, debt, hunger, and injustice. His teaching 'spoke to an immediate need in concrete terms' (Oakman 2008, 201). We too are called to work to transform the contemporary reality 'from lesser approximations of the heavenly city to ones that come nearer to the good that is their ultimate hope' (Hollenbach 2002, 128). This is, and has always been, an inherently political task: 'Christianity was, from the outset, an inherently political, economically active and profoundly social faith. The expression of Christian faith always challenges the present world order, but is, at the same time, prepared to work within it, regarding nothing as being beyond redemption' (Percy 2014, xx).

This transformation we are called to should not await the eschatological return, but rather will occur through practical, incremental steps to address injustice today, and propose 'changes toward what should be made possible by concentrating on identifiable concrete problems of justice that are capable of being dealt with at present' (Mott 2011, 174).

In a utilitarian-driven world we might decide to ignore the plight of a very small minority, as improving their outcomes will only trivially affect the overall picture. An example might be the health of the Australian First Nations who account for about 2 per cent of the Australian population. In this world, even though there is a large and tragic difference in health status for First Nations people compared to other Australians – a gap that has not significantly improved over the last half century (Wilson, Zhao, and Condon 2019) – improving the health status of First Nations people will have little impact on overall *average* Australian health status, or in utilitarian language, the good of the greatest number. However, this example again highlights the weakness of the utilitarian frame: there is no moral compass and no real consideration of the *distribution* of outcomes. Addressing the health status of First Nations Australians is a moral issue, one to do with justice and equity: who benefits is critically important.

A Christian contribution extends beyond the distribution of benefits, but starts at a different place: what are the overall questions that need to be addressed? What should motivate policy in healthcare? Christian ethics has a role to play in contributing to considerations of what questions to examine and how to weigh conflicting claims. A Christian voice, especially that of a Christian economist, should argue that community or society is something different from an economy and that there are decisions that need to be made for reasons other than a rational, economic calculus, conducted within a narrow economic frame. As Barton points out, 'Economic practices are not at all marginal to Christianity either in its originating moments or subsequently. They are not some kind of secondary, material epiphenomenon of something more fundamentally "spiritual". On the contrary, they are at the heart of early Christian self-definition, moral formation, and sociality' (Barton 2009, 56).

In a world where power is distributed unevenly, many individuals will feel powerless to protest, to challenge the orthodoxy of the distribution of resources, of a system treating people like numbers, or a system failing to be compassionate. Christians can call out these behaviours and help to mobilise support to signal the injustice that they see, providing the catalyst to establish a broader coalition to effect change (Lawford-Smith 2015; Sample 2016).

A Christian ethic of healthcare funding can contribute to public debate about health policy. It can offer a coherent approach to answering the value questions and the basis of value choices. Christian ethics can contribute in the area of health economics' greatest weakness: choices about goals and values.

This first reason for developing a Christian ethic to inform health policies is thus about the ability of Christians to contribute to secular debates. The second reason is an internally focused one – to speak to other Christians.

Many Christians feel called to work in the healing professions, mostly working in secular environments, or studying for the profession in secular programmes. This is appropriate, but it is also apposite to highlight to Christians the implications of their faith for the settings in which they work or will work.

Too often healthcare providers, especially large hospitals or residential aged care facilities, become impersonal. Staff working under pressure label the person as their condition ('the diabetic', 'the hip replacement'), their location ('the woman in 5B'), or as a number. All these practices erode human dignity and devalue the intrinsic contribution and personhood of every individual. The Genesis human creation stories are a fundamental part of Christian ethics: that humans are created in the image of God and so each should be valued accordingly. An important contribution of Christian ethics is to call out when the economic calculus shifts the dial away from recognising the intrinsic worth of individuals so that individuals become only a number in the economic evaluation machine. Lightbown (2014, 4) argued that 'the Christian faith offers resources, largely unknown even among Christians, which will help us create the ethical foundations that we need to put our economic house in order'.

Although he was writing about economics generally, the same conclusion can be argued about the 'health economics house', and healthcare funding specifically. The Christian ethics of healthcare funding should help to inform Christian health workers – and other Christians with an interest in health policy – about ways of thinking about health policy and, in particular, healthcare funding.

Gill (2006) has provided a frame to consider healthcare and Christian ethics but his work focused on the underpinnings of healthcare and so could not do justice to the more specialised field of the ethics of healthcare funding. Funding choices shape the way healthcare is delivered, and what healthcare is supported from the public purse. I will argue later that there is a theological underpinning that should inform the motivation for healthcare funding policies.

In the past Christian ethics shaped societies' approaches to rights and slavery (Witte and Latterell 2015). Christian ethics is a very broad field but, unfortunately, it has become typecast as being mostly about sexual morality, and more recently, about end-of-life issues. Today's healthcare or 'medical' ethics section of books on Christian ethics rarely have a section on healthcare funding, ignoring the bigger context that shapes access to, and quality of, care for so many. In many countries Christian voices have become dulled and delegitimised in part because of the churches' failures to deal with sexual predators in their own midst. Perhaps because of those failings it becomes more important for individual Christians to contribute to policy debates, bringing a Christian perspective, without necessarily overtly identifying the theological basis of their contribution. However, the Christian contribution to healthcare funding debates needs to be well-founded and systematic.

Towards a Theology of Healthcare Funding: Who Is My Neighbour?

There are many different approaches to Christian ethics (Gill 2012) – and potentially as many approaches to a Christian ethic of healthcare funding – but the most logical basis for a Christian ethic of healthcare funding is in the teachings of Jesus (Vaux 2010), not seeking 'detailed guidance' from the texts (Wilson 1997, 69), but rather for the texts to point to rules, principles, or paradigms (Hays 1996). The Bible should not be seen as a compendium of ethical instructions with directives of a moral teacher to be obeyed – Burridge (2021, 237) refers to that as a 'genre mistake' – but it can be used to establish directions for travel (Burridge 2021, 246).

In his book *Christian Ethics and Healthcare*, Gill discerns ethical principles applicable to healthcare from the teachings of Jesus of Nazareth through analysing the healing stories (Gill 2006). In this book I build on that approach to draw on the parable of the Good Samaritan to identify biblically grounded principles to inform healthcare funding policy.

Jesus nicely summarised his teaching when challenged to choose, from among the many laws in the Torah, 'Which commandment is the first of all?' He replied with the famous coupling:

> The first is, 'Hear, O Israel: the Lord our God, the Lord is one; you shall love the Lord your God with all your heart, and with all your soul, and with all your mind, and with all your strength.' The second is this, 'You shall love your neighbour as yourself.' There is no other commandment greater than these. (Mark 12:28–31; also, Matthew 22:35–40)

This critical linking of love of God and love of neighbour is one of the cornerstones of Christian ethical thought and behaviour. It raises the question, though, of who is your neighbour? In the Gospel of Luke, the Lukan Jesus answers that question through the parable of the Good Samaritan.

> Just then a lawyer stood up to test Jesus. 'Teacher', he said, 'what must I do to inherit eternal life?' He said to him, 'What is written in the law? What do you read there?' He answered, 'You shall love the Lord your God with all your heart, and with all your soul, and with all your strength, and with all your mind; and your neighbour as yourself.' And he said to him, 'You have given the right answer; do this, and you will live.'

> But wanting to justify himself, he asked Jesus, 'And who is my neighbour?' Jesus replied,
>
> 'A man was going down from Jerusalem to Jericho, and fell into the hands of robbers, who stripped him, beat him, and went away, leaving him half dead. Now by chance a priest was going down that road; and when he saw him, he passed by on the other side. So likewise a Levite, when he came to the place and saw him, passed by on the other side. But a Samaritan while traveling came near him; and when he saw him, he was moved with pity. He went to him and bandaged his wounds, having poured oil and wine on them. Then he put him on his own animal, brought him to an inn, and took care of him. The next day he took out two denarii gave them to the innkeeper, and said, "Take care of him; and when I come back, I will repay you whatever more you spend."
>
> Which of these three, do you think, was a neighbour to the man who fell into the hands of the robbers?' He said, 'The one who showed him mercy.' Jesus said to him, 'Go and do likewise.' (Luke 10:25–37)

In contrast to Mark and Matthew, in Luke it is the lawyer, presumed to be an expert in the (Mosaic) law (Strahan 2016; Hultgren 2017), rather than Jesus who enunciates the two Great Commandments. Jesus affirms this teaching but then uses the answer as a springboard for teaching unique to Luke (Fuller 1978, 42).

Jesus was a teacher and a storyteller. The parables were 'polyvalent', allowing multiple interpretations (Donahue 1988, 17), told 'leaving the mind in sufficient doubt about its precise application to tease it into active thought' (Dodd 1961, 5). Jesus' stories were meant to cause debate and discussion (Crossan 2012, 1992), and this one certainly would have.

We know nothing of the attack, as we are to suppose it is just one of those things that happen on the Jericho Road (Graystone 2022). The robbers have departed the scene, so the first character we hear about in the parable is the 'certain man of uncertain identity' (Clark 2014, 302), with the descriptor 'certain' adding 'strength and emphasis to the undefined quality' of the man, as it does in the birth stories of Samson and Samuel (Amît 2012, 162). We know nothing about the man except he was a traveller. He was stripped off his clothes, 'deprived not only of his possessions but also of his social location, for with his clothing he has lost vital external tokens of his social identity' (Spencer 2017, 98); his clothes might otherwise have helped passers-by identify whether he was a Jew, Gentile, or Samaritan (Donahue 1988; Knowles 2004). What we do know is he was left for dead but was not dead. He was the one in the gutter, cast aside by the robbers after they had picked him over. As it turns out, the wounded man becomes a central figure in the full story, and the basis of the value judgements at the end of the story (Crespy 1973).

The first two travellers in the story, the priest and the Levite, avoided any interaction, including helping, passing the wounded traveller by *on the other side* (Hoyer and McDaniel 1990, 329). For these two, 'the man on the roadside, bruised and abandoned, was a distraction, … he was hardly important. He was a "nobody", undistinguished, irrelevant to their plans for the future' (Francis 2020a, para. 101).

The priest and the Levite are sometimes distinguished in translations, with the former simply seeing the wounded man and walking on the other side of the road, but the latter is described as having 'looked on' the wounded man (King James Version) and 'crossed over to the other side' (Common English Bible). Drawing on a similar translation, Waldron (2003) suggests that both the priest and the Levite made an active decision to go out of their way not to help, or made an active decision to go out of their way to avoid making a decision to help.

Exegetes have often posited an interpretation that their passing the wounded traveller by was motivated by the desire of both these travellers to avoid ritual impurity, which touching a dead person may have involved. Bauckham (1998) builds on this to argue the story teaches that compassion should take priority over other legal obligations. However, this is all surmise. We know nothing about why the priest and the Levite passed by the wounded traveller; it could have been that they were in haste and not prepared to allocate time to care, or fearful the same fate may befall them. Certainly being in a hurry reduces compassion and helping behaviour, and hearing the story of the Samaritan does not redress that, even for seminarians (Darley and Batson 1973, but see Radant et al. 1985). We do know that the priest and the Levite determined they had no neighbourly relationship or obligation to assist, which may have surprised the listeners to the parable (Levine 2006, 145–146), and suggests that 'belief in God and the worship of God are not enough to ensure that we are actually living in a way pleasing to God' (Francis 2020a, para. 74). The priest and the Levite are blind to the needs they don't want to see: 'theirs is a one-way relationship, that takes account only of their own needs' (Graystone 2022, 5).

Hendrickx (1987, 85) suggests that we are not supposed to speculate about the motives of the priest or the Levite. Jesus does not draw out the 'ritual purity' interpretation; it is not necessary for the story's key message (Ryan 2021), and indeed it may not even be a proper reading of the place of ritual purity at the time (Esler 2000; Levine 2006; Saiman 2007; Blajer 2012; Akiyama 2018). The purpose of the first two passers-by is not to provide an opportunity to teach us about the place of ritual purity in Jewish law, but they are there as foils for the next traveller on the road, the Samaritan (Gourgues 1998), and to highlight the relationship between belief and action (Allport and Ross 1967; Hoyer and McDaniel 1990, 329).

Jewish society at the time was divided into priests, Levites, and other Israelites, each with different obligations under the law, including obligations to care for others. A story which started with the first two would be expected to follow with the third, but instead we have the Samaritan. The first two travellers are first described by their location (going 'down the road' or coming 'to the place') contrasted with the Samaritan who is first described coming to the wounded traveller (Bailey 1983, 48). The 'priest' and the 'Levite' are defined by their social category, but so too is the Samaritan, defined as the category of Other or Stranger (Ricoeur 1965, 99). To Jesus' Jewish audience, Samaritans were despised as enemies, evil (Esler 2000), and bastards (Hendrickx 1987, 87). Their position could not be clearer: they were not good people (but see Chalmers 2020 for an alternative view). And yet, in a way which would be totally confronting, the Samaritan in Jesus' story is the good person, with the listener forced to consider 'neighbour' and 'Samaritan' in the same sentence (Snodgrass 2008, 360). The Samaritan is moved by compassion, and cares for the wounded traveller, putting himself at risk as the robbers may still have been nearby.

The final player in the story is the innkeeper. Innkeepers at the time had an unsavoury reputation (Bailey 1983, 53; Donahue 1988, 133; Oakman 2008, 175), and there are tales where innkeepers were in league with the robbers on the road. However, the Samaritan could not care for the wounded traveller alone; he 'needed to have a nearby inn that could provide the help that he was personally unable to offer' (Francis 2020a, para. 165). The Samaritan trusted the innkeeper, contrary to the innkeeper stereotype (Longenecker 2009c), and this trust was reciprocated. The Samaritan pays some money in advance and commits to pay more on his return.

The dénouement occurs with Jesus' leading the lawyer to the interpretation: who is neighbour in all of this? The lawyer was explicitly seeking definition of an in-group of his neighbours, implicitly seeking to exclude others from any obligations (Esler 2000) by making a 'we-they' distinction (Hoyer and McDaniel 1990, 331). Jesus' answer would have surprised the lawyer: there is no clear definition of 'neighbour', rather an injunction for a continuing activity, and the person identified as a neighbour is, in fact, not the one in need (Van Elderen 1978, 114).

In answering the neighbour's question, Jesus directs our attention back to where the story started: the wounded traveller (Gagnon 1998; Clark 2014). Who is the neighbour *of* this person, to use a translation advanced by Strahan (2016, 84)? Which of them 'became a neighbour' (Bailey 2008, 285)? Who was it who stood nearby or next to the wounded traveller, to use the translation advanced by Ruden (2021, liv)? Who acted compassionately? By asking these questions, Jesus transforms the story from a series of events, into an expectation of a 'pattern for action' (Ricoeur 1965, 99).

At this critical teaching juncture in the story, we are invited to put ourselves in the place of the wounded traveller and look up from the gutter to who stretches out their hands. The parable invites us into the pain of the wounded traveller and their need for help, reminding us that 'neighbour' is an inherently reciprocating word (Proctor 2019). We are no longer a remote observer, but the traveller's pain becomes our pain as we too become moved by compassion. As Isasi-Diaz (1998) points out, love of neighbour invites us to be *in solidarity with* our neighbour and this is not some ephemeral attachment that 'one can have for a while, put it aside for whatever reason and then pick it up again' (Isasi-Diaz 1998, 31). Being called to solidarity 'is not a commitment to *working for* the poor in a paternalistic way, but rather involves *working with* and humbling *learning from* the poor' (Pope 1993, 165). Solidarity asks us to resist the temptation to isolate the 'vulnerable' but rather to incorporate all in community demonstrating what we have in common, including vulnerability, and to recognise what the weak and 'vulnerable' contribute (Kaveny 2002, 183).

In the conclusion of the parable, Jesus successfully shifts 'his audience's identification from the perspective of one who dispenses mercy to that of one who desperately hopes to receive it' (Clark 2014, 308). If we can truly understand what it means to be the wounded traveller cast aside by the robbers, then we have some chance of understanding what the realm of God is about, finding an answer to the lawyer's question of what must be done to inherit eternal life (Funk 1974), and understanding the 'essential qualities of discipleship' (Donahue 1988, 128).

The lawyer's question – about 'inheriting' eternal life – is inherently about limits: an estate to be inherited is bounded and involves trade-offs, what I inherit, you can't. Inheritance is usually confined to those who are near to us, but the gift of eternal life is a universal and generous one, the antithesis of a bounded inheritance. The lawyer seeks to limit his obligations, perhaps to other Jews – 'any of your own people' (Leviticus 19:18) – or, more broadly, to include 'the alien who resides with you' (Leviticus 19:34), both of which are specific examples associated with the injunction to love your neighbour in the Torah. But Jesus is having none of that limitation, broadening the targets to be widely inclusive.

The parable then becomes about character; it is not simply about deciding and doing, but rather is about *being*, specifically, being a neighbour. The priest and the Levite could pass by because they were able to rationalise the wounded man as not their problem, blocking any felt compassion. The wounded man's missing clothes meant that the 'natural compassion unblocker, bonds of shared identity, was unavailable' (Costello 2020, 53) and those passers-by did not feel a call to be a neighbour. But limiting compassion to those with whom one has bonds of shared identity converts the bonds into shackles, which prevents one from being a generous neighbour.

By placing ourselves in the position of the wounded traveller, we are now – as the lawyer was back then – asked to recognise that a neighbour is 'anyone whom you would want to act like a neighbor to you in your hour of pain and distress. [We are] commanded to act with the same love and mercy to another that [we] would hope to receive from that person if [we] were in need' (Gagnon 1998, 7).

The parable has had many interpretations – with early interpretations often being allegorical such as St Augustine's: the wounded traveller is the 'ādām, the band of robbers represents the Devil, the Samaritan is Jesus, and the inn is the Church (Roukema 2004; Blajer 2012).

Although a link can be made between the ethical and allegorical readings (Higton 2003; Stavrianos 2012; Clark 2014), contemporary interpretations emphasise the direct and obvious ethical implications of the parable. Jesus used the parable as a teaching moment for the lawyer, back then, and for everyone today, the lawyer was being asked 'not just to *obey* but to *care*' (Hoyer and McDaniel 1990, 330; emphasis in original). The ethical and policy implications of the Samaritan story are many and are used to support a variety of ethical and political positions (Spencer 2017), but with the love command especially seen as a 'timeless principle that has broad application both then and now' (Vaux 2010, 46). Here I will emphasise three core lessons relevant for a theology of healthcare funding: an emphasis on compassion; a call for inclusivity and social justice; and the need for stewardship and good management of resources.

Compassion

Importantly, the first that we are told about the Samaritan is that he was moved by compassion (verse 33, King James Version translation). This same word, ἐσπλαγχνίσθη, occurs a number of times to describe Jesus' emotions in the healing stories of Jesus (Gill 2006). It connotes a visceral, gut-wrenching feeling. It is part of the zone of 'emotion-fused thought'

(Pilch 2016, 204). Nussbaum (2013, 142) defines compassion as a 'painful emotion directed at the serious suffering of another creature or creatures'. Compassion is not a milquetoast emotion, but one of passion leading to action: in the Samaritan's case, picking up the wounded traveller, tending his wounds, and providing on-going care.

The parable is almost universally referred to as that of the Good Samaritan, a contemporary oxymoron, contrasting him with all other Samaritans, as a backhanded compliment or 'cryptoseme' (Ryan 2021, 9). It could also be referred to as the parable of the Compassionate Samaritan (Wink 1979; Esler 2000), as that is the motivating force in the Samaritan's actions. The parable is one which is a 'paradigm of the compassionate vision which is the presupposition for ethical action' (Donahue 1988, 132).

Compassion has an important place in Christian ethics: it is an emotion that involves action, the call is to go and *do* likewise (Strahan 2016). In the parable it transforms the Samaritan from observer to actor, from one who is not neighbourly to one who cares for and exhibits compassionate justice (Marshall 2012), attempting to rectify the harm done by the injustice of the robbers. The tale recounts a long list of actions by the Samaritan as he 'must make up for the actions of everyone else' (Bailey 1983, 41).

As Robbins (2004) has identified, the Samaritan was not simply moved by compassion but also took a number of compassionate steps involving all parts of his body: seeing the wounded traveller; being moved in his gut; walking with his feet towards rather than away from the traveller; using his hands to apply oil and wine, which happened to be elements of temple sacrifice (Derrett 1964; Hendrickx 1987; Donahue 1988); lifting the traveller onto the animal; and thinking about future needs, and paying for the wounded traveller's future care. Robbins highlights that the Samaritan's actions involved an interlinking of the two Great Commandments: by loving neighbour, the Samaritan was fulfilling the first Great Commandment: 'In an eightfold progression, then, the narration describes the Samaritan loving his neighbor with "his whole heart, his whole soul, his whole strength, and his whole mind"' (Robbins 2004, 262).

Compassion and love are multidimensional, and are, in essence, other-regarding, about extending oneself for the benefit of others, and active (Peck 1978, 81). The parable starts with an act of compassion. It is compassion, including the actions that flow from it, that distinguishes the priest and the Levite from the Samaritan. However, compassion – and neighbour love – are not the detached, disinterested feelings of separate autonomous beings, but rather involve passion, attachment, and engagement:

> The idea that we need to 'figure out' how we can best love our neighbor already presumes that we are in a position to dispense that love; it presumes that we occupy the role of givers, doers, performers. It risks completely overlooking the fact that all of us have been and will continue to be dependent in some way upon the very neighbor love we ourselves are commanded to show. (Clark 2014, 307)

The health worker is engaged with the neighbour for whom they care; all of us who support the caring endeavour are creating a society of reciprocity and neighbourliness, being neighbours to each other. Just as we support care for others today, we expect to be cared for by others tomorrow. The health system is not just a factory in which we engage with a time-limited purchasing or market relationship; caring in the health system is an expression of a caring and compassionate society, with ongoing relationships and bonds.

As well as benefitting the cared-for, compassion – with its emphasis on action – can benefit the healthcare professional by promoting resilience and reducing burn-out, and may contribute to reducing healthcare costs by reducing 'disputed' interventions and increasing the likelihood that patients will adhere to treatment regimens (Trzeciak, Roberts, and Mazzarelli 2017; Trzeciak and Mazzarelli 2019).

The parable starts with a question about how the lawyer might attain eternal life, but the answer is 'God's favor is not gained by some moral commitment or achievement, but is rather reflected in the passing on of the mercy through which God heals us' (Clark 2014, 308).

Compassion is a powerful motivating force. It moves and motivates front-line carers in their day-to-day work, but the intent of supporting compassion should also motivate policy. Front-line workers need to be paid and so the compassion of the front-line worker can only be effected if there is a funding scheme which allows compassion and which provides funding for staff to care for those in need. One of the critical contributions of the Samaritan was his time (Francis 2020a, para. 63), so any funding scheme must be such as to allow time for workers to care in a compassionate way.

Health policy debates often focus on the macro-policy settings: what is the role of private health funding vs public funding? What is the best way to remunerate health professionals?

However, policy should also be concerned about the micro-settings of care: all healthcare treatment involves interactions between individuals, most often in a treatment/care dyad between a professional and a patient/consumer, or care teams and the person they are caring for. In institutional settings interactions between the patient and all staff with whom they interact, including cleaners and clerical staff, are important parts of the care environment. This treatment/care interaction – be it in a dyad, with a team, or with the whole care environment – is critical to the patient experience. The patient needs to be valued, their concerns need to be heard, the patient's social and economic environment needs to be recognised and understood, and most importantly, they need to be cared for with compassion. Effective interventions to enhance compassionate care should be part of the curricula for the health professions and research targeted at learning how to facilitate compassionate care should be funded to develop a robust evidence base for this critical element of good care (Blomberg et al. 2016).

Promoting the conditions for compassion should therefore be part of what health policies do. Healthcare funding needs to be designed to create compassionate caring environments where compassionate caring staff are able to do their best. A Christian ethic of healthcare funding should be underpinned by compassion, and compassion should inform healthcare funding design.

Inclusivity and Social Justice

The dominant theme of the parable in contemporary exegesis is that 'neighbour' is inclusive, that it extends far beyond the boundaries of one's comfortable in-group (Esler 2000); it is a lesson about 'the boundless nature of love' (Van Elderen 1978, 114).

The phrasing of the teaching about neighbour is critically important. The initial question from the lawyer is 'who is my neighbour'? Here 'neighbour' is an object, one to whom help is offered. But Jesus reverses the question, asking who acted as a neighbour, so neighbour becomes subject, one who offers help (Crossan 1992, 58); neighbour 'becomes a behaviour in the first person' (Ricoeur 1965, 99). Jesus does not answer the question from the lawyer about who is the lawyer's neighbour, but directs the lawyer to question who the lawyer *is a neighbour to* (Furnish 1973, 40).

This change from object to subject converts the parable from a simple story of loving one's neighbour, to a more powerful story of Christian love:

> This kind of love of neighbor (love towards the neighbor) should not be called authentically 'Christian', even though there is no doubt that it entered our culture in the context of the Christian tradition. Rather what is specifically and characteristically Christian is that it is a neighbor who is loving. Also we can no longer talk here about a commandment to love, since anyone who is a neighbor exists as a neighbor, which means that this person loves. (Marxsen 1993, 97)

The 'commandment' to love one's neighbours and one's enemies 'no longer has the form of a commandment to be observed, but is an invitation to a way of acting that is bound to a promise. .... No one can really be a neighbor; we can only become neighbors over and over again' (Marxsen 1993, 106).

What Marxsen is arguing here is that the Samaritan story is not one of picking and choosing who is my neighbour, as the lawyer apparently seeks to do, nor about choosing who one helps and when. It is not about how to define or find a neighbour, but rather how to *be* a neighbour (Hoyer and McDaniel 1990, 331). If one is a neighbour, one exists as a neighbour to all in need; there is no conditionality. One demonstrates one's right to be called neighbour with each interaction, it is 'the *habit* of making oneself available' (Ricoeur 1965, 99, emphasis added).

The lawyer now is challenged not to think about (limit) his obligation to specific neighbours, but is forced to address 'what kind of action constitutes neighborly love' (Furnish 1973, 41). In the shift from object to subject, the parable shifts from being about 'a strict definition of neighbour [to being about] a generous definition of love' (Marshall 2012, 46), as 'the name neighbour is a relative one, and no one can be a neighbour except to a neighbour' (Augustine 2014, 1.31).

The Second Great Commandment is an injunction to love; it is a call about love of humanity and here 'Love raises justice above the mere equal treatment of equals: biblical justice is the equal treatment of all human beings solely for the reason that as humans they possess bestowed worth from God. God's people are commanded to do justice on the basis of what they themselves have received in the gracious acts of God' (Mott 2011, 53).

The love contemplated in the parable is an inclusive one, to all. It is a love which leads to action, but importantly it is a love which is about who we are and our context. The parable's teaching shows that the 'question of what I ought to *do* is actually about what I am or ought to be' (Hauerwas 1983, 117, emphasis in original), or as Stone phrases the same point: 'The story reminds us that help is a verb as well as a noun and that our actions make us who we are' (Stone 2008, 33).

The parable is not simply identifying that someone else needs help, but redefines social boundaries to bring the obligation closer: '"neighbor" is not a category that the lawyer is authorized to apply to others; instead, it takes the form of a challenge and recoils back upon him as a moral agent capable either of being or of failing to be a neighbor to someone else' (McFarland 2001, 60).

The parable is not only about the status of 'the other', the wounded traveller, important as that may be, but it is also about the status of the lawyer, and of the observer/listener as an actor or a person who defines away their obligations to others (McFarland 2001, 62). The listener, or target of the story, is as Clark (2014) has argued, no longer the remote ethical observer, but becomes part of a new reciprocal relationship with obligations to the broad community of those in need.

In the context of the rivalries of the time, it is also important that it is a Samaritan who is the neighbour. In Luke, immediately before the parable, Samaritans were seen as inhospitable (9:51–56). Although Samaritans and Jews shared much in terms of theology, they were in fact worlds apart (Knoppers 2013). Samaritans were said to have been involved in desecrating the Jerusalem Temple in Jesus' time (Pilch 2012, 75). In his answer to Jesus about who was a neighbour, the lawyer could not utter the word Samaritan, but rather used an 'evasive circumlocution' (Hultgren 2017, 75), and instead described the inclusive action: 'The one who showed him mercy'.

Thus the parable reinforces the teaching about loving one's enemies found throughout the Gospels (Gill 2020): if a Samaritan – 'an outsider in a hostile world' (McDonald 1996, 32) – can show neighbourly love to the wounded man, then so must all who heed Jesus' words show love to their enemies. Further, if *even a Samaritan*, the most unlikely source of succour (Raven 2012, 138), is so generous, paying the innkeeper to look after the victim, there should be an even higher expectation for the generosity of others (Furnish 1973, 40–44; Harvey 1990, 176–177).

Compassion and social justice are linked in this parable: compassion is a motivator that quashes limits on its scope: 'Compassion, which transcends legally sanctioned ethnic boundaries and discriminations when faced with real human need, is a superior form of human behaviour than continuing to live within their limits' (Esler 2000, 343).

The parable of the 'Good' Samaritan is about inclusivity: that being a neighbour involves demonstrating that, to everyone. It is about radically redefining who is 'like us' (Esler 2000) and thus who we should be neighbours to. We, like the lawyer, can no longer pick and choose who is in our neighbourhood. We can no longer simply discuss and emphasise the fine distinctions about who should be assisted. We must rather *provide* assistance, we must stop talking about the law and start living it (Stenhouse 2013). Neighbours are around us, but they are most importantly 'the least of our brothers and sisters. Neighbors are the poor, the oppressed, for whom we must have a preferential option. This we cannot have apart from being in solidarity with them' (Isasi-Diaz 1998, 31).

The obligation derived from the parable is thus a universal and extremely generous one: that we should be neighbours to everyone, and that 'everyone' is increasingly diverse and increasingly global (Jacobson and Jacobson 2017). It sets a very high bar, so much so that Cottingham thinks it 'untenable' and advocates a minimalist 'help your friends, and do not harm your neighbours' (Cottingham 1983, 98). But the parable teaches a radical inclusivity, which turns on its head narrow views that succour should only be provided to some who meet narrow inclusion criteria. Rather, the basis for support should be social justice, being a neighbour to everyone, equally.

A Christian ethic of healthcare funding should therefore incorporate this principle of being neighbour universally: healthcare funding should be underpinned by, and effect, social justice.

Are There Any Limits? The Issue of Stewardship

The innkeeper is an oft neglected but key player in the parable (Longenecker 2009c; Van Eck and Van Niekerk 2018). Jesus' story could have ended just as satisfactorily with the Samaritan loading the wounded traveller on his animal, but instead Jesus chose to introduce the inn and the innkeeper. There are two critical aspects of the innkeeper's role: trust and a monetary exchange, together they point to the critical issue of stewardship.

In the parable, the inn is the setting for extended healing: the Samaritan's restoration of the traveller's well-being goes beyond simple amelioration of the immediate needs of the wounded man and aims at full restoration of the man's capacity. It therefore suggests that a Christian response should go beyond the bare minimum, simply addressing presenting needs, and involve a more comprehensive response (Sagovsky 2008, 80). The Samaritan takes responsibility for full recuperation, which in contemporary policy might include preventive interventions or systematic responses to the causes of the harm.

The Samaritan mobilises the external resources of the inn and the innkeeper to assist the wounded traveller. He goes beyond meeting the immediate needs of the wounded traveller, paying money in advance for future needs – the two denarii would cover about a 7–14 day stay, probably long enough for the wounded man to recover (Oakman 2008, 44–45; Snodgrass 2008, 347) – and commits to pay more if necessary on his return. *Prima facie*, this suggests an obligation to a neighbour is unlimited – the Samaritan has apparently authorised the innkeeper to spend without limit (Hultgren 2017). Oakman (2008, 179) suggests that the parable might be better called 'The Foolish Samaritan', as the Samaritan placed himself at risk and would potentially be seen by Jesus' peasant listeners as over the top in terms of his generosity. This potentially unbounded generosity probably led Charles Dickens' Gradgrind to believe that the Good Samaritan was indeed a 'bad economist' (Gribble 2004).

However, a trust relationship has been created between the innkeeper and the Samaritan: the innkeeper knows that the Samaritan's resources are not unlimited, and the Samaritan trusts the innkeeper to be reasonable in the resources he outlays. The innkeeper also trusts that the Samaritan will return to the inn (Longenecker 2009c). Perhaps by committing two denarii the Samaritan was signalling what he anticipated the reasonable expenses might be. In any event the innkeeper is acting as a trusted agent for the Samaritan.

Trust is a multifaceted concept, In the parable we see that the Samaritan exhibits a characteristic of trust by making himself vulnerable (Castaldo, Premazzi, and Zerbini 2010): vulnerable to being attacked by the robbers too, and vulnerable to the innkeeper's behaviour. But in terms of the second aspect of vulnerability the Samaritan also shows, despite the reputation of innkeepers, he believes that the innkeeper with deliver on that trust and care for the wounded traveller, an example of what McKnight and Chervany (2000) refer to as 'institution-based trust'.

The trust between the Samaritan and the innkeeper may signal more than a simple contractual exchange – one encompassed by the transaction and about interests – but becomes a covenant, about a relationship which transforms the innkeeper from mere provider and contractor into a partner in the healing process. Covenantal relationships involve 'undertaking of responsibility for others, knowing that they too undertake responsibility for us' (Sacks 2020, 327), in this case the innkeeper undertaking responsibility for the wounded traveller, and the Samaritan showed his responsibility to the traveller, and committed to deal responsibly with the innkeeper.

A further lesson from the parable may be drawn from the innkeeper's management of the two denarii: that funding allocated for care must be spent wisely. Pope Francis summarised the lesson: 'Love of neighbour is concrete and squanders none of the resources needed to bring about historical change that can benefit the poor and disadvantaged' (Francis 2020a, para. 165).

Neighbour love is not limited to loving one's contemporary neighbour – excessive spending today may limit options in the future, especially if today's spending is from debt. Neighbour love thus involves stewardship over time – trading off needs and resources of today with an eye to the reality that similar trade-offs need to be made tomorrow.

Public funding for healthcare is not unlimited and spending on healthcare means money is not available to spend on some other purpose, either by the taxpayer or by government. Just as between the Samaritan and the innkeeper, there is a mutuality of trust between the health system and the wider society: the health system should call for funding support if and only if it can be justified.

Healthcare providers need to be careful stewards of the resources allocated to them. A key principle for healthcare funding must therefore be that there is careful stewardship of resources. Good stewardship in healthcare involves developing policies to ensure that healthcare investments are worthwhile, and a Christian ethic of healthcare funding should incorporate principles to ensure value for money, both now and into the future.

Conclusion: The Broader Implications of the Parable

The parable of the 'Good' Samaritan leads us beyond an anodyne interpretation of 'doing good', narrow obligations, and simply caring for the first order needs of the wounded. It fits well with the other parables of Jesus that are 'not earthly stories with heavenly meanings, but earthly stories with heavy meanings, weighed down by an awareness of the workings of exploitations in the world of their hearers' (Herzog 1994, 3).

The Samaritan story appropriately directs us to a more generous and systematic response to address the underlying causes of contemporary woundings. The organisational and systematic actions needed to respond to the Lukan injunction move Christian love from an individual ethic guiding an individual response, to one of support for a just allocation of resources. In the twenty-first century world, becoming and being neighbour involves joining a community of those who care, and those who are cared for. The full range of present and future needs cannot be met by an individual Samaritan or an innkeeper, but now involves a community of people from many disciplines and roles, and large institutions of care provision.

The utilitarian and consequentialist underpinning of contemporary economic practice sits uneasily – albeit not irreconcilably so – with the principles derived from the parable of the 'Good' Samaritan. Utilitarianism essentially values individuals, each with their own utilities, which, in aggregate, shape markets and determine prices. But economics and utilitarianism are challenged when decisions are to be made outside the traded goods sector, despite efforts to apply economics to areas such as marriage (Becker 1974, 1993); when the utility function of an individual is affected by another's, that is, recognising we are part of a community; and when an individual's basic needs are at stake (Häyry 2021). Economic, and indeed utilitarian, thinking still has an important contribution, but that contribution must be recognised as sitting within a wider, value-based, context.

As noted earlier, Camosy identifies many parallels between the secular, essentially utilitarian philosophy of Peter Singer and Roman Catholic moral theology. In Camosy's view, one of these commonalities is that 'Happiness is not indicated merely by 'feeling happy' but rather the long-term fulfillment which comes from achieving goals in a coherent life of meaning' (Camosy 2012, 243).

A 'life of meaning' might gain its coherence and have its foundation in a variety of places, including the principles which can be discerned in the parable of the 'Good' Samaritan. The economics project, including the application of economics to healthcare and healthcare funding, will be stronger if it recognises the importance of a 'coherent life of meaning', supplementing naïve utilitarianism by situating it within a principled framework, that accepts that an individual exists within a society or community, and is more than simply *Homo economicus*.

The needs of the poor, or the wounded traveller in the journey of life, require not only individual responses and individual charitable giving but also require creation and support of systems of social solidarity. Moreover, the needs of the poor are not addressed solely because of compassion – although compassion should still inform policy – needs are also addressed because that is just and inherent in the meaning of neighbour. The requirements of justice are social obligations of the whole neighbourhood of love. They are beyond what can be met by individual action towards individually known beneficiaries; requiring us to move from individual charity to social action.

Addressing need is important but is not the end of the parable's message. The radical inclusiveness of the parable calls us to remove the injustices that create these individual needs, and this requires the overturning of values, existing systems, and existing constraints, consistent with the broader Christian message of overturning of existing expectations: the first shall be last, and the last, first (Matthew 19:30; 20:16; Mark 10:31 and Luke 13:30). The parable of the 'Good' Samaritan is not simply a good example – the Samaritan as a model of good behaviour – but is also one which teaches about extreme generosity, even to enemies.

Martin Luther King used the parable in his challenge to the existing order:

> [We] are called to play the Good Samaritan on life's roadside, but that will be only an initial act. One day we must come to see that the whole Jericho Road must be transformed so that men and women will not be constantly

> beaten and robbed as they make their journey on life's highway. True compassion is more than flinging a coin to a beggar. It comes to see that an edifice which produces beggars needs restructuring. (King Jr 1967)

Compassion, social justice, and good stewardship all require a broader response than simply treatment. They turn our gaze upstream to prevention, to addressing the social, economic, and commercial determinants of health, at scale. A Christian ethic of healthcare funding also brings to the fore the moral determinants of health, which shape the values underpinning policies (Berwick 2020), and calls us to challenge what is accepted as a legitimate part of health policy discussion.

I have shown that one can distinguish three core ethical principles or lessons from the parable of the 'Good' Samaritan: compassion as a motivator, addressing the question of *why* we care; inclusivity or social justice as to benefits, *who* do we care for; and stewardship of resources required to achieve the ends of treatment and prevention, *what* should be provided. The parable is not a simple story of one person helping another but is a story of becoming and being neighbour.

As I have argued above, the parable must not only be read as being about an individual and their neighbourliness. It also calls us to think about neighbourhoods – not just as a collective of individuals but, as the sum is greater than the parts, a neighbourhood is a community that allows and facilitates broad social action. This broader social action should involve the same mix of compassion, social justice, and stewardship that we see in the parable itself. These same ethical principles provide an ethical underpinning far beyond healthcare funding but should shape the broader values of contemporary society. As the current Archbishop of Canterbury, Justin Welby, has argued:

> There is no better example of the expression of good values than in Jesus' parable of the Good Samaritan; a story deeply embedded in our collective understanding of what it means to be a good citizen, and which reminds us that our values have not emerged from a vacuum – but from the resilient and eternal structure of our religious, theological, philosophical and ethical heritage. (Welby 2016)

Although Welby is talking here about the United Kingdom, the same may be said of most countries of the white Anglosphere, and indeed beyond. These require us to commit to becoming neighbours, journeying together, and helping each other along life's Jericho Road as part of the very meaning of society. As we walk our Jericho Road together, we must seek to create a society where healthcare funding policy is influenced by compassion, social justice, and good stewardship.

In his exegesis of the parable of the 'Good' Samaritan in his encyclical *Fratelli Tutti*, Pope Francis argues that 'if we extend our gaze to the history of our own lives and that of the entire world, all of us are, or have been, like each of the characters in the parable. All of us have in ourselves something of the wounded man, something of the robber, something of the passers-by, and something of the Good Samaritan' (Francis 2020a, para. 69).

Francis has phrased that as about each person individually. It could equally be phrased as a challenge to each society: to what extent does society pass by the wounded traveller? To what extent is society contributing to the problems of people on the Jericho Road of life, acting as robbers? To what extent is society in disrepair so, like the wounded traveller, it needs external help – or looking to best practices in other places – to rectify its condition? To what extent does society exhibit the compassion, justice, and stewardship that we see in the Samaritan? And to what extent is society a good and trustworthy steward of its resources, like the innkeeper?

The same challenge might also apply to organisations: to whom is the organisation a neighbour? To whom a passer-by? To whom a robber, contributing to problems, and this may include sometimes exploiting staff? To what extent is the organisation like the innkeeper, trusting and being trusted, and being a careful steward? And to what extent does the organisation identify with – or act as – the wounded man, the man in the gutter?

Although the Samaritan parable has been used here to distil the three underlying principles, those principles are evident in many other places in the Bible – both in the Hebrew Scriptures and in the New Testament. The principles are not unique to the Samaritan parable, nor even to Luke, and are expressed in a variety of voices, from commands to other stories of paradigmatic behaviour, elsewhere in the canon. The fact that the same principles are found in multiple books, written in multiple places, gives one confidence that the coherence of the diversity of sources suggests that the principles identified are important and fundamental ones to highlight and apply to develop a theology of healthcare funding.

What Needs to Change?

The discipline of economics has made a remarkable and positive contribution to healthcare policy over the last sixty years. In many countries, in addition to showing a net clinical benefit, new healthcare interventions must demonstrate a net economic benefit prior to being approved for public funding. The public dollar, pound, or euro has been stretched further, increasing net social welfare. But, over the last sixty years, health economics has de-emphasised its moral foundation, compassion has become sidelined, not core to the discipline. Equity is often not central to discussion of net benefit with public funding decisions based on average incremental benefit, not adequately taking into account the distribution of those benefits. Economics may not have been seen as antithetical to religion, but at least it was seen as difficult to combine the two (Dean and Waterman 1999), economic and ethical rationality separated, and if seen as integrated, the latter is subordinated to the former: 'the "market principle" itself seems to be the guarantor of the moral principle' (Ulrich 2000, 46).

What I propose here is a new vision for health economics that builds on and extends the current dominant paradigm of health economics by identifying that economic evaluation needs to sit in tension with theologically grounded principles of compassion and social justice. It develops a new theology of healthcare funding, based on the teachings of Jesus, which will improve the application of health economics to healthcare. It advances a new theology that is not simply about hard choices in healthcare – although it recognises and addresses those – but aims to change the way health economics lives in the real world of patients, practitioners, and politicians, transforming health economics from a detached calculating machine to a discipline that engages with identifiable, rather than simply statistical lives, with compassion and justice.

In Chapters 2, 3, and 4, I will flesh out what these ethical principles of compassion, social justice, and stewardship mean for healthcare funding. Each of these chapters engages with the secular – generally what economics or health economics in particular has to say about the issue – and the theological, drawing on biblical texts. In Chapter 5, I will apply these Christian ethical principles to healthcare funding and payment. Chapter 6 returns to issues of public theology.

CHAPTER 2

The Call for Compassionate Action to Meet Needs

> But a certain Samaritan being on his journey, came near him; and seeing him, was moved with compassion.
>
> Luke 10:33, Douay-Rheims translation

What motivates an individual or society to provide healthcare? At first glance, the answer is obvious: we see a 'need' and we – society or an individual health worker – feel compelled to respond. In this chapter I start by exploring the concept of need and outline a Christian ethic – specifically, being a neighbour as demonstrated through compassion – that might underpin the desire to meet needs, and then I explore the implications of compassion for healthcare funding design.

Need 'represents the most immediate cause' (Andersen 1968, 17) and the 'stimulus or most direct reason' (Andersen, Kravits, and Anderson 1975, 6) for using health services; it is a 'central concern' of healthcare planners (Donabedian 1973, 58).

Although it is the starting point for considering and planning healthcare use, need is an ambiguous concept. In any given interaction it is shaped and defined not only by the consumer and the professional but also by society. Society may define some needs as eligible for public funding and support, and others as illegitimate (e.g. abortion in some countries).

Needology

There is an immense literature in economics, ethics, philosophy, and healthcare planning about defining healthcare needs. Economists are generally wary of the concept, deriding the study of need as 'needology' (Maynard 1979). Culyer (2005, 227) described need as 'arguably the most used and the least properly comprehended word in discussions of health. The meanings that attach to it are legion'. That view is more temperate than his 'possible conclusion' of a few decades earlier that 'the word "need" ought to be banished from discussion of public policy, partly because of its ambiguity but also because … the word is most frequently used in … "arbitrary" senses' (Culyer, Lavers, and Williams 1972, 114).

Mooney (1986, 75) had 'the feeling that use of the word "need" is designed deliberately to confuse the listener and to stifle rational thought and debate'.

As Clayton (1983, 215) points out: 'Statements about need are often used as though they refer to simple objective facts which can be clearly identified and planned for if only the right methods can be found to identify them. In practice, of course, this is not the case, for definitions of need inevitably incorporate certain value assumptions.'

She goes on to note that

> In general, use of the term need in the context of policy formation is complicated by the fact that it is used in so many different ways. It may be used, for example, as a descriptive, explanatory or predictive concept; as concerned with biological survival or in relation to a specific social culture. It can be individual or service-oriented, and focusing on causation, the circumstances of person's life, or desired end state. (Clayton 1983, 231)

A recent review of the concept of 'unmet need' found sixteen different definitions of that concept (Vreman et al. 2019). Even Bradshaw (1972, 81), a widely cited writer on need, suggested need is 'an area where precise thinking is needed for both theoretical and practical reasons'.

Most economists prefer to frame discussions about access to healthcare as being about demand, rather than need. In need language, demand is equivalent to Bradshaw's 'expressed need' (Bradshaw 1972, 73). However, although a central part of the economist's normal armamentarium, demand for healthcare is a much more contested concept, with market failure endemic in healthcare weakening the normal salience of the concept (Arrow 1963; Boulding 1966). In addition, from an ethical perspective, the most demanding people may not always be the people most in need.

Despite economists' scepticism, disentangling the concept of need is useful, especially in terms of who might define need and what types of need might be so defined. The starting point is often needs as exogenously determined by a professional, administrator, or social scientist; this is what Bradshaw refers to as 'normative need'(Bradshaw 1972, 72). Bradshaw's two other types of need are felt and comparative.

Although some economists use need language, when they do so they often accept that needs should be professionally defined (Cullis and West

1979, 85), sometimes qualified as being services that are effective in meeting this professionally defined health gap (Hurley 2000, 91). However, the professional determination of need, inherent in the concept of normative need, is not an exact science. Indeed, one writer suggested the related concept of 'medical necessity' was 'rarely defined, largely unexamined, generally misunderstood, and idiosyncratically applied in medical and insurance practice' (Bergthold 1995, 181).

Different health professionals both within the same discipline and in different disciplines may see the same person and yet identify different needs. The 'needs' identified by a professional may not provide a benefit to the patient, at least on average and as reported in clinical trials. The professional's lens may be informed by their own attributes (Boulding 1966), including, potentially, racism, sexism, and homophobia.

Contemporary economic thinking generally limits need to a capacity to benefit (Rodriguez Santana et al. 2022 (in press)), emphasising whether a service provides value, rather than who might determine need, with value in publicly funded systems being typically assessed as average societal-wide value for money, an issue to be canvassed in Chapter 4. A new science of identifying low or no value care has emerged, where low or no value care can be defined as 'care that is unlikely to benefit the patient given the harms, cost, available alternatives, or preferences of the patient' (Verkerk et al. 2018, 737).

Not all medical practitioners know the full range of available options for treatment, and some are more interventionist than others; so, although having seen the same person, some will perform a procedure, whereas others will wait and observe, so-called watchful waiting, and yet others might prescribe non-surgical treatment. In making treatment recommendations, medical practitioners may be influenced by the fees generated for a procedure, and so they may stimulate a lucrative response to a perceived need, a phenomenon known as supplier-induced demand (Wennberg, Barnes, and Zubkoff 1982; Richardson 1998; Bickerdyke et al. 2002; Pawson, Greenhalgh, and Brennan 2016; Evans 1974, 2016b), or by inducements to prescribe certain agents or use certain prostheses (Little, Lipworth, and Kerridge 2022). Variation in professional recommendations might also be a natural result of diagnostic uncertainty (Wennberg, Barnes, and Zubkoff 1982; Bhise et al. 2018). Public hospitals in Australia perform lower rates of low value care than private hospitals (Badgery-Parker et al. 2019; Chalmers et al. 2019), a difference unlikely to reflect patient selection or a comparative advantage of private hospitals in achieving better outcomes of care than public hospitals (Chandra and Staiger 2020). The combination of supplier-induced demand and the prevalence of low value care suggests that physicians are imperfect agents in pursuing patient preferences and needs (McGuire 2000; Stavropoulou 2012), further weakening the salience of normative need or professionally determined need as a useful construct.

Physicians in different communities can judge the need for interventions quite differently, as shown by very different rates of interventions in the pioneering Dartmouth Atlas of Healthcare Variation (Wennberg and Cooper 1996) and its successors, and also as seen in studies comparing nearby cities (Wennberg, Freeman, and Culp 1987; Gawande 2009a), and comparing countries (Aaron and Schwartz 1982).

The issue of different professionals identifying different needs is not the only challenge to normative need as defined by the professional. The emphasis on professional determination harks back to a time of 'medical dominance' (Willis 1983; Freidson 2007) and paternalism in medicine when (predominantly) male medical practitioners defined a patient's needs without challenge. The 'doctor knows best' attitude often ignored consideration of the social context and the role of social and environmental determinants of health (Evans, Barer, and Marmor 1994), with doctors sometimes narrowly focusing on 'clinical' signs and symptoms but in doing so failing to listen adequately to the patient (Waitzkin 1991, 2000; Stavropoulou 2012), particularly women patients (Dreifus 1977; Ehrenreich and English 2011), and dealing inadequately with mental health and use of alcohol and other drugs (Conrad and Schneider 2010).

Professional determination of need has also taken a battering in recent years with the emphasis on consumer measurement of value, particularly stimulated by the work of two Harvard academics on value-based competition (Porter and Teisberg 2006, 2004). They argue that healthcare would be improved if it focused more on value to the consumer, a view that is consistent with many other quality and technical efficiency approaches (Deming 1993; Liberatore 2013; D'Andreamatteo et al. 2015). Despite it having the attributes of a fad (Marmor 2004, 2007), value-based care is a useful corrective device that highlights the importance of a focus on patients and their priorities, rather than professional determinations of what is needed and what is not (Duckett 2019; Steinmann et al. 2020). There is now a plethora of generic and specific scales to measure patient-reported outcomes used as part of this refocus on individual patient assessment of need and reorienting services to focus more on patients' needs (Fitzpatrick 2009; Porter, Larsson, and Lee 2016; Organisation for

Economic Cooperation and Development 2019b; Churruca et al. 2021). At the very least 'the determination of needs should be a joint concern between the provider and the client' (Magi and Allander 1981, 51).

Studies, descriptions, and typologies of need often assume that it is dichotomous: a person or group is in need or not. But it is not so binary:

> In practice the distinction is not always clear-cut and it is perhaps the cut-off points upon which policymakers should be focusing. Rather than, by default, taking the clients' or experts' view as to where need begins, policy-makers might well discuss the circumstances of the people on the margins of need, and then make appropriate adjustments to provision. If marginal unmet need is really the focus of attention, either per se or in relation to other groups of people, then perhaps additional alternative investigatory techniques are necessary. (Clayton 1983, 227)

This focus on the margin is core to the discipline of economics and the profession's concern with the efficient allocation of resources. If a need is identified by planners, it evokes pressure for it to be met, and in publicly funded health systems that necessarily involves priority setting and choice, which comes back to the issue of value for money. Labelling a condition as an unmet need evokes priority choices by society. However, need often 'masquerades as an absolute term when it is in fact being used to describe circumstances considered incompatible with the resources and values of a society and period' (Clayton 1983, 231).

The final and critical player in the need determination triad is thus society. Walton (1969, 14) has helpfully suggested that societal recognition of a need of a person or group X involves three distinct steps:

i. X is in state Y.
ii. State Y is incompatible with the values held in society Z.
iii. Therefore, state Y should be changed.

Walton's formulation leaves open who identified X as being in state Y – it could be either a professional or the individual. The third step in the Walton formulation is also important, namely that if society accepts that state Y is incompatible with society's values, then state Y should be changed if possible, which suggests that interventions in response to need should be effective, aligning with the dominant view of health economists that need is related to the capacity to benefit (Allin, Hernández-Quevedo, and Masseria 2009).

Walton's third step does not have any qualification about for whom state Y should be changed, for example, that it should be changed only if X can afford to pay for the change in state. Implicitly, the determination of need in healthcare is an independent decision separate from any decision about how that need might be paid for. Walzer (1983, 20) has conceptualised this by assuming different spheres of society where recognition of a need existing in one sphere of society should not be contingent on the resources that a person has in another sphere (Kaveny 2002, 180).

The critical component of Walton's formulation is the second step, that state Y is incompatible with the values held in society or, more explicitly, that recognition of a need involves the broader community accepting that addressing state Y is meritorious and worthwhile (Hurley 2000, 91). The ethicist David Braybrooke also emphasises this linking of need to societal values (Braybrooke 1987). However, some states that an individual might judge as creating a need may not be so identified by society, cosmetic procedures being one example. Similarly, political, moral, and other forms of discrimination may mean that a need is recognised in some groups but not in others (Walton 1969, 14).

Need 'comprises both factual and value elements' (Walton 1969, 17) and, in particular, the formulation links identification of a need to the values held in a society. This linkage of needs back to values might explain why economists are need-averse. For economists, especially those working in countries with publicly funded health systems, resource allocation decisions, and by implication, identification of needs that should be publicly supported, are about social priorities and social values. These should not be determined solely by professional or individual judgements as naïve needology might prescribe. Stakeholders interviewed as part of a recent study of definitions of unmet need agreed that 'unmet need cannot be separated from the broader value framework' (Vreman et al. 2019, 1279). Need as provisionally identified in the first step in the Walton formulation is critically constrained by the second.

'Unmet need' has real implications. A person waiting longer for home care, for example, has a higher mortality rate than a person with a shorter wait (Visvanathan et al. 2019). Kröger, Puthenparambil, and Van Aerschot (2019) have argued that the concept of unmet need should be situated more directly in the broader welfare state literature by introducing the concept of 'care poverty': 'Care poverty is a question of the unequal outcomes of social policy, an insufficient level of care services and inadequate resources or opportunities in terms of organising care. It is an expression of inequality in the same way as poverty is' (Kröger, Puthenparambil, and Van Aerschot 2019, 488).

Kröger, Puthenparambil, and Van Aerschot (2019) introduce some state agency and accountability into the 'unmet needs' discourse – care poverty is the result of decisions not to provide adequate services, specific to the circumstances of the individual.

Walton's formulation, however, raises the question of why might state Y be incompatible with the values held in society Z, or rather what might underpin these values and where might these values come from. Beauchamp and Childress (2013), in enunciating their famous four key principles of biomedical ethics, gloss over this question and adopt a deontological stance, simply asserting that needs should be met. Their chapter on beneficence, for example, starts 'morality *requires* (beneficence)' and that 'positive beneficence *requires* agents to provide benefits' (Beauchamp and Childress 2013, 202, emphasis added). Apart from the vague assertion that (common) morality requires it, there is no clarity about the source of any moral principles that require beneficence (Christen, Ineichen, and Tanner 2014; Childress and Beauchamp 2021).

Beauchamp and Childress cited the parable of the 'Good' Samaritan as 'the most famous example of beneficence' (Beauchamp and Childress 1994, 261), although this was later weakened to simply 'an instructive and classic example' (Beauchamp and Childress 2013). They noted, 'In having compassion and showing mercy, the Good Samaritan expressed an attitude of caring for the injured man and also took care of him. Both the Samaritan's motives and his actions were beneficent' (Beauchamp and Childress 2013, 203).

Here they imply that beneficence is an overarching principle, with compassion an expression of it. By contrast, Childress (1986, 109) suggested that compassion might be the underlying virtue and that it 'leads to acts of beneficence'. However, it is not clear how labelling motives and actions as beneficent helps in interpreting the Samaritan story.

A Christian Ethical Basis for Societal Values

In contrast to the Beauchamp and Childress position, which has compassion as an expression of beneficence, it might be better to see compassion as the prime virtue, that is, compassion is the underpinning value that might be shown in beneficence, as the Childress (1986) phrasing suggests. A Christian ethical rephrasing of Walton's formulation might have the second step as 'state Y is incompatible with a compassionate society' and the third step rephrased as 'therefore, state Y should be changed through compassionate action'.

As discussed in Chapter 1, the parable of the 'Good' Samaritan provides a framework for considering the key principles that should inform healthcare funding decisions. That story explicates the teaching of the Hebrew Scriptures and articulates principles relevant to an everyday situation. The story calls attention to the injunction of the second Great Commandment and the implications of being a neighbour. This then leads to questions of what being a neighbour, being compassionate, taking compassionate action (Copeland 2018, 144), or living in a compassionate society, mean in healthcare and healthcare funding. The starting point of the Samaritan's actions is that he feels compassion for the wounded traveller, and that too should be a starting point for healthcare funding policy.

The Healing Stories of Jesus

Gill (2006) argues that compassion and care are two of the four virtues that should provide the basis for Christian ethics in healthcare. According to Gill, there is a reflexive relationship between these virtues: Compassion needs to be expressed in care, and care, in turn, needs to be shaped by compassion (Gill 2006, 127).

Gill's argument for compassion as a fundamental Christian virtue is based on his analysis of the healing stories in the Synoptic Gospels. Essentially, Gill counts the number of times a particular virtue or value occurs in each of the Synoptic Gospel healing stories. Gill also notes other mentions of these virtues (e.g. in parables), but these are not counted in his analysis. The stories and Gill's identified virtues are shown in Table 2.1.

The table orders the virtues in terms of their prevalence of occurrence. Gill (2006, 82) suggests that

> It might, though, be more logical to order these most characteristic features in terms of their sequence actually within healing stories. On this basis, mercy/compassion typically occurs at the beginning of stories, faith soon after the healing and reticent/restraint at the end. The remaining features – passionate emotion, touching and uncleanliness – tend to cluster in association in the middle of the healing stories. An overall four-fold pattern begins to emerge: an initial plea for mercy/compassion, followed by passionate emotion/unclean touching – then the healing itself – followed by a recognition of faith, and concluding with a command for restraint.

Faith plays an important role in the Synoptic stories, albeit one that is somewhat 'ambiguous' (Gill 2006, 86). Essentially, in the Synoptic stories, people have faith or trust, and through or because of that they are healed.

Gill does not analyse the healing stories in either the fourth gospel or in Luke's second volume, the Acts of the Apostles. There are four healing stories in John: the official's son (4:46–54); at Bethsaida pool in Jerusalem (5:1–18); the blind man (9:1–12); and the raising of Lazarus (11:1–45). The characteristics of these stories are shown in Table 2.2.

Table 2.1 *Virtues or features of the healing stories in the Synoptic Gospels*

Feature	Matthew	Mark	Luke
Passionate emotion *(18 occurrences)*	• Two blind men (9:30) • Blind/dumb demoniac (12:23) • Healing by Beelzebub (12:22–32) • 'Wondering crowd' (15:31)	• The man in the synagogue (1:27) • The leper (1:43) • The paralytic (2:12) • Power to forgive sins (2:3–12) • Man with withered hand (3:1–6) • The Gadarene demoniac (5:15) • Jairus' daughter (5:42) • Deaf mute (7:37)	• Widow of Nain's son (7:16) • Woman with 18-year infirmity (13:10–21) • Man with dropsy (14:1–6)
Faith *(15 occurrences)*	• Centurion's servant (8:10) • Two blind men (9:28) • Canaanite woman (15:28)	• Paralytic man (2:5) • Woman with a haemorrhage (5:54) • Failure to heal others (6:5–6) • Epileptic boy (9:24) • Blind Bartimaeus (10:52)	• Ten lepers (17:19)
Mercy or compassion *(14 occurrences)*	• Two blind men (9:27 and 20:30) • Canaanite/Syro-Phoenician woman (15:22) • Epileptic boy (17:15) • Stories of crowds (9:36 and 14:14) • Blind men at Jericho (20:29–34)	• Blind Bartimaeus (10:47) • The leper (1:40) • Jairus (5:22–3) • Syro-Phoenician woman (7:26) • Blind man at Bethsaida (8:22)	• Ten lepers (17:13) • Widow at Nain (7:13)

Touching or care *(12 occurrences)*	• Two blind men (9:29)	• Peter's mother-in-law (1:31) • Leper (1:41) • Jairus' daughter (5:41) • Some sick people (6:5) • Deaf mute (7:33) • Blind man (8:23) • Epileptic boy (9:27) • Woman with a haemorrhage (5:27) • Crowd at Gennesaret (6:56)	• Bier of the widow's son (7:14) • Woman with 18-year infirmity (13:13)
Uncleanliness	• Command to clean lepers (10:8)	• Man in the Synagogue (1:23 and 27) • Leper (1:41) • The crowd (3:11) • The Gadarene demoniac (5:2 and 5:13) • Syro-Phoenician woman's daughter (7:25) • Epileptic boy (9:24)	• Ten lepers (17:14)
Reticent or restraint *(10 occurrences)*	• Two blind men (9:30)	• Unclean spirits (1:25) • Cast out demons (1:34) • The leper (3:12) • Jairus (5:43) • Deaf mute (7:36) • Blind man (8:26)	

Note: Each story is only listed once against each feature or virtue, even though the story may occur in more than one gospel, Gill gives each of these other mentions a half weighting; stories are assigned to the gospel first listed by Gill. The names of the stories are Gill's. The number of occurrences is according to Gill's count (Gill 2006, 77–81).
Source: Author's summary of Gill (2006).

Table 2.2 *Virtues or features of the healing stories in the Gospel of John*

	Official's son	Bethsaida pool	Blind man	Lazarus
Compassion				
Care			Spread the mud on the man's eyes (9:6)	
Faith (trust)	The man believed the word that Jesus spoke to him and started on his way (4:50)			Yes, Lord I (Martha) believe that you are the Messiah, the son of God, the one coming into the world (11:27; also verse 40)
Reticence		Now the man who had been healed did know who it was, for Jesus had disappeared in the crowd that was there (5:13)		Jesus therefore no longer walked about openly among the Jews, but went from there … (11:54)
Faith in Jesus	'Unless you see signs and wonders you will not believe' (4:48) So he (the official) himself believed, along with his whole household (4:53)		'Lord, I believe' And he worshipped him (9:38)	Many of the Jews … had seen what Jesus did, believed in him (11:45)

Source: Author's analysis.

The four stories in John show little of the pattern that Gill identified in the Synoptics. The closest to the pattern is the Lazarus story where Jesus displays passionate emotion:

> When Jesus saw her weeping, and the Jews who came with her were also weeping, he was greatly disturbed in spirit and deeply moved (11:33)
> Jesus wept (11:35).

This passionate emotion may be the result of sympathy for Mary and Martha (Stibbe 1994, 53), but compassion is not explicitly recorded. The story continues with examples of faith and reticence.

Three of the four stories show a different meaning of faith, a faith in Jesus. The healing stories in John, indeed all the signs in that gospel, are meant to encourage belief – either to come to belief or to reinforce belief (Dennison 1976) – rather than occurring because of belief, faith, or trust: 'In the synoptic Gospels – Matthew, Mark, and Luke – Jesus performs miracles on account of the faith of his audience. In John's Gospel, however, it is the performance of miracles that elicits faith' (Harrison 2009, 493).

The distinction is perhaps not as clear cut as Harrison claims, as certainly some of the healing stories in Luke lead to faith (Achtemeier 1975). But in John the signs are meant to be interpreted symbolically (Carroll 1995), 'communicating the identity of Jesus himself' (Lee 2015, 101). This is most obviously seen in the Lazarus story, which is 'meant to be the climactic sign' (Stibbe 1994, 39), prefiguring Jesus' own death and resurrection.

Although there are more healing stories in Acts (Hardon 1954), most are very short indeed, often one or two verses, so there is little opportunity to assess whether the four-fold pattern Gill observed in Jesus' actions as told in the Synoptics is seen in the actions of the apostles. In a few of the longer stories one or two of the elements can be seen, for example, care in the healing by Peter and John of the man lame from birth (Acts 3:1–11) and in Ananias' restoring Saul's sight (Acts 9:10–21); and faith before the healing in Paul's healing of the crippled man in Lystra (Acts 14:8–11).

As with the fourth gospel, the stories in Acts tell the early communities that the healing power of Jesus did not die with His crucifixion but continued, and thus the stories helped to enhance the credibility of the message being preached by the apostles (Hardon 1954; O'Toole 1981). The stories also serve to emphasise that Paul has the same powers as the disciples chosen by Jesus in the Synoptics (Derickson 1998; Evans 2006). The healing stories in Acts may thus better be interpreted as part of the missional endeavour, as instrumental to bringing people to faith and to show Jesus' continuing power, rather than as acts of healing per se. The focus therefore is not primarily on the healing and its processes that we see in the Synoptics, but on the effects of the healing on the communities in which it occurs (Ferngren 1992; Warrington 2006).

The Contexts of the Healing Stories

Gill's analysis of the healing stories focused on Jesus' actions. Importantly, the contexts of these stories can also provide insight into the place of compassion. The contexts vary: in some cases it is the sick or afflicted person themselves who initiates the contact with Jesus, for example, the leper in Mark 1:48 (also Matthew 8:1–4 and Luke 5:12–14); the ten lepers in Luke 17:11–9; and the woman who suffered a haemorrhage (Mark 5:21–34, Matthew 9:20–22, and Luke 8:43–48). In others, it is the person's immediate family that draws the person's plight to Jesus' attention (Simon's mother-in-law in Mark 1:30 and Luke 4:38–39; the raising of Jairus' daughter in Mark 5:21–4 and Matthew 9:18–25; and the Syrophoenician woman's daughter 7:24–30). There is also a third category where people supporting the sick or afflicted person bring them to Jesus' attention.

There is a community orientation in many of the healing stories that involve people, other than family, bringing the person to Jesus' attention. In Mark there aree five such occasions in the stories of the healing at Simon's house (1:29–33, where the 'whole city was gathered around the door', also Luke 4:40–41); of the paralysed man (2:3–5, where 'some people came, bringing to (Jesus) a paralysed man, carried by four of them', also Luke 5:17–26); at Gennesaret (6:53–56); of a deaf man (7:32); and of the blind man at Bethsaida (8:22). We also see similar occasions in Matthew in the healings in Galilee (4:23–24); at Peter's house (8:16); of the paralysed man (9:2); and of the mute person (9:32) and in Luke, of the raising of the widow's son at Nain (7:11–15) who had 'with her a large crowd from the town'.

There is one example in these stories of what Gill would describe as 'passionate emotion' of the supporting people in the raising of Jairus' daughter who were 'weeping and wailing loudly' (Mark 5:38, also Luke 8:40–56).

What all of these stories show is that there is a community around the sick or afflicted person, a community which stretches beyond the family. The community is there, connected to and supporting the person afflicted, to bring them to Jesus and the possibility of healing. The community is also there to support the family of the person afflicted. These communities are exhibiting shared concern for the welfare of the person afflicted. Although not explicitly stated in the text, this shared concern can reasonably have been thought to be stimulated by compassion.

In these healing stories the virtue of compassion is therefore not simply a virtue shown by Jesus and the stimulus for the immediate care of the person, it is also the context within which the healing occurs. That is, the virtue of compassion is not just the initiating virtue, occurring at the beginning of the healing story, and driving the subsequent care and healing, but the individual person is supported by a community that exhibits compassion. These contexts point to a wider connectedness of the individual into a compassionate society around the healing act and that there is a community that is compassionate and that is seeking to support those in need.

In summary, the virtue of compassion is broader than the motivator for an individual health professional; it is also the motivator for wider community action in healthcare.

A Theology of Compassion

The average Israelite in Jesus' time existed not as an autonomous independent in the post-Enlightenment sense but as part of Israel. Pilch (2000, 5) identifies different aspects of values across cultures and, among other attributes, contrasts the primacy of individual goals over the goals of a 'collateral group (equals, other citizens, friends or kin)'. He suggests that the latter 'value preference characterises first-century Mediterranean groups such as the Judean peasantry and the Jesus group' and contrasts this with American individualism.

The Hebrew Scriptures write of humanity or, more precisely, the nation of Israel, only within 'the categories and boundaries of its own sense of Yahweh and Yahweh's partner' (Brueggemann 1997, 450). Humans live – and ought to live – within the covenant: 'Kind and compassionate in all His ways, the God of Israel chooses to bind His people in a covenant, in a reciprocal relation with Himself of rights and obligations' (Heschel 2001, 369).

Over Israel's history, the expectation of this covenant became increasingly formulaic, replacing the simplicity of the commandments (such as in Micah 6:8) with a set of rules and obligations. By Jesus' time, the compassionate underpinning Heschel describes had given way to exclusionary behaviours. Jesus challenged the strict observance of these rules on many occasions, including in the parable of the 'Good' Samaritan.

Borg (1998) argues that the defining characteristic of Jesus' ministry was to challenge the sophistry and hypocritical observance of the Holiness code of Leviticus 19, so named because it includes the injunction 'You shall be holy, for I, the Lord your God, am holy' (Leviticus 19:2), and emphasise instead a Compassion code enunciated in both Luke and Matthew (with the implicit common source, Q) as 'Be compassionate as God is compassionate' (Matthew 5:48, Luke 6:36, Borg's translation, page 139).

The Compassion code teaches a broad inclusiveness going well beyond the boundaries of those included in the Holiness code: 'Thus Jesus' understanding of God as compassionate implied showing compassion to those outside the covenant and to those considered to have forfeited their status within the covenant, the outcasts' (Borg 1998, 145).

For Jesus, compassion is thus a virtue that extends beyond the established boundaries of the Holiness code and Deuteronomistic law (Glanville 2018). Indeed it is a virtue of radical inclusiveness, and we should not limit the boundaries of our compassion to a narrowly defined neighbour (Snodgrass 2008, 358). The teaching of the parable of the 'Good' Samaritan is that compassion should be shown broadly, not just to those with whom we have a proximal relationship (Reader 2003; Waldron 2003; Sen 2009, 170–173).

Martha Nussbaum in her seminal article highlights the centrality of compassion, referring to it as '*the* basic social emotion' (emphasis added). Compassion, according to Nussbaum, has a utilitarian or egoistic basis, nevertheless it is a 'central bridge between the individual and the community; it is conceived of as our species' way of hooking the interests of others to our own personal goods' (Nussbaum 1996, 28).

Feelings of compassion are linked to identify with the sufferer and back to the potential that the same suffering might sometimes apply to the observer:

> in the temporary act of identification, one is always aware of one's own separateness from the sufferer – it is for another, and not oneself, that one feels; and one is aware both of the bad lot of the sufferer and of the fact that it is, right now, not one's own. If one really had the experience of feeling the pain in one's own body, then one would precisely have failed to comprehend the pain of another as other.
>
> While retaining awareness of her separateness, however, the (person exhibiting compassion) at the same time acknowledges that she has possibilities and vulnerabilities similar to those of the sufferer. She makes sense of the suffering by recognising that she might herself encounter such a reversal … She sees herself, in the process, as one to whom such things might in fact happen …
>
> The point seems to be that the pain of another will be an object of my concern only if I acknowledge some sort of community between myself and the other, understanding what it might be for me to face such pain. (Nussbaum 1996, 35)

Compassion, which is created by community, through solidarity, reflexively creates a community or solidarity. For Aristotle, who Nussbaum draws upon, community may be quite narrowly defined: 'Also we pity those who are like us in age, character, disposition, social standing, or birth; for in all these cases it appears more likely that the same misfortune may befall us also' (Aristotle 2014, 2208; Rhetoric 1386: 25–27).

This self-centred notion of compassion is challenged for Christians in the parable of the 'Good' Samaritan and in the strong teaching in the gospels about enemy love (Gill 2020) as 'compassion is a *social* virtue precisely because it involves an act of transcending the self-centred standards of judgments which Aristotle and Nussbaum rest their analyses on' (Carr 2001, 425; emphasis added).

The view of compassion as an other-regarding social virtue is supported in the psychology literature, which shows that empathy and compassion in humans are altruistic, ultimate goals rather than instrumental goals, as the self-centred basis of compassion might suggest (Batson 2017). The essence of compassion is 'an integrated flow involving compassion to others, becoming receptive to the compassion from others, and also self-compassion' (Gilbert 2019, 110).

Self-compassion here might also have an element of altruism too. Hordern (2013, 96) argues that caring for those who suffer should not involve taking on 'more responsibility than is good either for the self or the sufferer'. Self-compassion also means developing ways to manage the 'moral uncertainties' that compassionate care involves (Greenhalgh 2021).

Humans are, in essence, social creatures, we become a person by learning from others how to walk, talk, and interact. In Archbishop of Cape Town Emeritus Desmond Tutu's reading of *ubuntu* theology: 'I need other persons to become human myself … We are made for togetherness … to exist in a tender network of interdependence … . This is how you have ubuntu – you care, you are hospitable, you are gentle, you're compassionate and concerned' (Tutu as cited in Battle (2009, 65)).

For Tutu, 'a person depends on other people to be a person', emphasising sharing and interdependence, not independence (Battle 2009, 39). As Costello phrases it: 'Compassion accepts that we are not truly separate from others' (Costello 2020, 20).

Even if community is defined narrowly as those who are like us, compassion is not just an individual virtue, but it exists because there is this reciprocity of flows and a solidarity that exists between us and others, between Jesus and individuals in the healing stories, between the afflicted person and their supporters in those stories, between the healer and the sufferer, and between the community and the sufferer. The politics of compassion, as exemplified in a compassionate community, 'links the universal and the particular in that it assumes a shared humanity of interconnected, vulnerable people and requires emotions and practical, particular responses to different expressions of vulnerability' (Porter 2006, 99).

This shared humanity is most obviously displayed in how we respond to the 'vulnerable' and to suffering, and this is the essence of compassion. Compassion involves a generous reciprocity. 'Compassion flows inwards (self-compassion) and outwards, as well as reciprocally between individuals. Experiencing compassion fosters compassion to others' (de Zulueta 2021, 1).

Davies (2016, 18) summarises Nussbaum's definition of compassion as involving three elements 'in compassion we see another's distress (cognition), we feel moved by it (affectivity) and we actively seek to remedy it (volition)'.

All three elements are essential for true compassion. Mere observation (cognition) is not compassion, nor is simply observation and being affected, as this is 'simple pity' (Ricoeur 1992, 191), with pity being a form of hardening (Housset 2011, 83) or distancing. Zweig, in his novel *Beware of pity*, makes this distinction:

> But there are two types of Pity. One, the weak and sentimental kind which is really no more than the heart's impatience to be rid as quickly as possible of the painful emotion aroused by the sight of another's unhappiness, that Pity which is not compassion, but only an instinctive desire to fortify one's own soul against the suffering of another; and the other, the only kind that counts, the unsentimental but creative kind, which knows what it is about and it determined to hold out, in patience and forbearance, to the very limit of its strength and even beyond. (Zweig 1939, 184–185)

Pity here is a distancing emotion, connoting a desire to move on to less troubling thoughts. Although one might not accept that compassion is unsentimental, Zweig's description of compassion as 'creative' adds invention to the volitional element, which, together with his reference to the extent to which compassion requires us to go, further distinguishes compassion from mundane pity.

Borg (1998, 16) incorporates the volitional element into his definition of compassion: 'to be compassionate means to feel the feelings of another, and then to act accordingly'. Drawing on the quotation from Nussbaum above, our concern for another's pain creates a community of pain between the actual pain of people like I – Other I is the term used by Davies (2016) – and my potential or imagined pain, which helps I stand in community with the Other I.

The introduction to the *Oxford Handbook of Compassion Science* highlights the volitional element but also brings us back to the issue of need with compassion defined as 'a state of concern for the suffering or unmet need of another, coupled with a desire to alleviate that suffering' (Goetz and Simon-Thomas 2017, 3).

But the actions arising from compassion also involve discernment, 'a reasoning process of what is best to do' (Gilbert 2019, 109), sense-making (Kanov, Powley, and Walshe 2017; Worline and Dutton 2017; Cameron 2017b), and a 'distinct appraisal process' (Goetz, Keltner, and Simon-Thomas 2010). Compassion is a 'pre-moral' emotion if it is just an observed experience of suffering; it only becomes a moral emotion 'at the moment when the other person's misery is *consciously accepted*' (Leget and Olthuis 2007, 618–619, emphasis added). Compassion is thus not simply an automatic or rote response, but involves a complex interweaving of the cognitive, affective, and volitional elements. As we see in the parable of the 'Good' Samaritan, it involves discerning what is right not just in the immediate term, by assisting the traveller, but discerning and acting in the medium term, by taking the traveller to the inn and paying for future care.

Community, solidarity, or connectedness is essential for compassion, and compassion itself is an outgrowth of the 'liberating power of connectedness' (Johnson 1992, 270) and an outpouring of our shared humanity and our closeness to those in need (Collins, Cooney, and Garlington 2011). Compassion, then, is not simply one person being connected to another, but it points to a broader societal connection, addressing the needs of a community of pain. It is not just a 1:1 relationship, with the person I am being neighbour to, but it is a 1: many relationship, being in solidarity with, and being neighbour to, many. Johnson highlights this solidarity or community connectedness in attributing the victory of the resurrection as stemming from 'the awesome power of compassionate love, in and through solidarity with those who suffer' (Johnson 1992, 159). She also argues that 'Compassion is an empowering power, and efficacy, a blazing fierceness, rather than an interior emotion' (Johnson 1992, 284).

Several writers have suggested that organisations can create compassionate cultures (Kanov et al. 2004; Worline and Dutton 2017; Cameron 2017b), an issue to be discussed later in this chapter. Cameron's attributes of compassionate organisations apply equally to compassionate societies. They involve 'not only sensitivity to suffering and a desire to respond, but also a coordinated response aimed at assisting or supporting others in coping with the pain or distress that they experience' (Cameron 2017b, 422).

This coordinated response needs to be nurtured and promoted by leaders in the community who can highlight the nature of the suffering and build space for a society to exercise compassion (Worline and Dutton 2017). Consistent with the definition of compassion, coordinated compassionate social action should be taken because society defines some needs as 'incompatible with the values held in society' (Walton 1969), and is moved by that suffering if those needs are not met. A compassionate society supports inclusion of minorities and eschews creating 'outcasts'; in addition to a rights basis for inclusive policies, exclusion and stigma lead to poorer health outcomes (Saxby, de New, and Petrie 2020).

A particular role of leaders is to mobilise and catalyse a society's compassionate action, shaping society so it responds in valid and meaningful ways to identified needs (Worline and Dutton 2017, 443).

Leaders can build solidarity and inclusiveness or can exclude: they can portray suffering as 'bad luck', engage in victim blaming (Crawford 1977), or, alternatively, point to the systemic factors that might have created the suffering (Horsell 2017). A compassionate society will embrace rather than blame the outcasts and move to redress the preconditions which create the conditions of suffering.

Compassion, then, is not an anodyne armchair feeling of an individual, but rather must be directly and viscerally linked to a tangible response to suffering, both by the individual healer, as we see in the Jesus healing stories, and by society as a whole, as we see in the contexts of many of those stories. Certainly, it should motivate the individual, but it should also shape society, and motivate societal action. Compassion is a 'social good', a good that only exists by sharing and where 'the more we share, the more we have' (Sacks 2020, 18), and the more we have the more society as a whole is compassionate with compassionate policies and actions.

Compassion and solidarity should be inextricably linked to action, and without action, it is difficult to demonstrate either compassion or solidarity. Our attitude to compassion – be it as an individual or society – defines us, and reflects who we are: 'The motivation for compassion can … give rise to a sense of identity, a self one tries to become and live by; a compassionate self' (Gilbert 2019, 110).

Although Gilbert here is writing about individuals, the same phrasing can be used to describe a compassionate society.

The essence of an appropriate, compassionate societal response to suffering involves solidarity with the sufferer (Isasi-Diaz 1998), which in turn requires 'compassionate action'. Although the word compassion connotes suffering with or alongside, the volitional element of compassion is central and so that suffering alongside needs to be translated into some form of action.

Gill (2006, 94) also highlights the linking of compassion and action:

> Within the Synoptic healing stories compassion is not simply about feeling sorry for the vulnerable, nor is it even just about empathy, a preparedness to identify with the vulnerable. Rather, compassion is both a response to the vulnerable *and a determination to help them*, sometimes at the expense of principled scruples. (emphasis added)

The Acts of Compassion

Compassion is the motivation for both individual and social responses to need. Compassion should shape the reasons why a particular need is incompatible with the values of a society. It should also shape an individual carer's response to need and how society as a whole responds to need. Compassion provides a coherent underpinning motivation for both individual and societal responses to need.

Compassion evokes a call to action. In the parable of the 'Good' Samaritan, acts of caring, altruism, and rehabilitation to full restitution to health are involved. But in telling the story, Jesus is demonstrating another type of action – trying to reshape the very way society thinks about who is included and who is not. This is an example of a different type of action arising from compassion: 'radical compassion', which is preventive in its orientation and seeks to change the underlying conditions that cause the suffering (Lampert 2014, 170–175). The compassion that is core to the parable of the 'Good' Samaritan is to be exercised through solidarity with sufferers (Isasi-Diaz 1998).

Radical compassion involves the typical cognitive and affective components, but the volitional component of compassion is different. It is no longer simply ameliorative or restorative but seeks to change the underlying dynamics of the source of suffering. Radical compassion involves a focus on the broader situation of an individual's suffering, not only addressing the immediate need but also taking steps to reduce the likelihood of a return of suffering by addressing the underlying social, economic, and commercial determinants of ill-health (Isasi-Diaz 1998).

Compassion for the individual's plight and addressing the immediate care needs should only be one element of the compassionate response, which should involve an element of redressing the injustice that has caused or contributed to the suffering (Reilly 2008, 27–29).

The Implications of the Virtue of Compassion

Compassionate action plays out in the clinic in the way in which care is provided (Kitson et al. 2013; Shea and Lionis 2017; Kitson 2018); staff are paid to provide care, and this can involve them engaging fully with those they are caring for, providing 'emotional labour' (Hochschild 2012) or 'emotional practice' (Erickson and Stacey 2012). Although I have argued that compassion is not only a virtue for the healer but of a community too, the health team interacts with an *individual*. Compassion entails being affected by and responding to the individual's pain. It goes beyond just sharing; compassion involves being with.

In his work on the theology of compassion, Davies (2016) argues that the very essence of being is one's self identity as I, and recognising the boundaries with not-I, which includes identification of other people like I, Other-I. Davies goes on to argue that an 'ethical community' is one which seeks 'to propagate in others the intrinsic good of the affirmation of the other' (Davies 2016, 35), without consideration of which specific Other-I are valorised and which are not. All I and Other-I are bound together, with the 'highest expression [as] compassion, where I enters into the suffering of Other-I, offering companionship by acknowledging the encroachments of alien suffering into the self and seeking to alleviate the suffering of the other' (Davies 2016, 36).

For Davies, compassion is the 'epiphany of being' (Davies 2016, 36), and

> compassion stands at the heart of the Christian response to God … the presence of God with us is known to us through his acts of liberating compassion and that this insight is given by God himself and is therefore of fundamental importance in our thinking about him. We have also suggested that the theological language of compassion serves … to remind us we can only think about God in depth, and draw near to him in understanding where we re-enact within ourselves the conditions of his own being, which is to say dispossession of the self for the sake of other. (Davies 2016, 253)

As Farley phrases it in her Madeleva Lecture: 'Compassionate love is not dependent always on sharing the feeling of misery, but on feeling in some way the misery itself' (Farley 2002, 73–74).

Compassion is therefore not so much a distant and somewhat superior relationship, 'there but for the grace of God go I', but rather is about identification with the suffering, 'there go I', recognising that the suffering of the other will change me (Francis 2020b, 3).

Farley perhaps presents the ideal case: that we are so close to the person in the gutter that not only do we feel compassion, but we also feel that pain. It is too easy for us to look down on the penitent tax collector and rejoice in our own health, wealth, and happiness. Our distance creates a hardness of attitudes, inviting us to separate the deserving from the undeserving, setting ourselves up as the ones to sort the sheep from the goats.

Our reality, though, is that we are (mostly) not the ones in the gutter and so our ability to be them is constrained. Can I truly understand racism, sexism, or socio-economic oppression as I walk the world with the experience of a white professional male? Can I understand what it is to be denied the benefits of safe housing, enough food, the ability to read a form, to access the medical help I may need at some point? My lived experience has not been (to date) as a person experiencing cancer, depression, or a missing limb. So, what is required is '*imaginative* dwelling on the condition of the other person, an active regard for his good, a view of him as a fellow human being, and emotional responses of a certain degree of intensity' (Blum 1980, 509, emphasis added).

The imaginative reconstruction of someone's condition, which is part of compassion, means I have to imagine Other-I's need and suffering and be close to feeling that; it involves I being with Other-I, rather than above Other-I. But compassion calls us to be close – both as individuals and as communities (Wilson 2012), not to be mere curious spectators, 'far from making a contribution to a politics of pity or compassion' (Banner 2014, 90–91). Rather we are to attempt to understand and to stand as close as possible to the other, perhaps not becoming the one in the gutter – for that involves 'identity confusion' (Blum 1980, 509) – but certainly laying alongside them and enveloping them in our compassion, showing 'the mutual grace of the Samaritan and the victim, who give and receive care as equals' (Graystone 2022, 5).

The compassionate interaction with the individual has been described as shedding 'light on the individual patient in her concrete situation in all of its particularity and complex embodiment; it also illumines the situation of sickness, reveals the form of relationship needed between caregiver and patient, places in relief structural deficiencies in the providing of care' (Farley 2002, 42).

These structural deficiencies may be gaps in care for an individual, but they may also be gaps in the compassionate society. Just as the healing stories take place in a community context, so too do healthcare interventions today. The individual in need is in a context, a family, and a broader or narrower network of relationships, and if in residential care, a context of paid staff. The exercise of compassion itself creates a community; because compassion is about shared suffering, it creates an equitable, sharing community: 'Suffering is the great equalizer, but compassion reaches up and down and across, assuring a kind of equal respect – the kind that is part of what compassion gives. Or at least part of what compassion can offer' (Farley 2002, 66).

The issue of equity is discussed in more detail in Chapter 3 but suffice to say now that although compassion is to be exercised equitably for all, the exercise and interpretation of compassion is different for each (Porter 2006, 113). Compassion calls for a health system response that is sensitive to the needs of each individual in their own situation. In a compassionate society that response is not a paternalistic, hierarchical response of charity reserved for the deserving, but rather the response should be a generous outpouring because I identifies with all the Other-I and shares the Other-I's pain; I is being a neighbour to all.

Compassion and care involve understanding, being moved by, and acting on an individual's suffering. However, suffering and pain is very personal. Wilkinson (2005, 16) argues that '[s]uffering is common to all of us, yet can only be known uniquely as our own'. Eberl agrees 'that no person can enter into the psychological state of another person who is suffering and facing death' (Eberl 2012, 259). So as much as compassion involves identifying with the person in need, it is still the individual's pain or suffering that is being experienced. A person's pain might arise from multiple different causes with different impacts on a person's life. People get frustrated when healthcare doesn't recognises and take into account these differences (Tuzzio et al. 2021). Compassionate care must therefore respond to the specific circumstances and context of the individual and to how the individual frames their own need.

Returning to the three vertices of need determination – individual, professional, and societal – compassionate care calls us to accept an individual's definition of need, and therefore respect the individual's autonomy in terms of treatments they want. This means working with individuals and their carers to identify what their goals of care are (Kaldjian et al. 2008; Thomas et al. 2014). At this stage of their condition are the goals full restoration of function? Or maintenance of their current state? Or the avoidance of further pain? Truly recognising an individual's goals of care can be difficult: professional prejudices and aspirations can sometimes get in the way of hearing what an individual wants to work towards (Murdoch et al. 2020). Decline is inevitable; compassionate care is about the trajectory – steep or gradual, and what abilities the individual desires are maintained and protected along the way (Gawande 2014).

Compassionate and patient-centred care can sometimes be wrapped up in the language of 'consumer choice' and markets (de Zulueta 2013). This language is often antithetical to compassion stemming from a motivation of being a neighbour, commodifying the stimulus to care as simply being driven by a market relationship. The language of 'choice' assumes that people have the knowledge and resources to exercise choice and that there are options from which they can chose (Gabe, Harley, and Calnan 2015) and the opportunity to do so (Boulding 1969). Unfortunately, choice is often illusory – consumers do not have information about the consequences and outcomes of a choice, with their choices effectively determined by a health professional acting as their agent. Choice options – across a range of service systems – are particularly constrained for the most at risk, with the least power in the system (Beck 2018). In these circumstances the rhetoric and the offer are insincere (Latimer, Roscamp, and Papanikitas 2017).

Compassionate Care at the End of Life

Care at the end of life brings the nature of compassionate care and the need for person-centred care into sharp focus. Heroic interventions, by the hero professional, may make the last days of life difficult for the patient. Health professionals, trained to cure, may find it difficult to move to supportive caring and they may continue to recommend treatments that provide little or no benefit to the patient in terms of life expectancy but at great cost, limiting communications between the patient and their families and carers. Pressure from families for more treatment, especially treatment that the treating team knows will have a low likelihood of changing the patient's prognosis, can be stressful for clinical teams, especially when they know that the treatment for this patient means that another patient with a better prognosis will be denied access to a scarce resource such as an intensive care unit bed (Workman et al. 2003; Chamberlin et al. 2019; Lambden et al. 2019).

Compassionate care requires honest communication (Olson et al. 2021), perhaps facilitated by development of an advance care directive (Lewis et al. 2016; O' Mahony 2016; Johnston and Beckman 2019; Thomas et al. 2020) and a better connection between general care services and palliative care (Jordan et al. 2020). It recognises that pain and suffering, especially toward the end of life, is a 'profoundly personal and subjective experience' (Dees et al. 2010), and so compassionate care must also be profoundly personal.

Over the past few decades, the question of inappropriate or 'futile care', ostensibly aimed at extending life, has risen in policy prominence.

Definitions of the concept(s) abound (Aghabarary and Dehghan Nayeri 2016), drawing on a range of concepts (Morata 2018). Schneiderman (2011, 125) defines 'futile care' as care with an unacceptably low 'likelihood of achieving an effect that the patient has the capacity to appreciate as a benefit', highlighting the importance of the patient's perspective in assessing benefit. The issue here is whether aggressive interventions are appropriate, judged by some combination of the outcome in terms of patient survival, the cost to the patient's comfort and dignity and interactions with family and friends at end of life, and the resources consumed in the care provided (Esserman, Belkora, and Lenert 1995; Löfmark and Nilstun 2002; Downar et al. 2015; White et al. 2016; White, Willmott, and Close 2020). Unfortunately, when patients are not in a position to make their views clear, substitute decision-makers may not appreciate the limitations of treatment or may not be willing to accept a patient's prognosis (Downar et al. 2015).

Investigations may be ordered right up to the last few days of the person's life (Ong et al. 2017; Mitchell et al. 2021), sometimes slowing referral of the patient to palliative care. Early referral to palliative care has been shown to extend life (Temel et al. 2010).

An Australian three-hospital study found the incidence of 'futile care' in the hospitals ranged from 6 per cent to 20 per cent of admissions, with the mean length of stay after initiating 'futile' treatment of 15.1 days, composed of 9.8 standard ward days and 5.3 intensive care unit days (Carter et al. 2017). Somewhat higher estimates – more than one-third of patients – occur when specific non-beneficial treatments are measured (Cardona-Morrell et al. 2016; Cardona-Morrell et al. 2017). There is no consistency in the methods used to define non-beneficial care, so estimates vary widely and make a fair estimate of prevalence difficult to determine (Gabbay et al. 2010; Cardona-Morrell et al. 2017).

Patients who expect to live longer have more intensive treatment (Phillips et al. 1996), even though this may not actually prolong their life (Weeks et al. 1998). Patients consistently overestimate their prognosis (Hole and Salem 2016), and 'hope' plays an important and complex part of palliative care conversations (Kirby et al. 2021). Patients' and their surrogates' spiritual beliefs and belief in miracles are associated with more intensive treatment at the end of life (Phelps et al. 2009; Rosoff 2019; Bibler et al. 2020; Jones 2020; Torke et al. 2020), although, at least in the Roman Catholic tradition, artificially prolonging agony is not consistent with human dignity and the 'moral duty to accept death' (Taboada 2002, 64). Conflict within families and treatment teams is associated with higher rates of non-beneficial treatment (Carter et al. 2019), highlighting the importance of early discussions with families and within teams about the likely prognosis associated with various treatment options.

Compassionate care should mean identifying what is important to the patient as an individual in their specific circumstances, for example, celebrating a milestone event for them or their family – but it may also be maintaining their dignity or their communication so they can say their last goodbyes (Rosenberg 2020). Although estimating clinical prognosis will always be an inexact science (Meadow et al. 2014; Hui, Maxwell, and Paiva 2019), the clinical team needs to ensure that patients and their carers appreciate and understand the most likely clinical trajectory and the uncertainty around that, and understand whether or not treatment is likely to be beneficial, with the associated additional uncertainties.

'Futile care', 'clinically inappropriate care', or 'non-beneficial treatment' is not, as the terms may be taken to imply, a dichotomy: futile, etc., or not. As with all healthcare there is a balance: what is the likelihood of benefit, what is the likelihood of harm, how certain are the estimates and views of the treating team, and how clear the wishes of the patient and the patient's carers? The term 'disputed care' has been advanced as a way of signalling this uncertainty (White, Willmott, and Close 2020).

Compassionate care does not require provision of disputed care (Rosoff 2019), and, as with all healthcare, treating teams cannot be forced to provide care they think is inappropriate. However, the role of the treating team is as a partner in compassionate care:

> Doctors must realise that when the decision is at least partly an ethical one (namely, whether the treatment is in the patient's best interests, or is 'worth doing'), they do not have privileged access to the truth. They have relevant information and their opinions, while potentially illuminating, should not be determinative. (Downie, Willmott, and White 2014, 38)

The care provided sits in a social, clinical, and institutional context. The options presented by the treating team, and the management of disputed care generally, should not set up 'unattainable utopias' of unlimited options, some with vanishingly small prospects of improving outcomes, but rather should be about 'encouraging deliberation, genuine, shared decision-making' (Misak, White, and Truog 2014, 1672). Misak and her colleagues argue that this shared decision-making takes place within 'the context of an implicit and evolving social contract among patients, physicians, and societies at large' (Misak, White, and Truog 2014, 1668).

The way forward for treating teams, patients, and carers, as well as for institutional decision-makers, is to make clear what are the relevant values that impinge on these decisions – patient autonomy, fairness, and distributive justice (Downie, Willmott, and White 2017) – and to engage in a 'compassionate dialog' (Rosoff 2019, 136) both with the patient and their carers, and, prior to that, within the institution to develop policies about these issues. Institutional frameworks for managing responses to disputed care may need to be developed both within services and by the relevant – state/province/national – legal jurisdiction (White et al. 2017).

A compassionate dialogue can only succeed if there is trust between the patient, their carers, and the treating team (Leland et al. 2017). Trust is required so that the concerns and goals of the patient are fully heard and understood and the estimates of prognosis and the alternatives to the disputed treatment accepted. Strategies to improve communication at end-of-life are complex and evolving (Turnbull, Bosslet, and Kross 2019), but trust will always be core and reducing the areas of disagreement about facts/estimates can help clear the air for an open dialogue about values and priorities. A key attribute of compassionate care will be these authentic dialogues, working with the patient and family to help them understand the prognosis and being clear about the available alternatives to the disputed care to manage symptoms consistent with the goals of care.

I revisit this issue in the context of potential rationing of care in Chapter 5.

Compassion and Healthcare Funding

The fundamental attribute of a compassionate society is about ensuring access to care and the type of care one has access to. Compassion calls for a response to every suffering, that every person can get care. This does not mean that every conceivable intervention should always be provided, without regard to the cost to society, an issue addressed in Chapters 4 and 5. Rather it means that an appropriate and proportionate response to suffering is available to everyone, with healthcare professionals not over promising and patients not demanding too much. Gill (2006, 195) describes these attributes as the meaning of 'humility', another of the virtues he identifies in the stories of Jesus' healing.

Consistent with the argument that compassion 'is not simply a virtue for individuals' (Borg 2014, 226), a Christian ethic or virtue of compassion calls for compassionate *social* action, recognising there is a social or collective interest in ensuring that people have access to healthcare.

In a compassionate society access to healthcare is not simply an individual responsibility; society has a shared responsibility to ensure everyone can have access to care. The issue of equity and financial barriers to access is discussed in Chapter 3, but financial barriers are not the only ones that inhibit access – people may not get access to care because of their geography, race, sexuality, or gender.

As the parable of the 'Good' Samaritan teaches, we are to be neighbours to everyone. Although the lawyer asked, 'Who is my neighbour?' (Luke 10:29), clearly attempting to limit the obligation to a specific person or group, Jesus' answer was about *being* a neighbour (Luke 10:36), which is about being there for everyone, waiting the opportunity to show our neighbourliness.

The writer of Matthew tells the story of the judgement day when the Son of Man will separate people just as a shepherd separates sheep from goats. The commendation to 'the righteous' is that 'just as you did it to one of the least of these … you did it to me' (Matthew 25:40) and the criticism of those charged heavily is that 'just as you did not do it to one of the least of these, you did not do it to me' (Matthew 25:45). The point of the story is that Jesus is to be seen in the face of the poor: 'the poor remain entrusted to us and it is this responsibility upon which we shall be judged at the end of time' (Pontifical Council for Justice and Peace 2004, para. 183).

It is this trust which is to be fulfilled through compassionate social action. Compassion may be defined as recognising, feeling, and acting on suffering. It is not bounded to only be compassionate to some, rather compassion should be unbounded to all. What is required to fulfil this mandate 'can be addressed only by reforming the structure of society' (Collins 2019, 209), including a universal programme supporting access to care.

The Challenges of Effecting Compassion

The parable of the 'Good' Samaritan calls for a broad definition of neighbour, to be compassionate to all. But healthcare is not available equally to all, with barriers erected by geography, race, power structures, financial means, and other factors.

Although clearly not every service can be made available in every location, the tyranny of geography needs to be recognised in healthcare policy. Policy design may include additional payments to encourage health professionals to live and work in remote areas or to support fly-in-fly-out professionals (strategies to bring services in person to those areas) or implement licence restrictions to encourage work in remote areas; it might also involve strategies to overcome the geographical barriers using contemporary technology such as tele-health, bringing a virtual rather than a physical presence. Tele-health is now a well accepted and proven technology across a range of areas of healthcare as diverse as cardiac rehabilitation (Rawstorn et al. 2016), management of chronic conditions (Totten et al. 2016; Jin et al. 2019; McFarland, Coufopolous, and Lycett 2021), obstetrics and gynaecology (DeNicola et al. 2019), and autism spectrum disorders (Ferguson, Craig, and Dounavi 2019). It became even more accepted during the SARS-CoV-2 pandemic. Support for patient (and carer) travel – bringing the individual to the service – should also be part of a policy mix.

Geography is an identifiable and relatively politically neutral barrier to be addressed. Health services that are culturally appropriate for the majority or dominant culture may not be so for minorities and may indeed be so culturally intimidating that they are culturally unsafe and create a real barrier to access to care.

Health services in Australia, for example, exhibit systematic institutional racism (Bourke, Marrie, and Marrie 2019), and there is now widespread evidence of poor outcomes for First Nations Australians even after they have access to care (Dwyer et al. 2016). A truly compassionate society will recognise, empathise with, and act on the poor health status of people of racial minorities in all countries, and develop policies to ensure that every health service addresses implicit racism and attempts to ensure that its services are culturally appropriate.

Similarly, health services may not be welcoming for women, or people outside the heteronormative culture. One ameliorative strategy has been to develop specific health services to provide access to care in a culturally acceptable environment, such as women's health services (Broom 1997, 1991; Norsigian 2019), First Nations' controlled community health organisations (Bartlett and Boffa 2001, 2005), and gay men's services (Kayal 2018). These are of course a necessary response to the marginalisation experienced in general healthcare provision and can provide models for incorporation into all health services to make them accessible to all. However, ideally all services will address the issues that lead to cultural exclusion, including by embedding specific services for marginalised groups within their business as usual (McClain, Hawkins, and Yehia 2016; Tuller 2020).

Although many staff have dedicated their careers to providing care to the excluded, care for minorities and the excluded is often second rate – power exercised by excluding options for care from even being on the agenda; staff of services for the poor or minorities being less well-trained; equipment being old or faulty; and the general amenity of care being poorer (Institute of Medicine Committee on Understanding and Eliminating Racial and Ethnic Disparities in Health Care 2009; Elliott et al. 2015; Patel and Rushefsky 2015). This is not what should occur in a compassionate society. The teaching in Matthew 20:16 is that the last shall be first, not that the last will always be at the end of the queue for equipment, good staff, and the best evidence-based treatment. A compassionate society should ensure there is no systematic difference in process or outcomes of care for people who are on the margins of society.

Health funding design in a compassionate society should be pro-poor, and consciously consider the impacts of funding formulae and incentives on marginalised groups, an issue explored more fully in Chapter 3.

The Challenges of Compassionate Funding Design

Quality care – in particular, compassionate care – cannot be provided if policies, politics, and culture conspire against it (Flynn and Mercer 2013; Fotaki 2015), and if austerity and budget cuts trim bone as well as fat. Although I argue in Chapter 4 that stewardship requires that organisations be efficient, cutting budgets is not synonymous with improved efficiency, nor is it necessarily consistent with an ethical approach to funding healthcare (Hellowell, Appleby, and Taylor 2018), an issue also discussed in Chapters 5 and 6. Cost control can go too far, impeding innovation, to the detriment of efficiency, properly defined (Chen et al. 2021).

The context within which healthcare staff do their job has to be such that they have time to be compassionate. Compassionate care requires that clients or patients are treated as humans, made in the image of God, not as commodities; they are subjects not objects (Moore 2017). The contemporary marketisation trend in social care (including aged care and disability support) is ostensibly designed to empower clients (Ottmann, Allen, and Feldman 2013). This objective is to be welcomed, but it requires an effective market and market regulation. Marketisation may have perverse effects if creation of markets with supposedly empowered consumers results in increased power for poorly regulated providers and consumers – lacking the resources and information to enable them to be effective market participants – have no effective choice and are offered 'efficient' provision, with compassion defined out of the efficiency definition (Dowse 2009; Miller and Hayward 2016; Moore 2017; Shuttleworth 2017; Davidson 2018; Henderson and Willis 2019).

Narrow austerity policies can mean staff lose their professional autonomy and compassion is crowded out through work intensification and unrealistic workloads (Henderson et al. 2016; Kerasidou 2019) and not giving time for the professional to 'feel with' the patient or client (Dougherty and Purtilo 1995). Staff are forced into the invidious position of trading-off an appropriate professional response to one patient to provide an appropriate professional response to another (Kitson et al. 2013; Tanner 2020). Staff feel devalued (Winant 2021) and those who cannot show the compassion they would like to are at risk of 'moral distress' and of consequent burn over burnout and leaving the organisation (Whittaker, Gillum, and Kelly 2018; Atashzadeh-Shoorideh et al. 2020). As West (2021, 42) points out, 'Being forced to go against their moral compass undermines professionals' feelings of integrity, their sense of self worth and their well-being.

Crowding out of time for compassion may be counter-productive as compassionate care leads to faster recovery (Trzeciak and Mazzarelli 2019).

Changing the organisation of care may inadvertently change the ability to care, and inhibit compassionate care:

> Along the way something else happened too. Encouraging a patient to eat, listening to a patient's story, making a joke, patting an arm–such acts lost importance. They were absent from the medical charts. And these days, 'if something isn't on the charts', as one observer noted, 'it didn't happen'. Emotional labor became invisible.
>
> That didn't mean nurses and aides didn't continue to do it. They did, but from inside a care system in disrepair. As frontline workers, nurses and nurse's aides now had to put a good face on emotion-deaf arrangements. Given fewer nurses to go around, they rushed. They skimped. They were prevented from giving their best. Some tried to detach themselves from the new scene while others managed a loss of pride. We could call this the emotion work of a broken care system. (Hochschild 2012, Preface to the 2012 edition)

These small acts of caring, not in the chart, are diminished, seen as 'immaterial, unproductive, unskilled and outside of the labour process' (Bolton 2009, 76), and devalued in both their importance and in the pay rates of the caring workers because of masculinist views of what is important in health and social care, as if people displaying compassion are not also entitled to justice (Hendrickx 1987, 95). Compassionate conversations, especially at the end of life, require time and committed staff (Olson et al. 2021), neither of which might be available in the face of mindless budget cuts. Narrow and mindless 'austerity' is not 'efficiency' in the sense that economists use that term, and is often simply untargeted cost-cutting, unfortunately, 'cutting tangible costs at the expense of intangible benefits' as Mintzberg (2017, 70) so nicely puts it.

Austerity and swingeing cost cutting are not consistent with a Christian ethic of healthcare funding. Compassion must always be front and centre of health policy and management, with staff and patients valued as humans not 'human resources' or management's widgets. But healthcare management can too easily lose sight of this

> medical care [has] been recast in our society as if it took place in a factory, with doctors and nurses as shift workers, laboring on an assembly line of the ill. The new people in charge, many with degrees in management economics, believe that care should be configured as a commodity, its contents reduced to equations, all of its dimensions measured and priced, all patient choices formulated as retail purchases. The experience of illness is being stripped of its symbolism and meaning, emptied of feeling and conflict. The new era rightly embraces science but wrongly relinquishes the soul. (Groopman 2009, 27)

Austerity and work intensification can create unhealthy tensions between a nurse's professional identity and their being treated as an 'organisational commodity' (Harvey et al. 2016, 522), with the caring role of the nursing professional being diminished and viewed simply as a contribution to 'nursing hours' (Toffoli, Rudge, and Barnes 2011). Healthcare funding policy can too easily lose its soul and forget the importance of those who need care and compassion, in pursuit of 'efficiencies' that are not efficiencies at all, as they have redefined the care out of healthcare, and the 'product' becomes something very different indeed, and care settings are no longer places where compassionate carers want to be.

Compassionate care requires both skills and a commitment or affinity to the work role: not all people will want to engage in 'emotion practice' day in day out, and it becomes even harder when the systems in which they are called to work devalue their work, and make their work harder:

> This all means that many emotional laborers face a great paradox. Though they may come to work hoping to take pride in a job well done, low pay, understaffing, rigid rules, and devaluation can set up circumstances which prevent that. Sadly, their main job becomes protecting patients from the harm of life in a broken, globalized, over-bureaucratized, or profit-hungry system. A tragic cycle is set in motion. The more broken the system, the more disheartened its emotional laborers. The more disheartened they become, the more detached they are from their work, the higher the turnover rates, and the more broken the system. (Hochschild 2013, 30–31; 2009)

The solution to this vicious cycle is partly to be found in funding design and accountability. Policymakers involved in funding design should be aware of the consequences of their funding design decisions – and may benefit from training to help them understand that (Harding 2015). Policymakers should always be able to demonstrate that the funding formula and funding rate are capable of providing compassionate care, and that the funding rate is not set arbitrarily but reflects and allows provision of high quality of care to all.

Accountability, too, needs to focus on the marginalised. Performance indicators often simply report averages, ignoring the distribution. Is waiting time for people caring the same for people from wealthy neighbourhoods as poorer neighbourhoods, for white people compared to people of colour, for people with or without a disability, for rural compared to metropolitan residents, and for people from a culturally or linguistically diverse background compared to those born into the dominant culture? In a compassionate society, all key performance indicators should be reported by the key cleavages in society to highlight the need for action to address these gaps. Where pay-for-performance is used, as discussed in Chapter 5, the design of the metrics should not simply 'standardise away' the effect of race, for example, but services should be held accountable to ensure processes and outcomes are as similar as possible for all. Measurement should point to where action is necessary, not be used to absolve decision-makers of responsibility – it is true that poorer people have worse health outcomes, but that should be a call for action, not used as an explanatory variable to suggest that society can move along, with nothing to be seen here (Dijkstra and Horstman 2021).

Finally, decision-makers need to keep reminding themselves that quantitative measures need to be balanced with qualitative measures (Mintzberg 1975; Case and Given 2016), and both need to be seen as part of a holistic assessment of ensuring compassionate care:

> There are two lexicons in use in public policy. There is the language of metrics, and value added, of growth and resource allocation, of regulation, and of impact. And there is the language of kindness and grief, of loneliness, love and friendship, of the ties that bind, our sense of identity and of belonging. … Both these vocabularies have strengths, but each is deeply dangerous on its own. (Unwin 2018, 9)

Compassion and responsible stewardship can co-exist, but this requires careful selection and use of metrics (Mannion 2014), and abandoning excessive austerity so that environments of kindness and compassion can flourish.

Compassionate Leadership

Environments of compassion need to be nurtured. Compassion should be

> accomplished and reproduced at all levels of the healthcare organisation, from 'bedside to Board'. Compassionate care emerges from the routine enactment of behaviour, dialogue and decisions, much of which takes place far removed from frontline care delivery but which may nevertheless have a profound impact on the ability and motivations of frontline staff to behave in a compassionate way towards the patients in their care. (Mannion 2014, 116)

Leaders play a crucial role in nurturing a compassionate context or compassionate culture. Indeed, Schein (1992) argued that the most important thing that leaders do is create and manage the culture of an organisation.

Leaders in any organisation may have the role of guiding their organisation through times of suffering thrust on them – when the organisation itself has been impacted by trauma (Dutton et al. 2006). However, compassionate leadership is not just about stepping up in times of trouble: the compassionate leader develops a compassionate organisation, one which makes it easy for staff to show compassion as part of their caring roles all the time. Compassionate organisations require a leadership which 'catalyses, fosters and sustains compassionate healthcare' (de Zulueta 2021, 4).

West (2021, 111) has suggested that compassionate leadership has four key attributes: it is effective (including having a clear, shared, inspiring purpose, or vision); inclusive; collective (that is it involves shared leadership); and systemic (pursuing long-term objectives, and providing mutual support across boundaries). What West is pointing out here is that compassion is not suffused through the health or social care organisation because of the label on its entry way. Compassion requires particular behaviours in leaders – behaviours which encourages teamwork and collective leadership, and learning and growth (de Zulueta 2016). Compassion in an organisation is also fostered by signalling its importance through measuring the right things and adapting practices to implement compassionate care (Dewar, Pullin, and Tocheris 2011; Dewar and Nolan 2013).

Conclusion

The starting point for healthcare funding design should be ensuring access to care and meeting the needs that society recognises, and that staff can provide high quality care. According to Walton (1969), recognition of a need means that society has accepted that if a person or group were to remain in the relevant state, it would be 'incompatible with the values held in society'.

Societies' values should have compassion at their core and respond compassionately to the cries of those in suffering in solidarity, with systems of funding and provision that change the state of the sufferer and reduce the likelihood that the suffering will recur. This requires that good quality care is available to all, and that the person who is suffering is treated as an individual, with their needs, aspirations, and priorities heard and respected. This may involve well developed systems of performance monitoring and rewarding superior performance. A funding system should also be such that compassionate care is able to be provided.

Identifying compassion as an underlying societal motivation affects how care and policy are evaluated. Policies that exclude, or treat the 'least of these' differently, and create barriers to access would surely fail when evaluated against the criterion of promoting compassionate care. It is not enough for society to delegate its obligations for compassionate actions to individual healthcare workers, expecting staff to show compassion in every interaction, all day, every day. That individual compassion is welcomed, but the individual behaviour takes place in a context that is facilitated or hindered by societal (and organisational) policies, including healthcare funding policies.

In his famous sermon, John Donne writes:

> No man is an island,
> Entire of itself;
> Every man is a piece of the continent,
> A part of the main.
> ...
> Any man's death diminishes me,
> Because I am involved in mankind.
> And therefore never send to know for whom the bell tolls;
> It tolls for thee. (Donne 1624, Meditation XVII)

We are all linked as humans, involved in humanity (mankind), each should be neighbour to all. Any person's pain diminishes us all, but a compassionate society should recognise these links and our collective humanity and solidarity in design of healthcare funding policy.

In Chapter 3, I argue that this solidarity should also be underpinned by a principle of social justice.

CHAPTER 3

The Call for Social Justice in Healthcare Funding

> [Jesus asked] 'Which of these three, do you think, was a neighbour to the man who fell into the hands of the robbers?' He [the lawyer] said, 'The one who showed him mercy.' Jesus told him, 'Go and do likewise.' (Luke 10:36–7)

Policy is about choices and trade-offs. There is rarely an obvious and simple answer to a policy question where a single option is clearly superior on every relevant criterion, and this raises the question of how much weight should be applied to each. The relative weights for criteria are shaped by underlying values and priorities: how much emphasis on gender equity? How much emphasis on cultural issues? How much emphasis on individual autonomy? How much emphasis on efficiency?

These choices play out at the broad societal level as well as within the health sector. A fundamental choice involves a trade-off between individual rights and autonomy against collective or government action (Buchanan 1981; Golding 1981). One way of framing this is to consider it a balance between a focus on justice for an individual – or an individual's rights – and the importance of considering community concerns and social justice; between 'individuation'/separation and connectedness (Barton 1998; Allin, Hernández-Quevedo, and Masseria 2009). Donabedian (1973) refers to these contrasting values as libertarian and egalitarian.

In the first section of this chapter, I will argue that a Christian ethic of resource allocation calls us to favour and emphasise the importance of social justice and concern for the outcasts as compared to more individualistic emphases. This emphasis is referred to in Roman Catholic social teaching as the preferential option for the poor (Worland 1991; Byrne 1993; Pope 1993; Twomey 2005, 2006).

The second main section in this chapter analyses the implications of a concern for social justice for healthcare financing. A critical decision in health system design is how healthcare is financed; in particular, to what extent is financing to be mutualised, collected through taxes or other universal compulsory contributions such as social insurance, and to what extent is it to rely on an individual's direct contribution, either through voluntary insurance or out-of-pocket payments. These choices might differ for different aspects of healthcare such as hospital care or dental care. I will argue that a Christian ethic of healthcare funding should emphasise mutualisation, specifically through tax or compulsory contributions, and should minimise the use of out-of-pocket payments that hinder access to care for the poor.

Robin Hood or Piggy Bank?

Barr (2001) characterised social welfare schemes as either favouring a Robin Hood principle – taking from the rich to give to the poor – or as a piggy bank, where an individual makes contributions in good times and draws on them in bad times or at different stages of their life cycle. Contemporary social policy is not quite that simple, and there is probably no pure example of either in most countries. The critical policy issue is how much mutualisation of finance should there be? Some argue that a high degree of mutualisation saps individual responsibility and leads to 'unsustainable' levels of taxation. This individualistic philosophy leads to either no mutualisation at all, or the piggy bank theory of welfare policy design: individuals should be encouraged to take responsibility for their own present and future needs across all dimensions of policy.

The alternative position – the Robin Hood principle – emphasises a society's collective responsibility where a just society involves calling on those with greater means to support those with greater needs. We have the Marxist 'from each according to his abilities, to each according to his needs' (Marx 2010, 87) and the contrasting libertarian philosopher Robert Nozick who poses a framing which emphasises voluntarism and individual choice: 'from each as they choose, to each as they are chosen' (Nozick 1974, 160).

A values orientation closer to Nozick's preferred frame deemphasises the role of government in supporting the needy, emphasises lower taxation, greater self-reliance, and talks up the risks of 'welfare dependency' and creating what economists call 'moral hazard': the risk that insurance might adversely impact on individual behaviour. *Ex ante* moral hazard posits that insurance leads individuals to take risks they would normally avoid, and so insurance increases the risk that the insured event occurs (Culyer 2005, 219). This, it is argued, means that health insurance leads to people being less concerned about looking after their own health, as they do not have to bear the cost of healthcare themselves. The Nozick or libertarian approach leads to neoliberal policies of limiting the size of the welfare state and social provision, and an emphasis on market-based solutions in health and social policy (Terris 1999; McGregor 2001). It played out in the SARS-CoV-2 pandemic in prioritising individual freedom over collective public health measures, and a rhetoric of 'personal responsibility', with devastating consequences in terms of the spread of the virus, particularly among disadvantaged groups (Cardona 2021; Giroux 2021; Warf 2021).

In contrast, an egalitarian frame emphasises the importance of ensuring access to care for everyone and recognises that ill-health is not evenly distributed, with poorer people having poorer health (Townes 1998; West 2006; Lago et al. 2018; Nolan and Valenzuela 2019), and a person's *perceived* lack of resources magnifying this effect (Sommet and Spini 2022). The egalitarian frame has been adopted by international organisations such as the United Nations through the International Covenant on Economic, Social and Cultural Rights which creates a right to healthcare (Schoukens 2008) and its pursuit of Sustainable Development Goals, goal 3 of which relates to health and healthcare (United Nations 2016), and the World Health Organisation in its goal for Universal Health Coverage (Garrett, Chowdhury, and Pablos-Méndez 2009). There are many variants of the more egalitarian 'from each according to-to each according to', all of them having some links to New Testament phrasings, see, for example, Acts 4:35 and Romans 2:6 (Bovens and Lutz 2019).

Perceptions of what is fair varies among countries. People's acceptance of healthcare inequality depends on the prevailing status quo in their country, and is also associated with the extent of public financing: the greater the proportion of health expenditure met from public sources, the more inequality is seen as unfair (Immergut and Schneider 2020).

Arrow and Mutualisation

Although an emphasis on mutualisation of financing is often made on social justice grounds, it can also be made on technical or economic efficiency grounds. Nobel Laureate Kenneth Arrow advanced such a case in his seminal paper on the welfare economics of medical care (Arrow 1963).

Arrow argued that the very characteristics of healthcare lead to market failure, as does Culyer:

> Markets in healthcare are notable, not because they failed to satisfy any one of the standard assumptions required for competitive markets to [*work*], but because they failed every single one of them: there is enormous asymmetry of information between producers (medical professionals of all kinds) and consumers (patients actual and potential); the agency relationship [*where a*

> *doctor is supposed to work on behalf of patients*] works imperfectly and can be distorted by systems of physician pay; there is little evidence that patients behave in accordance with the axioms of rational choice theory; … In addition much of healthcare has the character of a public good and generates externalities both physical (as with communicable disease) and psychic (as when you derive comfort from knowing that your neighbours are insured). [Italicised words in square brackets are mine, non-italicised words in brackets are in the original]. (Culyer 2005, 207)

In the presence of inevitable market failure, government intervention in the market is welfare enhancing. Arrow focuses on the nature of risk in healthcare and argues the appropriate response to managing risk is insurance and the mutualisation of risk. He refers to the demand for medical care as being 'irregular and unpredictable' (Arrow 1963, 948) and hence access to healthcare should be underpinned by insurance against the two kinds of risk he identifies: 'the risk of becoming ill, and the risk of total or incomplete or delayed recovery' (Arrow 1963, 959). According to Arrow, individuals are risk averse and would prefer to take out insurance to manage these risks, and there would be an individual welfare gain as a result. More importantly, he also argues there will be a social gain on the reasonable assumption that the insurer is not running at a loss.

Arrow does not use the term 'community rating' – where an individual's insurance premium is not based on the individual's actuarial risk, but rather on the overall risks of the population or community insured – but he argues the merits of this approach. Specifically, 'If a plan guarantees to everybody a premium that corresponds to total experience but not to experience as it might be segregated by smaller subgroups, everybody is, in effect, insured against a change in his basic state of health which would lead to a reclassification' (Arrow 1963, 964).

Although Arrow also does not argue explicitly for compulsory insurance, he does allude to the fact that individuals benefit from care being available to others:

> The taste for improving the health of others appears to be stronger than for improving other aspects of their welfare. In interdependencies generated by concern for the welfare of others there is always a theoretical case for collective action if each participant derives satisfaction from the contributions of all. (Arrow 1963, 954)

The tenor of Arrow's case is thus that all should be insured, and he sees community rating as part of that. Arrow's article has been widely cited and provides the theoretical justification for the mutualisation of healthcare financing we see in most high-income countries. In the next section of this chapter, I will argue that there is also a moral justification for mutualisation, through God's concerns for social justice.

Biblical Conceptions of Justice

The balance between individual rights, such as the right to set one's own priorities for spending, and communitarian concerns can be thought of as different conceptions of justice. Is justice primarily to be thought of as about justice for an individual, or is justice more about social justice, and a set of mutual obligations between one and another?

In this section I will argue that the overwhelming emphasis in the Hebrew Scriptures and the New Testament, especially Luke, is an emphasis on justice as social justice, founded on the fundamental 'theological commitment to the equality of all people before God' (Hicks 2000, 167).

The Hebrew Scriptures

The Hebrew Scriptures tell the tale of God's relationship with Israel, commencing with the primeval history of Genesis 1–11 and moving on to the stories of the great leaders, starting with Abram/Abraham. Genesis 18 recounts God's thoughts that Abraham will form a great and populous nation. As part of that same reflection, God mused on the conditionality of Israel:

> No, for I have chosen him, that he may charge his children and his household after him to keep the way of the Lord by doing righteousness and justice; so that the Lord may bring about for Abraham what he has promised him. (Genesis 18:19, Revised Standard Version)
>
> For I have singled him out, that he may instruct his children and his posterity to keep the way of the LORD by doing what is just and right in order that the LORD may bring about for Abraham what He has promised him. (Genesis 18:19, Jewish Study Bible translation)

So, Abraham is 'chosen' with a specific purpose, a purpose about justice and righteousness, which also binds future generations. Thus, right at the start of the story of Israel we have this centrality of justice, with this issue of justice woven through the Hebrew Scriptures: 'The two crucial Hebrew nouns, *tsedeq* and *mishpat* will continue to reverberate literally and in cognate forms … through the story of Abraham and Abimelech that follows' (Alter 2019a, 58).

Similarly, Weinfeld (1995, 7) notes that 'Israel's prophets saw the fulfilment of this goal [performing righteousness and justice] as the basis of the nation's existence'.

Mishpat is used over 400 times in the Hebrew Scriptures and so it is clearly a central concern of the whole of the Tanakh. The two versions cited above use slightly different translations of both nouns, to do righteousness versus doing right, and to do justice versus doing what is just. But in both cases, *mishpat* is an action word, with a connotation of obligations to others. Justice here is not about individual rights but is rather an action towards others.

Brueggemann also highlighted these external-facing calls for justice as critical:

> Israel is to listen to the commands of Yahweh and to respond in obedience. While the commands in the tradition concerning listening are many and varied, we may say in sum that *Israel's obligation is to do justice*. Israel is a community put in the world, so the testimony suggests, for the sake of justice. The justice commanded by Yahweh, moreover, is not the retributive justice of 'deeds-consequences' wherein rewards and punishments our meted out to persons and community according to conduct. Rather, Israel understands itself, in its unsolicited witness, as a community of persons bound in membership to each other, so that each person-as-member is to be treated well enough to be sustained as a full member of the community. (Brueggemann 1997, 421, emphasis in original)

There is some academic debate about whether the moral commandments and teachings of the Hebrew Scriptures were meant to apply only to Israel (and Judah) or all people, with notable theologians arguing that quite famous injunctions were narrow in their application: Barth (2004, vol II, part 2, page 572), for example, restricts Micah 6:8 to Israel.

It is clear that much teaching in the Hebrew Scriptures reflected the context of the time, including the specific injustices inherent in the social structure of ancient Israel (Esler 1998b), and the contemporary social mores and conceptions of justice. However, the teachings in the Hebrew Scriptures go further in concern for the most disadvantaged than was common in the contemporary ancient near East (Evans 2016a, 23). These wider lessons of the Hebrew Scriptures are still relevant today (Evans 2016a, 23–26, 29–31; Birch 1991; Malchow 1996; Hiers 2009, 212–218). Most of the Hebrew Scriptures' teaching about social justice is of this wider kind. As Barton notes:

> When the prophets speak out on behalf of the poor, it is probably not from a kind of proto-socialist attitude to society, but on the contrary out of a sense that the existence of people whom others exploit and harass is contrary to the peace of society in this sense. Justice will make good the disequilibrium caused by the oppression of helpless people. (Barton 2014, 107)

Ethical principles, including the concerns for social justice, come in part as direct instructions from God phrased in the imperative, the Decalogue being an example; in part as 'conformity to a pattern of natural order'

(Barton 1978, 60); and partly because the readers of the Hebrew Scriptures were aiming to imitate God.

In terms of direct instructions and the natural order, the Torah includes the Decalogue (Exodus 20:2–17 and Deuteronomy 5:6–21) and three early enumerations (Law Codes) of the expectations of how people might live and work together: the first is in the Book of the Covenant (Exodus 20:22–23:33); the second in the Deuteronomistic codes (Deuteronomy 12–26); and the third in the Holiness code (Leviticus 17–26) with each successive version increasing the number of references to social justice and also broadening the application and expectations (Birch 1991, 157–163; Malchow 1996, 21).

The Holiness code includes the command in Leviticus to 'Love your neighbour as yourself: I am the LORD' (Leviticus 19:18b). This was drawn on by Jesus to form the second Great Commandment. Although well known today, and certainly consistent with the strong social justice teaching that characterises the Hebrew Scriptures, love of neighbour was probably not as common a phrasing of moral teaching in ancient Israel as it became subsequent to Christ's command (Kelly 2017).

The Nevi'im continues this theme of justice – in particular justice for the 'quartet of the vulnerable' (Carroll 2016). The prophets Amos, Micah, Hosea, and Jeremiah especially focus on issues of justice with Amos, in his prophetic call, crying out to

> let justice roll down like waters,
> and righteousness like an ever-flowing stream. (Amos 5:24)

This imagery of justice and righteousness rolling down the river alludes to both the life-giving power of water and the power of rivers to reshape the landscape. Justice here cannot simply be thought of as individual justice but is portrayed as a mighty life-changing force.

This emphasis on a broader conception of justice is also present in the Ketuvim (Boda and Baines 2016). Proverbs, a book of individual instruction applicable to all people, not just the people of Israel, starts with a set of objectives for the book. This includes instruction in 1:3 about the importance of acquiring the discipline of 'righteousness, justice and equity'.

Imitation of God is phrased as an injunction in a number of places (e.g., Leviticus 19:2, 'You shall be holy, for I the LORD your God am holy'; see also Deuteronomy 10:17–19). Barton argues: '… the task of human beings, and especially the Israelites, is to do as God does: to take God's character as the pattern of their character and God's deeds as the model for theirs' (Barton 1995, 17).

Imitation of God distinguishes the ethics derived from the Hebrew Scriptures from other contemporary systems, possibly because the other gods 'do not exemplify the conduct they command' (Barton 2003, 167). This is most obviously seen in Psalm 82, where God (Elohim) judges other, lesser gods:

> God has taken his place in the divine council;
> in the midst of the gods he holds judgment:
> 'How long will you judge unjustly
> and show partiality to the wicked?
> Give justice to the weak and the orphan;
> maintain the right of the lowly and the destitute.
> Rescue the weak and the needy;
> deliver them from the hand of the wicked.'
> They have neither knowledge nor understanding,
> they walk around in darkness;
> all the foundations of the earth are shaken.
>
> I say, 'You are gods,
> children of the Most High, all of you;
> nevertheless, you shall die like mortals,
> and fall like any prince.'
>
> Rise up, O God, judge the earth;
> for all the nations belong to you!

What we see clearly in this Psalm is both God's commitment to social justice, but more importantly, God's condemnation of those gods who do not practise social justice for the poor, the orphan, the lowly, and the destitute. This Psalm is one of the transitioning places in the Bible, from the mythological, polytheistic world to monotheism, but here God (Elohim) is the pre-eminent one in a constellation of gods, the God who can pass judgement on the other gods. These other gods could potentially be representatives of the wider world beyond Israel, showing that here the God of Israel is enforcing justice on the wider world. Alter (2019b, 200), in his commentary, also implicitly accepts that the Psalm has universal application, noting that the 'poem is concerned with the infuriating preponderance of injustice in the world'.

The Quartet of the Vulnerable

'A striking feature', as Wolterstorff (2008, 75) puts it, of the Hebrew Scriptures' discussion of justice is its connection to what he calls the 'quartet of the vulnerable': widows, orphans, resident aliens, and the poor. Evans (2016a, 14–22) adds a fifth group, slaves; and Hiers (2009, 184) a sixth, people with disabilities. These are 'the bottom ones, the low ones, the lowly (and thus are) especially vulnerable to being treated with injustice' (Wolterstorff 2008, 76). However, being labelled as 'vulnerable' may contribute to that injustice – vulnerability may be seen as a result of endogenous attributes of the person, rather than being created exogenously by the policies of society. Labelling a group as 'vulnerable' potentially creates a negatively framed deficit narrative de-emphasising the structural causes of their 'vulnerability' (Munari et al. 2021).

Justice for the 'vulnerable', and indeed justice in the Hebrew Scriptures generally, needs to be understood in the context that the Hebrew Scriptures were 'the product of a community and also designed to create and perpetuate a community' (Wenham 2000, 102) and thus are important in the 'formation and maintenance of a particular community character' (Birch 1991, 165). One consequence of this is that concerns for the poor are not to come at the expense of justice for others in the community. Justice for the most disadvantaged is to be considered within the context of fairness for everyone:

> You shall not follow a majority in wrongdoing; when you bear witness in a lawsuit, you shall not side with the majority so as to pervert justice; nor shall you be partial to the poor in a lawsuit. (Exodus 23:2–3)

> You shall not render an unjust judgment; you shall not be partial to the poor or defer to the great: with justice you shall judge your neighbour. (Leviticus 19:15)

> You must not be partial in judging: hear out the small and the great alike; you shall not be intimidated by anyone, for the judgment is God's. (Deuteronomy 1:17)

The individualistic principle of 'equal before the law' – to use a modern phrasing – is a given, a minimum standard. Imitation of God imposed a higher ethical obligation that goes significantly beyond the legal minimum requirements (Sagovsky 2008, 80). Laws simply 'define the floor of tolerable behaviour. Break them and punishment follows. But that does not mean that simply keeping the laws is sufficient … Ethical duty involves much more than keeping the law' (Wenham 2000, 104).

The ethical duty of communities and their members is set at a very high bar indeed – they 'must exhibit divine virtues in their behaviour' (Wenham 2000, 105). This expectation is one of extreme generosity and redistribution:

> It is important that we recognise with some precision the quality and intention of Mosaic, Yahwistic justice, for it is easily misunderstood given the easy and careless use of the term *justice*. The intention of Mosaic justice is to redistribute social goods and social power, thus it is distributive justice.

> This justice recognises that social goods and social power are unequally and destructively distributed in Israel's world (and derivatively in any social context) and that the well-being of the community requires that social goods and power to some extent be given up by those who have too much, for the sake of those who have not enough. This enormously radical principle is constitutive for revolutionary Israel and for Yahweh, as it is evidenced in various traditions. (Brueggemann 1997, 736–737)

Justice in the Hebrew Scriptures, then, is a distributive and redistributive justice, pointing us to more than justice as an individual concern or an individual right, but being about a radical, redistributive social obligation of all the nation of Israel. This is consistent with identifying justice as affecting a class, the 'quartet of the vulnerable'. It is Israel collectively that must address the problems of the class, not only individual people responding to the individual circumstances of other specific individual people. The solution to a social problem must be a social justice.

An example of the extent of divine generosity, thus showing the extent of generosity expected in communities and their members, is in the foundation narrative of Israel – the escape from Egypt – told in Exodus. The story is obviously one of God's concern for God's chosen, but the story is also a striking demonstration of the extent to which God is prepared to go in order to liberate the oppressed, and provides a 'prototype of God's concern for the poor' (Lohfink 1995, 27). This sets the standard that imitation of God requires. Lohfink (1995) points out that this narrative shows that there were multiple attempts to rectify the injustice faced by the Israelites before the Exodus. These included:

- an *individual act of charity*, when Pharaoh's daughter rescued and adopted the baby Moses (Exodus 2:1–10);
- Moses 'begins his career as a liberator soon afterwards with *counter-terror* when he kills an especially brutal oppressor' (Lohfink 1995, 34, here referring to Exodus 2:11–15);
- Moses and Aaron attempt, unsuccessfully, to *negotiate* with Pharaoh with the unfortunate outcome being more burdens (Exodus 5:1–23);
- a series of *plagues* (Exodus 7:1–11:10).

All these are to no avail. They all represent different strategies of amelioration, counter terror, negotiation, and catastrophes:

> All of these events represent, then, other ways by which one could try to put an end to a situation of oppression and impoverishment. According to the book of Exodus, they are of no use. God has another way of dealing with the situation. He leads people out of the system. (Lohfink 1995, 35)

Lohfink goes on to point out that the scale of this divine solution surpasses human imagination. However, it also highlights the breadth of the expectation of social justice in the Hebrew Scriptures. Simple individual charity, and amelioration of the immediate circumstances of the 'quartet of the vulnerable', is not what social justice in the Hebrew Scriptures is about. It points to social justice at scale, with the force of a powerful stream, taking people out of the whole system that creates the injustice. The message of the Hebrew Scriptures is one where YHWH comes to liberate the oppressed in a quite dramatic and radical way (Tamez 1982). Social justice in the Hebrew Scriptures points us to system transformation, not a simple rescue and recovery response, but one of prophetic transformation (Stivers 2011).

Social Justice and the Lukan Jesus

Jesus lived and taught the covenant, as it was delivered by YHWH, and he was learned in the law. It is no surprise that the social justice concerns of the Hebrew Scriptures appear with equal, if not amplified force, in Jesus' teachings. In this section I will explore Jesus' teaching about social justice, drawing initially on the Gospel of Luke where these teachings are described most sharply, but then showing that these same issues are common in the New Testament.

It is well recognised that Luke is a 'justice gospel', with a stronger emphasis on justice compared to the other Synoptics and John. Apart from the 'scandalous book of James' (Tamez 1990), there is probably no other book in the New Testament that has stronger teaching on money, on the rich and the poor, and on justice generally. We see 'particularly in the unique sections of Luke's own source material and his redaction of others' in his gospel, a clear and consistent ethic about the "option for the poor" with warnings for the rich' (Burridge 2007, 263).

Luke includes a number of parables about wealth, stewardship, and other issues relevant to justice which are not found in the other gospels including the parables of the two debtors (7:40–43); the Good Samaritan (10:25–37); the friend at midnight (11:5–8); the rich fool (12:13–21); the lost coin (15:8–10); the prodigal son (15:11–32); the shrewd/dishonest manager (16:1–13); and the rich man and Lazarus (16:19–31). This is not to say that Luke's concerns are absent in the other gospels, indeed all gospels contain teaching about poverty and riches. According to Mealand

> Compared with Matthew and Mark, Luke does appear more severe. But this impression is largely due to the inclusion of more material by Luke. We must also allow for Matthew's tendency to soften some of the harder

> sayings. The apparent severity in Luke is therefore largely to be attributed to his sources, and to the tradition which they contain. (Mealand 1980, 19–20)

Although Luke is sharper in writing, Jesus' preoccupation with 'this-worldly material reality' (Brueggemann 2016, 185) is seen in all the gospels and the teaching in Luke is thus representative of the other gospels.

That justice is a theme in Luke is a given. But the critical question is whether the justice that is required is an individual responsibility – an act of charity that individual Christians should practise – or whether the remit is broader: that more than individual charity is required, and that justice has the communal favour we saw in the Hebrew Scriptures. Although most of the parables in Luke are about individual behaviour and individual stewardship, the call to a social justice is a major theme of Luke and this can be discerned most clearly from two of the great teachings in Luke: the Sermon on the Plain (6:20–49) and the parable of the 'Good' Samaritan (10:25–37).

However, there is another call to justice right at the start of Luke's gospel. Here there is a dramatic reversal in Mary's glorious hymn, the Magnificat, where the proud, the powerful, and the rich are cast down and the lowly and hungry lifted up:

> He has shown strength with his arm;
> he has scattered the proud in the thoughts of their hearts.
> He has brought down the powerful from their thrones,
> and lifted up the lowly;
> he has filled the hungry with good things,
> and sent the rich empty away. (Luke 1:51–53)

Brueggemann (2016, 198) suggests that 'The parallels (in the Magnificat) clearly assume a class analysis of the powerful and lowly who are, inevitably, the rich and the hungry respectively.'

Mary's song of praise is about what God has done, with subsequent Christian theology arguing that humans should imitate God as seen in Christ and behave likewise. But the Magnificat also presages what is to come: it is sung 'thirty weeks before Bethlehem, thirty years before Calvary and Easter' (Wright 2014, 14). For this promise to come to fruition, the world will need to be turned upside down, a new realm proclaimed, and a new ethos, with a particular sort of love, dominating. What is anticipated is a very different sort of love from what was taught heretofore. What is called for is a love of all, including enemy love (Gill 2020). We see in Luke – and in the other books in the New Testament – the same calls for broader, rather than narrower, expectations as we saw in the Hebrew

Scriptures, leading us towards mutuality rather than an individual orientation in policy.

The Magnificat contrasts the fate of two groups: the proud and the powerful compared to the lowly and hungry. The emphasis here is that there is a problem for a whole class who is to be sent empty away and a need to benefit a whole class who is to be filled with good things. It may be possible to think of this scenario as one of individual justice at play, but it is more logical to read the Magnificat as social justice occurring, overturning, and changing the lives of whole classes.

Sermon on the Plain

The Sermon on the Plain has been described as Jesus' manifesto (Montero 2019). It is sharper, shorter, and more directed than the Matthean Sermon on the Mount. Although some exegetes have argued that the poor in Luke has the same meaning as the poor in spirit in Matthew (Meadors 1985) or that poor has both an economic and a spiritual meaning (Barrera 2013, 205), consistent with the emphasis on the poor throughout Luke, these references to the poor more likely 'signify persons with economic and/or physical need. Further, the common association of "the poor" with other terms of low status and marginalization significantly connects them as a group to those on the outside of the social order' (Dyer 2016, 110).

The good news is for the poor, which can be broadly interpreted to include 'any person of low status and on the fringe of society' (Dyer 2016, 110), and the dispossessed. This good news will set the oppressed free: 'For Luke, "good news to the poor" is nothing less than God's gracious word of invitation and welcome to the dispossessed' (Green 2014, 177).

The Sermon on the Plain (Luke 6:20–49) has three main components: the blessings and the woes (verses 20–26); the ethics (verses 27–38); and the parables (verses 39–49). Clark (1996, 432) suggests that appropriate subheadings for the three sections are *reversing earthly values*, *reflecting heavenly values*, and *responding to the teacher*.

Unlike the Sermon on the Mount, Luke's account of the blessings (and the woes) is phrased in the second person – blessed are *you* who are poor – compared to the more remote third person phrasing in Matthew. They are thus more personalised than Matthew's version, reflecting both Jesus' audience and his mission as he announced it in his inaugural sermon (Luke 4:18–19). The blessings address the poor (cf. the rich); the hungry (cf. those who are full now); those who weep (cf. those who are laughing now); and those who are hated because they are Jesus' followers (cf. those of whom all speak well). The first three address 'the real poor and the actually hungry'

(Burridge 2007, 261) with the blessings and warnings 'distributed according to class, and the outcome is more or less set in stone: the underclass is getting the blessing, and the privileged class is getting the woe, end of story' (Montero 2019).

The blessings and the woes contemplate an eschatological reversal of the traditional order, as we have already seen in the Magnificat. In this first section of the Sermon, Jesus is clearly identifying a concern for the poor and foreshadowing, with the parallel warnings, both that the needs of the poor and hungry will be met, and that there will be a reversal, as Clarke's 'reversing of earthly values' label suggests.

Jesus' sermon thus 'foreshadows a reversal of fortunes that unfolds in his ministry' (Matera 1999, 68). The first blessing foreshadows that this overturning will be a consequence of the reign of God, without further explanation. The Hebrew listeners to the sermon may well have inferred this to be a requirement to live the covenant fully, to

> return to the justice of the prophets, which required equality in sharing the resources and good things of the earth. (Grassi 2003, 177)

An explicit injunction to love one's enemies in the second section of the Sermon is labelled by Clark (1996) as being about 'heavenly values'. This section points to how the blessings for the poor and the hungry are to be realised. In addition to the sharper blessings in the Sermon on the Plain (compared to the Sermon on the Mount), the 'heavenly values' include teaching to love one's enemies, and this teaching is more explicit and somewhat stronger in the Sermon on the Plain, compared to its Matthean parallel.

Jesus' teaching to love one's enemies is a dramatic extension of the Torah injunction to love one's neighbour as oneself (Leviticus 19:18), and is expressed as 'an extreme and unconditional formulation' (Harvey 1990, 107). In Matthew the reasoning is essentially that loving one's neighbour is easy, expected, and simple reciprocity: 'for if you love those who love you, what reward have you?' (Matthew 5:46).

We see the same reasoning in Luke (versus 32–33). However, in Luke we also see an important rephrasing of the reasoning – not only are you not doing anything out of the ordinary if you just love your neighbour, but your *Christian* love should go beyond reciprocity because it should be done 'expecting nothing in return' (verse 35). Yet, paradoxically, even if you love/give and expect nothing in return, you will be rewarded greatly (verses 35 and 38).

The sermon has a nice wordplay against reciprocity, which is lost in translation:

> The Greek word translated 'credit' is *charis*, and it is possible that there is a wordplay intended. The word *charis* can mean both 'thanks' and 'grace'. People who offer only love that depends on the hope of getting something back deserve no *charis* ('thanks') because they showed no *charis* ('grace', that is 'undeserved kindness'). (Clark 1996, 430)

The Sermon on the Plain is addressed to collectives of the poor and the rich using plurals, suggesting collective responsibility and collective reversals, again pointing to a social rather than individual justice.

The Parable of the 'Good' Samaritan

Jesus returns to the theme of neighbours and enemies in the parable of the 'Good' Samaritan (Luke 10:25–37). The parable reinforces the teaching about loving one's enemies found in the Sermon on the Plain: if even a Samaritan can show neighbourly love to the wounded man, then so must all who heed Jesus' words show love to their enemies.

The teaching in the parable goes beyond the Second Great Commandment:

> True love of neighbor, moreover, demands more than a negative respect for the neighbor's right not to be harmed, which is the primary intention of Leviticus 19:18. It also requires a positive dedication to restoring the well-being of those who have been injured by the deeds of others, regardless of their social identity or status. (Marshall 2012, 46–47)

Jesus' command to the lawyer was not for him to talk or think but to *do*, it was a call to act, and continue to act, like the Samaritan. Hornsby-Smith (2006), writing in the context of the tradition of Catholic social teaching concludes that:

> The Christian imperative to love our neighbour as ourselves is best developed through a *social action cycle* that consists of four successive and interlinked stages:
>
> - the identification of the social reality: needs and social injustices;
> - the social analysis of their causes and the concrete reality;
> - theological reflection on these in the light of scripture and the developing social thought of the Church and its members; and
> - the social action response to the needs and injustices in the light of the social analysis and Christian reflection. (Hornsby-Smith 2006, 7, emphasis added)

Hornsby-Smith (2006) is here recommending actions for individuals, but as Hollenbach (2002, 196) has noted, this same social action cycle is relevant to communities and nations: needs and social injustices should be identified, the causes determined, and a social action response developed and implemented. Social justice is core to the other forms of justice – distributive, contributive, and commutative – which go to create the common good (Hollenbach 2002).

Luke Is Not Unique

Although Luke's writing is sharper than in the other New Testament writers, the same emphasis on social justice can be seen in many other places in the New Testament.

The parable of the 'Good' Samaritan is the Lukan explication of the second of the two Great Commandments, which appear as explicit teaching of Jesus rather than as voiced by another party in the other two Synoptics (Matthew 22:35–40, Mark 12:28–34). The Lukan Sermon on the Plain is the more focused parallel of the Matthean Sermon on the Mount found in Chapters 5–7.

Not surprisingly, the Synoptic Gospels share many commonalities (Aland 1982), and concerns for justice are woven through both the Gospels and the other books of the New Testament. In Matthew 23:23 and Mark 12:40 Jesus calls out hypocrisy, contrasting following the minutiae of the law but neglecting what Jesus – and the Jewish tradition (Weinfeld 1990) – see as 'the weightier matters of the law: justice, mercy and faith' (Matthew 23:23). The expectation from Jesus here is that justice and mercy, along with faith, is an inherent expectation.

Much of Jesus' justice teaching appears in parables that might appear in only one of the Synoptic Gospels, although the same teachings often appear in the others. For example, the parable of the labourers in the Vineyard is unique to Matthew (20:1–16) and has lessons about justice (Caponi 2018) and systematic injustice (Crossan 2012, 95–98). The Matthean pericope ends with the dramatic eschatological upheaval of a new order where justice prevails: the last will be first and the first will be last (Matthew 20:16). However, although the parable is unique to Matthew, this same foreshadowing appears in Mark (10:31) and Luke (13:30).

This eschatological overturning is critical to the understanding of biblical teaching on social justice. As Mott points out

> Biblical justice is biased in favor of the poor and the weak of the earth … The first principle of justice in distribution is the correction of oppression. This is the first concern; others follow. In assessing the level of justice in society, the needs of the least advantaged member must first be identified; it is from that person's position that the social system is then evaluated.(Mott 2011, 59)

Mealand's conclusion about the teaching on poverty in the Gospels is an apposite summary of this aspect of the Gospel message:

> Jesus and his immediate disciples ... saw the sufferings of the poor as part of the evil of the present order which was in need of being transformed. Jesus and his disciples led no political revolt, but they did sharply criticize accumulation of wealth and neglect of the poor. Some of the sources go further than others in this respect, but both the Hebrew Bible and the New Testament are highly critical of any state of affairs in which some have plenty while others starve.... The New Testament gives no comfort to those who think that religion or morality can turn a blind eye to oppression, injustice or flagrant inequalities. The teaching of Jesus and of the Gospels is rather to call people to participate now in a new order in which love both includes and exceeds the demands of justice. (Mealand 1980, 98)

Paul

The Pauline corpus has had an immense influence on Christian, especially Protestant, thought. Paul is undoubtedly one of the most significant figures in the development and shaping of Christianity; Borg and Crossan (2009, 2) describe Paul as 'second only to Jesus as the most important person in the origin of Christianity'.

For Paul, 'Christian life is life in the Spirit' (Bowe 2017, 173). Paul's spirituality involved a complex interweaving of elements, including pastoral care (Hardin 2015), and a concern for the poor (Longenecker 2010). Paul's dominant message was one of grace and life with Christ, and many of his epistles also preached a message of justice as part of this new life.

Romans, Paul's longest and one of his most important epistles, has justice interwoven through the whole letter, where it is 'a central and pervasive theme' (Harink 2020, 1). Most importantly, the gift of grace – a concept which is core to Romans – is a gift of justice: 'Jesus' own justice proceeds from divine abundance and is given abundantly to all' (Harink 2020, 78).

Paul *assumed* a justice message and a concern for the poor. Paul's letter to the Galatians describes in verse 2:10 the discussions that took place prior to Paul's departure where the only requirement asked of him by the other church leaders in Jerusalem was to 'remember the poor' (Longenecker 2010). Paul saw this as part of his essential being; he was 'eager' to remember the poor (Galatians 2:10), other translations use the word 'zealous'. Although Paul held the view that 'works' were not necessary for salvation, it was nevertheless Paul's view that concern for 'the poor' was an expected part of life.

In 2 Corinthians Paul identified the need for balance:

> I do not mean that there should be relief for others and pressure on you, but it is a question of a fair balance between your present abundance and their need, so that their abundance may be for your need, in order that there may be a fair balance. (2 Corinthians 8:13–14)

Borg and Crossan (2009) extend this to support a call to contemporary equity and justice applying it

> not just to the original situation of Paul's collection, but to the present situation of our modern world. It is, then, now, and always, about a 'fair balance', or a distributive justice, in which God's family all get an equitable share God's world. (Borg and Crossan 2009, 224)

James

The call to social justice, and explicitly action, is most prominent in the book of James, where almost half the verses have 'an economic theme' (Davids 2005, 355). James was dubbed an 'epistle of straw' by Martin Luther (George 1986), who wanted to excise it from the canon. James focusses on 'intensely practical' issues (Johnson 2016, RG551) addressing the behaviour which ought to be seen in followers of Christ (Johnson 2016, RG552). Importantly, this expected behaviour explicitly links followers of Christ to action: 'For just as the body without the spirit is dead, so faith without works is also dead' (James 2:26).

Gotsis and Dodd (2004) suggest that the authentic works contemplated in James should involve generalised reciprocity, a giving (or works) that benefits all, with no expectation of direct reciprocity. This contrasts with the condemned exploitative relationships of the rich who practise negative reciprocity.

James' strong rhetoric is one of the intertwining of faith and works – not one or the other (Dowd 2000). James is an epistle with a strong emphasis on praxis, and a 'concern for integrity, consistency between theory and practice' (Tamez 1990, 54). In James 2:14–16, there is a direct call for faith to be demonstrated in action. Faith or prayer is important, but James highlights the importance of the faithful being secondary agents through whom God can work to address needs.

A Social Justice Spine

So Luke, traditionally thought of as sharp on poverty and wealth (Hays 2010), is not so much a different gospel as a different phrasing: Jesus' concern for neighbour and concern for a new way where justice triumphs suffuses the

New Testament. Throughout the Synoptic Gospels, Jesus identified himself with the outcasts and the poor, and those oppressed by the political structures of the time. The message is a consistent one: a concern for justice; that the justice is broad in its focus, so a social rather than simply an individual justice; and the need to live justice not just talk it.

Similarly, the early Christians practised an ethic of inclusion, where they

> did not simply keep the poor at arm's length through a charitable gesture. Instead, the poor were welcomed into the very heart of those communities of fellowship. Accordingly, they seem often to have imagined their miniature acts of generosity to be part of a much grander narrative of the structural reform that would eventually change things forever, through the power of God. (Longenecker 2009a, 310–311)

Social justice, then, appears to be a spine running through the New Testament in the same way it ran through the Hebrew Scriptures, leading to specific actions and behaviours of the followers of Jesus and the Torah. But this spine is not of indefinite or infinite length, with its endpoint the eschatological reversal. Jesus' concerns were inherently practical, talking to the immediate concerns for bread and forgiveness of oppressive debts (Oakman 2008). Following that example, Christians today must advocate social justice and not compact it into an issue that need only be addressed with the full experience of the realm of God.

Contemporary Catholic Social Teaching

The 'preferential option for the poor' and the call for social justice is clearly seen in explicit church teaching, most notably in Catholic social teaching. The modern reinvigoration of Catholic social teaching started 130 years ago with the publication of Leo XIII's encyclical *Rerum Novarum* (Leo XIII 1891), which 'decisively shaped social teaching down almost to the present day' (Walsh 1991, 3). Its focus was more on justice in labour relations, including fair wages (Yuengert 1999), and this theme continues to be a focus in documents issued by subsequent pontiffs (Sasiadek 2017). *Rerum Novarum* acknowledged a role for the state and 'moderate taxes, equitably levied' (para. 33). Overall *Rerum Novarum* was a cautious document, railing against socialism (paras 3–5), and seeing redistribution as much stemming from individual obligations for almsgiving (paras 20–22) as from the role of the state.

There have been a number of encyclicals and other authoritative documents issued by the Vatican building on, and influenced by, *Rerum Novarum*, including a number of encyclicals named after anniversaries of its release: *Quadragesimo Anno* in 1931; *Octagesimo Adveniens* in 1971 and *Centesimus Annus* in 1991. *Laborem Exercens*, released in 1981 was also an 'anniversary' encyclical (Hornsby-Smith 2006).

Pius XI explicitly addressed social justice in *Divini Redemptoris*,

> there is also social justice with its own set obligations, from which neither employers nor workingmen can escape. Now it is of the very essence of social justice to demand for each individual all that is necessary for the common good. But just as in the living organism it is impossible to provide for the good of the whole unless each single part and each individual member is given what it needs for the exercise of its proper functions, so it is impossible to care for the social organism and the good of society as a unit unless each single part and each individual member – that is to say, each individual man in the dignity of his human personality – is supplied with all that is necessary for the exercise of his social functions. If social justice be satisfied, the result will be an intense activity in economic life as a whole, pursued in tranquillity and order. (Pius XI 1937, para. 51)

Social justice, thus, involves ensuring no one is left behind and that each individual can live with dignity. Pius went on to argue, along the lines of previous teaching, that social justice could not be achieved if workers 'are denied a salary that will enable them to secure proper sustenance for themselves and for their families' (para. 52).

More recently, John Paul II brought his own priorities to the social magisterium informed by his context of the demise of communism in Europe and his emphasis on human freedom. John Paul II also emphasised subsidiarity (of which more later) and this in turn led to an emphasis on the role of the church in serving those in need. He criticised state action on social justice decrying what he saw as the 'social assistance state', with even the welfare state referred to with negative connotations:

> In recent years the range of such intervention has vastly expanded, to the point of creating a new type of State, the so-called 'Welfare State'. This has happened in some countries in order to respond better to many needs and demands, by remedying forms of poverty and deprivation unworthy of the human person. However, excesses and abuses, especially in recent years, have provoked very harsh criticisms of the Welfare State, dubbed the 'Social Assistance State'. Malfunctions and defects in the Social Assistance State are the result of an inadequate understanding of the tasks proper to the State. Here again the principle of subsidiarity must be respected: a community of a higher order should not interfere in the internal life of a community of a lower order, depriving the latter of its functions, but rather should support it in case of need and help to coordinate its activity with the activities of the rest of society, always with a view to the common good.

> By intervening directly and depriving society of its responsibility, the Social Assistance State leads to a loss of human energies and an inordinate increase of public agencies, which are dominated more by bureaucratic ways of thinking than by concern for serving their clients, and which are accompanied by an enormous increase in spending. In fact, it would appear that needs are best understood and satisfied by people who are closest to them and who act as neighbours to those in need. It should be added that certain kinds of demands often call for a response which is not simply material but which is capable of perceiving the deeper human need. (John Paul II 1991, paras 48–49)

Although 'welfare dependency' is regularly raised as a risk associated with expanded social provision, the concept is more a rhetorical device rather than supported by evidence (Fraser and Gordon 1994a, 1994b). John Paul II's criticism of the so-called 'social assistance state' falls into that trap. His criticisms seem more to be setting the ground for his subsidiarity-based alternative, namely social and material assistance organised through the church 'capable of perceiving the deeper human need', rather than a well-thought-out critique of government social provision.

The papal teaching of the twenty-first century, particularly that of Pope Francis, is stronger in language but reflects a continuity with the earlier teaching of the previous 100 years. Papal teaching is influenced by the character and experience of the pontiffs, most obviously seen in John Paul II's concern about communism and freedom; the pastoral background of Francis is also shaping his teaching (Duncan 2014, 2017; Moccia 2017; Massaro 2018).

There is a strong economic tone to many of Francis' pronouncements (Duncan 2014, 2017; Ramirez 2017) and, indeed, about 15 per cent of his speeches include economic references, although there is a higher proportion of media interest focussed on those issues (das Neves 2017). Documents issued under Francis's authority and name (Francis 2013a, 2015, 2020a) place much greater emphasis on the damage capitalism might engender compared to documents from previous pontificates. But interestingly, Francis is not arguing for equality *per se*, but rather emphasising the consequences of inequality:

> Another aspect is equality, which many commentators consider one of the main political platforms of Pope Francis. Nevertheless, it is curious to note that his use of the word equality is very rare in this context. It is actually five times less frequent than the use of the word inequality, which is his real concern … Pope Francis is not an economist occupied by income distribution. He is a pastor concerned with suffering. … Economic structures, both national and international, are unequivocally considered to be responsible for the unjust pain of the poor and distressed. (das Neves 2017, 164)

Francis' message is primarily a challenge to the contemporary outworking of an unjust economic system focusing on what Moccia (2017) describes as the 'four noes'; No to an economy of exclusion; No to the new idolatry of money; No to a financial system that rules rather than serves; and No to the inequality that spawns violence. None of these noes specifically address social justice, but rather they all draw attention to how economic structures impact adversely on human dignity.

A major difference between Francis and his predecessors is his more adept use of language. He uses 'new, colorful, and engaged language' (das Neves 2017, 168) to highlight contemporary application of traditional church teaching. His teaching, as he himself affirms, is consistent with and draws on the fundamental aspects of Catholic social teaching as expressed, with varying degrees of emphasis and differences in strength of language, since *Rerum Novarum* (das Neves 2017, 160–161; Ramirez 2017, 1246). Francis' teaching is also made more vivid by his actions in reaching out to serve the marginalised (Krames 2014).

There are four key 'principles of Catholic social doctrine' relevant to social justice: the dignity of the human person; the common good; subsidiarity; and solidarity (Pontifical Council for Justice and Peace 2004, 81).

The dignity of the human person underpins much of Catholic teaching and Catholic bioethics. It is based on the concept that human beings are created in the image of God, *imago dei*, and each human has an intrinsic dignity. The other three principles are more specific to Catholic social teaching. In essence, Catholic social teaching argues that

> A society that wishes and intends to remain in service of the human being at every level is a society that has the common good – the good of all people and of the whole person – as its primary goal. The human person cannot find fulfilment in himself, that is, apart from the fact that he exists 'with' others and 'for' others. (Pontifical Council for Justice and Peace 2004, para. 165)

There are two important components of this summary. Firstly, there is the goal articulated for every society that it pursues the common good. Secondly, there is a concept that humans are social – they exist in a society, with and for others: everyone is to be a neighbour, existing in a social milieu, contributing to society, alongside everybody else. Although not explicitly referenced, the concept of humans as social beings is based on 'a Trinitarian understanding of personhood as relatedness to others in a politically inclusive community' (Simons 1995, 72).

This concept of person-in-community is reinforced in *Fratelli tutti* where Francis argues that one cannot

> reduce my life to relationships with a small group, even my own family; I cannot know myself apart from a broader network of relationships, including those that have preceded me and shaped my entire life. (Francis 2020a, para. 89)
>
> The human person, with his or her inalienable rights, is by nature open to relationship. Implanted deep within us is the call to transcend ourselves through an encounter with others. (Francis 2020a, para. 111)

Although we are all to contribute to society as neighbours, the state is now seen to have a critical role:

> The responsibility for obtaining the common good, besides falling to individual persons, belongs also to the State, since the common good is the reason that the political authority exists. (Pontifical Council for Justice and Peace 2004, para. 168)

However, the common good goes beyond horizontal equity (equals treated equally); vertical equity is also a critical element of Catholic social teaching (unequals treated unequally). This is given expression in the concept of the 'preferential option for the poor', which for Stephen Pope:

> constitutes a radical Christian commitment to work with the poor and oppressed for the sake of their empowerment and integral liberation (i.e., not simply or even primarily material, of course). Rather than simply extend charity universally, in an outward radiating series of concentric circles, the preferential option reverses the usual priorities whereby the nearest are given priority and needs of the most distant are secondary. Special devotion and priority is given to those to whom we are least bound by ties of affection, blood, class, etc. (Pope 1993, 163)

The preferential option for the poor, also referred to in Catholic social teaching as the preferential love of the poor, and by an Anglican bishop as a 'bias to the poor' (Sheppard 1983), provides a significant motivator for the fight against poverty (Pontifical Council for Justice and Peace 2004, para. 449), and by implication, the quest for social justice in healthcare. The preferential option leads to a conclusion that amelioration is insufficient, rather the call is one to social justice (Hornsby-Smith 2006).

The third principle, of subsidiarity, underpins or is explicitly referenced in almost every encyclical or teaching on social justice since *Rerum Novarum*. Essentially subsidiarity builds on the concept of human dignity and freedom to assert that dignity and freedom are maximised if decisions affecting people are delegated to the level of agency in closest proximity to the individual. Concomitantly, it assumes that local voluntary agencies are core to this delegation.

The argument is that:

> The principle of subsidiarity protects people from abuses by higher level social authority and calls on these same authorities to help individuals and intermediate groups to fulfil their duties. (Pontifical Council for Justice and Peace 2004, para. 187)

It is this principle of solidarity that underlies John Paul II's criticism of the 'social assistance state' because of its assumed 'centralisation, bureaucratisation … and to the unjustified and excessive presence of the state and public mechanisms' (Pontifical Council for Justice and Peace 2004, para. 187).

However, the principle of subsidiarity needs to be held in tension with the fourth principle, solidarity: 'Solidarity highlights in a particular way the intrinsic social nature of the human person, the equality of all in dignity and rights and the common path of individuals and peoples towards an ever more committed unity' (Pontifical Council for Justice and Peace 2004, para. 192).

The only way of reconciling the principles of subsidiarity and solidarity is to assume overall universalist programmes with delivery delegated to more local, perhaps contracted, organisations.

The principle of solidarity rests on the assumption that all humans are equal, that all can contribute, and that all are neighbours. Public policies informed by the principle of solidarity must therefore ensure that services are available to all in need, recognising both the differences between individuals and the commonality of humanity. Solidarity recognises that people live in, and benefit from, community, with stronger social support being a mediating factor in reducing the health impact when people fall on hard times (Singh, Contreras Suarez et al. 2021).

The principle of solidarity links explicitly to the Lukan teaching about love of neighbour. The preferential option for the poor is not simply about considering the poor person as an individual, but consistent with other aspects of Catholic social teaching, it situates the poor person in their context:

> Social and political charity is not exhausted in relationships between individuals but spreads into the network formed by these relationships, which is precisely the social and political community; it intervenes in this context seeking the greatest good for the community in its entirety. In so many aspects the neighbour to be loved is found 'in society', such that to love him concretely, assist him in his needs or in his indigence may mean something different than it means on the mere level of relationships between individuals. To love him on the social level means, depending on the situations, to make use of social mediations to improve his life or to remove social factors that cause his indigence. It is undoubtedly an act of love, the work of mercy by which one responds here and now to a real and impelling need of one's

> neighbour, but it is an equally indispensable act of love to strive to organize and structure society so that one's neighbour will not find himself in poverty, above all when this becomes a situation within which an immense number of people and entire populations must struggle, and when it takes on the proportions of a true worldwide social issue. (Pontifical Council for Justice and Peace 2004, para. 208)

What we are seeing here is an explicit recognition of a link between the needs of individuals and the social structures within which they are embedded, and the need to change those social structures if the life of the poor is to be improved significantly (Longley 2014). Thus, Catholic social teaching again emphasises a social justice as necessary to achieve improvement in the outcomes of individuals. The particular issue of Catholic social teaching, the principle of subsidiarity, is one of the means, the use of delegated agencies and in particular faith-based agencies, not one of the ends, which are to achieve universal improvement, which in turn can only be achieved by social action.

The Roman Catholic Church has a magisterium, able to develop and promulgate an authoritative position. Its teaching, however, is not unique, indeed the development of Anglican social theology and Catholic social teaching followed similar trajectories (Rowlands 2014), come to similar conclusions, and point to similar policy prescriptions (Suggate 2014). The same is true of the other Abrahamic religions (Carney 1981).

The Implications of the Teaching

Brueggemann (2016, 198) argues that 'The Gospel of Luke is, from the outset, good news that both challenges present economic arrangements and anticipates alternative arrangements.'

So, what are the 'alternative arrangements' anticipated? Jesus time and time again talks of the need to change now and to recognise present (economic) realities, including giving to Caesar what is Caesar's. The implications of Luke (and the other Gospels) are not simply about a future eschatological reversal but are about changed practice in the current world.

As with the other gospels, Luke is written to tell the story of Jesus and the reign of God. The text has a balance of imminence and presence of God's realm, with a call for repentance and changed life priorities, including a request to show love (Luke 7:42). A theme of Luke is a principle of unequivocal love, love which is total and unambiguous, without any conditionality: as God has loved God's followers, so the follower must love others, even enemies (Gill 2020).

Oliver (2019) has argued that a fundamental basis of functioning societies is reciprocity, even citing Luke 6:31 (Do to others as you would have them do to you) as evidence of the universality of reciprocity and that 'the importance of this so-called golden rule as an ethical imperative is as old as the history of recorded thought' (Oliver 2019, 1). However, in Luke there is no simple reciprocity:

> (Jesus) emphasises the importance of loving others, especially those who cannot, or will not, return such love in kind. (Matera 1999, 90)

Indeed, the context of the Lukan formulation of the golden rule suggests that Jesus is not endorsing its simple utilitarian ethic, but rather challenging it (Ricoeur 1995, 36).

Charity as the Response

There is now an extensive economic literature about altruism (Simon 1993; Gérard-Varet, Kolm, and Ythier 2000; Stark 2000), 'pro-social' behaviour (Meier 2006), the utility of sharing (Margolis 1984), and charitable giving, often with an underlying theme of reciprocity (Oppenheimer and Olivola 2011; Scharf and Tonin 2018; Kolm 2000). Even if one thinks that charity is about pure altruism, the evidence appears to be that people who give charitably or altruistically are happier, and happier people give more (Anik et al. 2009; Anik et al. 2011). Phrased differently, although *prima facie* charitable giving is giving without thought of reward, those who give are indeed individually rewarded with additional happiness. Downs has gone further and argued that the biblical injunctions for giving – and teaching in the early church – have an element of future heavenly reward to it that some giving can be conceived of as 'atoning almsgiving' referencing early scriptural traditions 'that present care for the poor as having the potential to secure future reward, and even the cleansing of sin, for those who practice mercy' (Downs 2016, 273).

Charitable giving choices are personal, with donors' criteria being subjective and quite different from, for example, governments' criteria about effectiveness (Caviola, Schubert, and Greene 2021). Charities find it easier to raise money if there are identifiable, tangible, single targets for giving, often promoted in the past by letters and photos from the recipient to donors (Cryder and Loewenstein 2011; Kogut and Ritove 2011; Sharma and Morwitz 2016; Cameron 2017a; Smith, Ottoni-Wilhelm, and Scharf 2018). These strategies presumably increase the extent to which donors feel they are 'doing good' and thus increase the reward to the donor. Similarly, donors feel more rewarded and are more generous when donating to identifiable individuals or groups whom they can feel empathy towards (Kogut and Ritove 2011; Kogut and Ritov 2005; Andreoni, Koessler, and Serr-Garcia 2018) or with whom they have a relationship (Small 2011). The more specific this identification of the object of charity, the less the giving is without thought of reward. The corollary is that the more giving is to groups rather than individuals, and the more the groups are unidentified or indeed unidentifiable, the more the giving is truly expecting nothing in return.

If there is a spectrum, from giving to identifiable individuals through to giving to unidentifiable groups, then the latter is closer to an expression of the Christian love of enemies taught in the Sermon on the Plain and in the parable of the 'Good' Samaritan. However, there are still benefits for the individual: where the group is an unidentified group within the same community or country, the benefit is a diffuse one of living in a better society. When the unidentified group is outside one's own country, the benefit may still be perceived as living in a better world.

Giving to unidentified groups is not how individual charity works. Charitable donations are made to specific organisations, working with specific groups of specific types of recipients. The advertising campaigns of most charities are designed to evoke an identification with the recipient, whether the identification is one of pity, concern, or sympathy for people who are somewhat like the donor (Small 2011).

The argument here is that while individual giving is worthy and important, it is not showing Christian love of enemies. It is not where the implications of the obligation to love one's enemies ends. Rather, love without hope of earthly reward is about showing love to people who are unknown. As in the parable of the 'Good' Samaritan, such love and giving arises because one exists as a neighbour to all who are in need and are seeking help, be they friends or enemies.

There is a fundamental difference between charity and social justice as the Christian ideal. Charity is a volitional act: it is the outcome of a preference that is expressed by an individual. In contrast, social justice has a rights rather than a preference basis – it is based on intrinsic worth of the individual (Wagstaff and van Doorslaer 2000), and the recognition that the individual in need is a neighbour.

The 'benefit' of charity is that the donor can pick and choose who to support, limiting their giving and compassion to people like them and other 'worthy' recipients, and in addition managing 'compassion fatigue' (Cocker and Joss 2016; Coetzee and Laschinger 2018). The crux of donor compassion fatigue is how can one manage the multiple demands of Christian love in the face of the teaching to be a neighbour again and again, and not be paralysed by so much suffering and need (Francis 2020b, 11)? How do we 'not grow weary in doing what is right' (Galatians 6:9)? How do we manage 'obligations to millions, indeed billions, of others' (O'Neill 2000, 187)?

> The problem is that we are confronted with too many demands for support and solidarity – from victims of unjust war, detention, and violence; to those who suffer and die from the diseases of structural poverty; to workers struggling to organise in fields and sweatshops around the world; to movements for civil and political rights near and far; and so on, and so on. No single demand is excessive. To the contrary, each is eminently reasonable: people's lives and livelihoods are on the line, and we hear the call, and they are entitled to expect our help .... Yet taken in the aggregate, these demands could drive each supporter to exhaustion ....
>
> Aggregation can address these problems – not by magically solving them, unfortunately, but by putting people in conversation with one another enabling them to light a moral course through. Once we take the demands in the aggregate we can understand them as a single demand that the duty of solidarity makes upon us. (Kolers 2016, 148–149)

Aggregation is what societies do; they create the mechanism for mutuality through solidarity, facilitating a collective response to individual needs, not requiring or allowing other individuals to pick and choose who is deserving and who is not for mutualised support. Aggregation and mutualisation in its weak form is through financial mutualisation, a sharing of risks for the technical reasons that Arrow (1963) identifies. But in a stronger form, aggregation and mutualisation can be about solidarity, as Kolers (2016) mentions, with solidarity entailing a commitment to address causes as well as symptoms, and solidarity being both a mechanism to achieve social justice and a necessary part of it (Puyol 2018). What aggregation and solidarity may achieve is to overcome individual 'compassion fatigue' or a hypothetical 'altruism budget' (Gee and Meer 2020), allowing for more generous societal responses, and, potentially, more generous individual pro-social responses by appealing to this solidarity (Costa-Font and Machado 2021).

The Christian injunction about giving, and recognising the needs of the poor, is not simply about charitable giving by the wealthy distributing their surplus, nor reciprocal giving among the poor (Schellenberg 2018), but rather is generosity because it is the right thing to do, and an obligation of the whole nation of Israel – or today, the whole community – not simply of individuals.

As I argued in Chapter 1, the parable of the 'Good' Samaritan calls us to be with the traveller in the gutter; radical solidarity, not simply individual charity is the call. Isasi-Diaz (1998, 31) picks up this theme of solidarity and goes further, arguing that solidarity 'must replace charity as the appropriate Christian behavior – ethical behavior – in our world today'. She looks to a 'paradigmatic shift' which sees 'solidarity as the appropriate present-day expression of the gospel mandate that we love our neighbor'.

Isasi-Diaz (1998) challenges us here to walk in *solidarity with* the other, our neighbour, and to build the common good through the work of 'active, equal agents' (Hollenbach 2002, 189). To do this we must build *solidarity among* us – the distinction is from O'Neill (2002) – to accept all as neighbours and work to overcome the injustice that our neighbours face, displaying that we recognise the other as neighbour, that we have mutual concern and collective responsibility for the other, and that we want to limit the inequality that we see in our society (Miller 2017, 64).

Solidarity is not a given in any society; it does not emerge spontaneously but has to be developed, nurtured, and championed (Banting and Kymlicka 2017, 33). It can be challenged and undermined by political actors anxious to label and exclude 'the other', but the converse is also true: it can be promoted and encouraged as the Christian call to social justice demands.

A focus on social justice and the 'preferential option' is not a theoretical endeavour; it is an action-oriented concept, aiming to change the lived experience of those in poverty:

> With typical concreteness, the Bible does not engage with an abstract problem like poverty or pauperism, but with poor people, and their lot and standing in God's eyes. The poor are people, made in the image of God, with claims and contributions to make. Instead of being labelled as a problem, the poor are treated as people who have gifts and claims to bring into the interactions of society. Indeed, it is more common in Scripture for the wealthy to be seen as in a problematic situation. (Forrester 1997, 104–105)

For Christians, concern for social justice is to be a real one, leading to real actions, hopefully with real consequences for people. It is based on people with rights, claims, capabilities, and contributions, who should be partners in the endeavour of achieving equitable access to healthcare. The response is to be a generous one, as 'solidarity is not the sharing of crumbs from the table, but to make space *at* the table for everyone (Francis 2020b, 110, emphasis added).

A Christian ethic of social justice should be seen in listening to the voice of people in poverty, engaging in co-design to develop responses, and addressing social, economic, and commercial determinants of ill-health, not simply developing ameliorative strategies (Stivers 2011).

Beyond Charitable Responses

In the past, communities of faith could support each other, hold goods in common, and meet the needs of the poor in their communities by collective action. But both the Sermon on the Plain and the parable of the 'Good' Samaritan call Christians to offer support beyond their own Christian communities. The radical message of these teachings is that individual love expressed towards those who are like us is no longer enough. The implication of the teachings is that individual action needs to be supplemented by love more broadly directed to unknown groups in need. A Christian ethic prioritises neediest over nearest (Hallett 1998).

The contemporary alternative to the ancient model of individual giving within the Christian community must be one of giving that reallocates funding on a broader scale. It is here that the reversals in both the Magnificat and the Sermon on the Plain are relevant. In the reversed order, the lowly and the poor are lifted up and the rich are sent empty away. This language is not of picking and choosing who is my neighbour, nor who will I choose to assist when they are wounded. Rather, it is language that this overturning ought to occur because it is right – that is, the poor are to be in their new position because it is just.

Much charitable giving is an immediate response to an immediate need, invoked by a natural disaster or some other precipitating event (Kogut and Ritov 2005; Smith, Ottoni-Wilhelm, and Scharf 2018). It has an immediate amelioration/restoration focus. Few charities address the underlying causal factors of poverty and continued disadvantage. However, the reversals contemplated in the blessings and woes, and in the Magnificat, are not presented as one-off responses, rather they are systemic overturnings. The rich are indeed sent empty away. Systemic change and systemic overturnings require responses that are broader than individual charitable actions, and point again to societal-wide social action. 'Jesus' call to love is fundamentally also a call to justice because justice is the necessary medium of love; precisely because love is hyper moral, it enters the practical and ethical sphere only under the aegis of justice' (Ricoeur 1995, 36–37).

The Lukan message is that:

> Jesus' leadership is not concerned primarily with establishing a new local community organisation with a patronising concern for the poor. Rather a renewed intimate covenantal alignment between God and all humanity is being announced and realized .... Jesus does not simply preach an ideology but rather models a response of openness, transparency, nonviolence and passive resistance. (Kitchen 2014, 49)

There was a strong expectation as part of the covenant and the explicit teaching of the Hebrew Scriptures that communities would look after the 'quartet of the vulnerable': widows, orphans, resident aliens, and the poor (Wolterstorff 2008, 75). This was a model of communities looking after their own and was carried over in the early Christian church, which extended so that distant churches would 'remember the poor' in the church in Jerusalem (Galatians 2:10), although the contemporary consensus that this verse was indeed so geographically limited is contested (Longenecker 2009b). Many of the parables are silent as to whether almsgiving was to be limited to those within the Christian community (Kim 1993, 233–255). This ambiguity signals a change that intra-community giving may not be enough, an expectation made explicit in the parable of the 'Good' Samaritan.

The needs of the poor and the hungry cannot be met by individual action from love towards the individual wounded on the side of the road, but rather must be addressed by the action of being a neighbour. In particular, the neighbour must be a good citizen to all, contributing to society, especially contributing to society through taxation-based redistribution. The 'amount prescribed' to be collected (Luke 3:12–13) needs to be set to allow a more just society, and one which allows social need to be met by social provision.

What is radical about Lukan teaching – especially in the parable of the 'Good' Samaritan – is that love should no longer be limited to within the community, and/or people with whom one can identify. Rather, love needs to be shown more broadly and universally to unknown recipients. This is not a challenge that can be met simply by more individual charitable donations. In contemporary society a more organised and systematic response is required and is available.

The overturning of the social order contemplated in Luke is given contemporary effect through just taxation, historically supported in both Catholic social teaching (Curran 1985) and in Protestant traditions, the latter going back to Martin Luther (Shriver and Knox 1985). There is no clear biblical support for a particular form of taxation but

> [The] moral logic with its consistent willingness to use taxation to support the least advantaged runs like a red thread through Jewish and Christian history. … But the red thread emerges again in modern affirmations of the 'preferential option for the poor' and in the widespread acceptance of progressive taxation in informed statements by modern religious communities. Thus, we can say that while head and proportional taxes have had their place in Jewish and Christian thinking, the advocacy of progressive taxation as a means of serving the least off and promoting social equality and opportunity is a leitmotif of these traditions. (Green 2020, 142)

Redistribution of income on a fair basis, with more levied on wealthier people through a system of progressive taxation, is a contemporary secular exemplar of the overturning taught in Luke. Progressive taxation, however, is a necessary but not sufficient condition for equitable financing of healthcare. Even with a substantial proportion of healthcare funded through taxation, the overall incidence of funding might depart from progressivity because of proportional social insurance contributions or the regressive incidence of out-of-pocket payments (van Doorslaer et al. 1999; Wagstaff et al. 1999; Asante et al. 2016; McIntyre and Kutzin 2016; Ataguba et al. 2018).

Although even the most progressive taxation system does not lead to a complete overturning of society (Piketty 2020), public funding, shared public responsibility, and social justice need to be the key underpinnings of any just health and welfare provision. Jesus' command to 'go and do likewise' (Luke 10:37) is not only about individual actions of charity, but also about Christians being neighbours to everyone, which in turn means supporting systems that support everyone, and these necessarily involve public funding underpinned by progressive taxation and principles of social justice.

Further, it appears that mutualised funding in a country – which contributes to social solidarity – is associated with higher public satisfaction with the health system, possibly because 'citizens in countries with a publicly financed health care system are more likely to believe in the fairness of the system and they have an easier and more affordable access to health care services than their counterparts in privately financed health care system' (Yuan 2021, 1364).

Although the emphasis in this discussion has been on the progressivity of taxation, and hence how funding healthcare in this way contributes to a more equitable society, taxation, properly structured, can help to achieve other societal benefits. McCoy, Chigudu, and Tillmann (2017), for example, identify benefits of taxation in improving democratic accountability, and in increasing prices for harmful products; this latter issue is discussed further later in this chapter.

A Christian ethic of social justice requires a move beyond individual charity or individual justice, whether the latter means justice for individuals or justice by individuals. It points to breaking the link between what healthcare I get and what I can afford to pay (Hellowell, Appleby, and Taylor 2018).

Applying a Christian Ethic of Social Justice to Healthcare Funding

Both the Hebrew Scriptures and the New Testament place more emphasis on a social justice rather than they do on individual justice. I have argued that an implication of this is support for progressive taxation.

Contemporary Catholic social teaching argues that public policy should be inclusive and universalist, informed by the principle of solidarity, and again this leads to policies which support equitable taxation. In this section I explore the implications of an ethic of social justice for funding healthcare specifically.

An ethic of social justice immediately raises the question: equity about what (Allin, Hernández-Quevedo, and Masseria 2009)? Is the objective of funding to achieve equitable access? Equitable care? Equitable outcomes? Each goal requires more than just decisions about healthcare funding: equitable access requires decisions about ensuring services are equitably distributed geographically and culturally acceptable; equitable care requires addressing variations in quality of provision, which may have gender, income, sexual identity, or racist causes; equitable outcomes requires addressing social and economic determinants of health (National Academies of Sciences Engineering and Medicine 2017).

The focus in the remainder of this chapter is cast narrowly – equity of access – not because the broader issues are not important, they are, but rather because one cannot achieve any of the others while financial barriers exist, and people cannot get access to care (Levesque, Harris, and Russell 2013). But this narrowing is solely about which dimension of equity, not about how equity of access is bounded. Equity of access is not simply about horizontal equity, equal treatment of equals, but a Christian ethic of social justice must conceive of equity generously, as vertical equity – the equity required to address need or dessert (Forrester 2012).

'Social justice' is an essentially contested concept (Gallie 1955), and its meaning can change over time, and incorporate new dimensions. I argue in this section that even though the term can be interpreted differently, applying an ethic of social justice must lead to specific policies, in particular policies that promote solidarity through mutualisation of healthcare funding and reduce financial barriers to access to healthcare. Voluntary approaches to sharing the financial risks of healthcare create inequity, fail to protect the poor and the most disadvantaged, and lead to financial barriers to access to healthcare. A preferential option for the poor is one that eliminates such barriers through universalist approaches.

A strong theme of the Hebrew Scriptures is the protection of the identity of the people of Israel, emphasising and building a strong sense of community. This emphasis on social solidarity is heightened by Jesus' teaching in the parable of the 'Good' Samaritan where all are called to be neighbours, and an ethic of inclusion is preached. This social rather than individualistic orientation in Jesus' teaching leads to valuing social solidarity and collective responses to healthcare financing, including mutualisation.

In the introduction to this chapter, I phrased the key trade-off as a dichotomy: mutualisation versus individuation. In practice life is more complex with the choice better placed along a spectrum rather than at the endpoints. The policy choices are not whether mutualisation or not, but rather how much mutualisation, what are the consequences of different degrees of mutualisation or financial protection (Mirelman and Cookson 2020), and how that fits into a society's value frame.

Mutualisation through taxation impinges on individual rights – taxpayers no longer have autonomy about how they spend a proportion of their money. Those who advocate a low tax argue that government spending is often wasteful, that high taxes sap incentive, in the long-term reduce the size of the economy, and that the ability to control one's own spending is fair and just. This view of the world eschews a 'Robin Hood' approach to taxation and, where some form of mutualisation is seen as appropriate, favours social insurance or 'piggy bank' approaches to social provision, which emphasise individual contributions and individual benefit (Barr 2001).

In healthcare there is not one simple spectrum of mutualisation. The World Health Organisation has identified three dimensions of mutualisation: the population covered (breadth), the services covered (depth), and the extent of costs covered (height). The World Health Organisation, which promulgates this model as part of its goal of universal coverage, portrays this as the 'coverage cube' (Busse, Schreyogg, and Gericke 2007; World Health Organization 2010; Kutzin 2013). The cube focuses on coverage and mutualisation and does not address other dimensions of needed reform such as quality of care, health literacy, and institutional structures.

Unfortunately, even in high-income countries, the cube is not fully completed. In almost all wealthy nations, there is a mutualisation core: funding for hospitals and medical services is mutualised. The United States is the standout exception in terms of breadth of coverage of medical and hospital care. Despite the Affordable Care Act (Obamacare), population coverage for healthcare in the United States is still a patchwork of age-based eligibility (for Medicare), means-tested access (for Medicaid), and employer-sponsored and employer-tied coverage, together with a small population who need to negotiate their own insurance, and some people still lacking any coverage at all (Frean, Gruber, and Sommers 2017; Sommers, Clark, and Epstein 2018).

In terms of depth, coverage varies with different types of services having different levels of mutualisation. For example, although there is a government commitment to full coverage of pharmaceuticals in Canada, that is to be phased-in and so at the time of writing, coverage is low (Advisory

Council on the Implementation of National Pharmacare 2019). Dental services are covered in some countries, not in others (Allin et al. 2020).

However, the key gap in the coverage cube in most high-income countries – other than the United States – is height: the extent of costs covered, and the extent of allowable or compulsory personal contributions (co-payments) that are designed into healthcare financing.

If we are to follow an ethic of social justice, we need to consider all aspects of the coverage cube. Issues of depth – what services should be covered – will be discussed more extensively in the Chapter 4. Here we will first consider the issue of breadth – who should be covered – and height, the extent of costs to be covered, particularly the role of patient contributions.

The Structure of Mutualisation

Mutualisation is core to achieving access to healthcare informed by principles of social justice. It involves a community sharing the costs of healthcare so that cost is no longer an insurmountable barrier to needed care. Countries differ on how mutualisation is effected, with a fundamental choice being between voluntary insurance, typically private, compared to compulsory, universal coverage. Voluntary, private insurance is both inequitable and inefficient.

Voluntary systems inevitably lead to lower levels of coverage: the breadth dimension of the coverage cube is smaller. Although some wealthy people may choose to self-insure, those who are left uncovered in voluntary systems are overwhelmingly the poorer and near poor in the community. Means-tested programmes, the equity-oriented policy response in systems based on voluntary insurance, leave gaps for the near poor, with people in greater need often not able to navigate the complexities involved in claiming eligibility for means-tested support or living in cycles of being eligible and then ineligible. The result is people miss out on coverage and care. The evidence from the United States – which is the only high-income country without universal coverage – continues to be that incentives and means-tested programmes are insufficient: people still face huge healthcare costs and bankrupt themselves seeking needed care (Himmelstein et al. 2009; Burtch and Chan 2019; Himmelstein et al. 2019). Despite theoretical arguments for a voluntary approach to social justice (Baker 2012), justice in access and coverage can only occur with government intervention to require it, not just encourage or subsidise it (Deeble and Scotton 1968).

Although Hurley (2001, 236) distinguishes between those types of private insurance that are or are not publicly subsidised, there is no high-income country that relies entirely on private voluntary insurance, unsubsidised by public funding, to achieve its mutualisation objective. Private insurance is inefficient compared to public coverage on a number of grounds, including the high administrative costs involved in marketing and rate-setting; and information asymmetries between buyers and sellers that can lead to adverse selection, where people with high healthcare needs are more likely to take out insurance compared to people with low needs, creating a skewed risk pool with resulting very high premiums (Hurley 2001, 237).

In summary, private insurance is 'grotesquely inefficient, expensive, and unfair' (Evans, Barer, and Stoddart 2016a, 258).

Public Compulsory Options

Other than the United States, all high-income countries have recognised that compulsory insurance is the only way to ensure universal health coverage. There are two main types of public systems for universal health coverage: systems with multiple insurers – in some cases competing for members but in many with membership determined by employment or place of residence – and systems where there is a single tax-financed insurer or National Health Service. The former group of countries is often described as following a Bismarckian 'social insurance' system, stemming from the pension systems of the nineteenth-century German Chancellor von Bismarck, with unified systems named after the U.K.'s post-World War II social reforms recommended by William Beveridge (Cuadrado et al. 2019).

Although the two archetypes are quite different, it is not clear that one system is unequivocally better than the other (Wendt and Kohl 2010; van der Zee and Kroneman 2007; Weale 2015). Overall, single-payer or tax-financed systems provide universal coverage for a lower cost – saving about 0.75% of Gross Domestic Product (Bichay 2020) – but perform less well on other dimensions. Or et al. (2010, 290) conclude that 'in terms of cost containment and affordability Bismarck-type systems appear to be less successful than the Beveridge type. In contrast, Beveridge-type systems appear to be less successful in terms of access, defined as availability of services when required.'

Possibly in response to this historic weakness in cost containment, Bismarckian countries are paying relatively more attention to this dimension of policy, while all countries continue to focus on access (Tenbensel, Eagle, and Ashton 2012).

Given the mixed evidence, a Christian ethic of resource allocation should focus on the ends of equitable access and outcomes, and social justice, and be less concerned about the mechanisms of achieving that end, as both social insurance and a public National Health Service approach appear equally able to achieve the universal mutualisation called for in an ethic of social justice.

Undermining Social Solidarity with Private Options

I have argued for a public, universal response rather than a private voluntary response for ensuring access to healthcare. Again, however, these are not alternatives as public and private can coexist. This is the situation in Australia, which has an extensive system of private funding through private insurance operating alongside a system of public funding. Membership of private insurance is encouraged by a complex array of carrots and sticks subsidising and coercing participation into private health insurance (Hall, De Abreu Lourenco, and Viney 1999; Robson and Paolucci 2012; Duckett and Nemet 2019).

The Australian system is characterised by muddled policy thinking, with the supporters of private funding sometimes arguing that private funding is for services that both complement the public system (e.g., better amenity) and serve as a substitute for public care, taking demand off the public system (Duckett and Nemet 2019). However, in Australia areas and specialties with higher levels of private activity also have longer public waiting times (Duckett 2005, 2018b). Supporters of private insurance also rhetorically diminish universality of the public system by referring to it as a 'safety net'. The debate about the role of private health insurance in Australia is ongoing and reflects division about underlying values in the healthcare system, in particular the degree of emphasis on social justice and public, compulsory mutualisation (Duckett 2008a).

Although private funding is often portrayed as simply being about freedom of choice, supplementary private funding as exists in Australia presents a challenge to an underlying principle of solidarity. Very often freedom of choice for some, typically wealthier, people will come at the expense of poorer services for others. Private funding and freedom of choice is often exercised to provide faster access to services, creating a second track or second tier that bypasses public sector waiting lists or other public sector constraints. This shifts private funding from simply being a complement, providing better amenity, to being a substitute, now providing inequitable (faster) access to care.

Färdow, Broström, and Johansson (2019, 521) recently neatly summarised the challenge of private funding as:

> introduction of the (private funding) model is difficult to square with a broadly agreed-upon commitment to equality of opportunity. It is true that the goal of the publicly funded healthcare system … is to provide good

> healthcare for all in the society. However, this goal may be viewed as utopian, and certainly the public commitment could never guarantee equality of health. More realistic, perhaps – and a more obvious normative cornerstone in this kind of healthcare system – is a commitment to provide healthcare to all on equal terms. A common interpretation of this commitment, albeit not necessarily the only one is that everyone should have access to care on the basis of need only. In other words no special treatment should be given to some individuals if the very same treatment is denied to others in the same need.

A second track for access to care provided by private funding creates 'a controversial symbol of inequality' (Färdow, Broström, and Johansson 2019, 522). If wealthier people can buy their way out of a constrained public system, then not only is solidarity undermined but political pressure to ensure that the public system provides good quality care is also reduced. We all will no longer be in the same boat facing healthcare storms, but some will be in luxury liners and some on leaky rafts (Barr 2020).

Co-payments

A second critical issue for access relates to the height dimension of the coverage cube: the extent of costs covered. Here there is a fundamental trade-off: all healthcare funding comes from some combination of taxation or compulsory social insurance contributions, private insurance payments, and individual contributions through patient out-of-pocket payments. Out-of-pocket payments can have different attributes:

- payments for every visit or service, such as each prescription or diagnostic test. These will be referred to as co-payments;
- individual out-of-pocket payments only up to a threshold amount ('deductible' or 'excess'); and
- mutualised support after a threshold amount is accumulated ('safety net').

Both deductibles and safety net arrangements presume co-payments: that is, they are designed to ameliorate the problems associated with the cumulative effect of co-payments made by people with high use of services.

The argument for co-payments rests on two intertwined bases. Firstly, that any service which is 'free' – for which there is no requirement for an individual monetary contribution – risks moral hazard: individuals using services inappropriately. Secondly, that government funding is tightly constrained and that sharing of funding, between individual and collective, reduces the amount needed to be found from the public purse. Both arguments fail and a Christian ethic of healthcare resource allocation should eschew use of co-payments.

Moral Hazard

The pejoratively named concept of moral hazard – which people will consume more of a product than appropriate if it has a zero price (and also neglect health improving behaviours if they do not bear the costs of ill-health) – has shaped policy discussions, about co-payments for the last fifty years (Whitford 2008), particularly in the United States. Moral hazard has a confused intellectual history, marked by differing underlying assumptions about if and why it exists (Grignon et al. 2018).

Arguments for moral hazard are more easily made than proved – there are many costs of using healthcare other than monetary costs, including the opportunity cost of a person's time. The physical environment of a medical clinic is also not one where most people would want to spend unnecessary time. Further, it assumes individuals are totally autonomous when deciding to use healthcare, which in turn assumes, for example, that patients' decisions are not shaped by the physician in terms of calling them back for a second visit.

A systematic review of effects of the introduction of health insurance in low income countries did not find evidence of moral hazard effects (Ekman (2004); but see Einav and Finkelstein (2018) for a contrary view of the existence of moral hazard), and even where moral hazard might exist its effect appears to be small and maybe even health enhancing (Nyman 2004; Pauly 2004).

Although the initiating primary care visit is a consumer choice, subsequent healthcare interventions, including diagnostic tests ordered and medications prescribed, are the decisions of agents. In these circumstances, the risk of consumer-side moral hazard is mitigated because the patient's consumption is mediated by decisions and recommendations of the agent. It is the agent, usually a physician, who decides that the referral to a specialist, the diagnostic test, or the prescription for medication, is necessary. Imposing co-payments on individuals for these secondary, referred services is thus anomalous as the consumer is not the effective decision-maker.

However, moral hazard may well be at play in the consumer's decision to initiate the first visit – to the doctor, nurse, emergency room, or other healthcare provider. Here, the moral hazard argument for co-payments fails on pragmatic grounds: co-payments are not cost free, and the net cost of a co-payment policy may be greater than the net benefits.

There is now an extensive literature on the effects of co-payments summarised by Kiil and Houlberg (2014, 825) who confirmed the adverse equity impacts: 'vulnerable groups, including individuals with low income and in particular need of care, reduce their use relatively more than the remaining population in consequence of co-payment'.

Although it has been criticised on methodological grounds, including underestimating the impact of co-payments on the poor (Nyman 2007), the classic study of co-payments is still the 1990s Rand Health Insurance Experiment in the United States (Newhouse and the Health Insurance Experiment Group 1993). Three critical conclusions can be derived from this extensive controlled experiment:

- 'Use of medical services responds unequivocally to change in the amount paid out-of-pocket' (Newhouse and the Health Insurance Experiment Group 1993, 40);
- sicker people were more responsive to price than the healthy (Newhouse and the Health Insurance Experiment Group 1993, 49) and use declined more among poorer people (lowest third of the population income distribution) than richer people (Newhouse and the Health Insurance Experiment Group 1993, Table 3.4; page 46); and
- 'Cost sharing does not have a differential effect according to the effectiveness of care; it is just as likely to lower use when care is thought to be highly effective as when it is thought to be only rarely effective'. (Newhouse and the Health Insurance Experiment Group 1993, 162).

The Rand study found that the reductions in utilisation did not lead to increased health costs in the long run, at least as monitored during the period studied. However, more recent research has found that co-payments can lead to long run cost increases. Indeed, the senior author of the Rand study and another colleague concluded, very cautiously, that

> These empirical findings are strongly suggestive that some individuals, especially those with certain chronic diseases, can be induced by *less* cost sharing to take actions today that will reduce their future use of medical services and/or improve their future health. (Newhouse and Sinaiko 2008, 96; emphasis added)

The second conclusion from the Rand experiment, supported also by more recent literature, draws attention to the inequitable nature of co-payments. In taxation-funded healthcare systems, costs of healthcare are funded in line with the progressive basis of that taxation so the rich pay proportionately more. Because of the incidence of illness, benefits of healthcare accrue mainly to the poor and sick and so the system achieves a redistribution of income from richer to poorer. Co-payments disrupt that, falling mainly on higher users of healthcare, often the poor.

Not surprisingly, these distributional consequences shape the politics of co-payments:

> Thus, one finds, for example, that people with higher incomes are more likely to favor greater reliance on user charges as a source of system finance, and less use of general public revenues. A priori it should be pretty obvious that, whereas tax liabilities tend to be more or less proportionate to income, illness is not. For any given level of expenditure on health, more will come out of the pockets of wealthier individuals if the system is tax-financed, and less if it is user-paid. (Evans 1997, 445; Evans, Barer, and Stoddart 2016b, 207)

The distributional consequences go further than regressive income redistribution to, as Evans argues, regressive redistribution of health outcomes as well:

> If user charges are as likely to discourage 'needed' as 'unneeded' contacts, and if they serve not to reduce overall use but to reallocate services from those with less ability to pay to those with more, and if at least some of the services thus reallocated are not only 'needed', as judged by clinicians, but actually effective, then user charges will reallocate health outcomes as well.... User fees may redistribute not only money and access to care, but health itself, from lower to higher income groups. (Evans, Barer, and Stoddart 1995, 381; 2016b, 179)

In addition to officially mandated co-payments, voluntary co-payments – either officially sanctioned or as part of informal payments and bribes – are endemic in many countries (Habibov and Cheung 2017; Pourtaleb et al. 2020). Such payments are almost invariably regressive as richer people are much more able to afford these payments (Kankeu and Ventelou 2016). Even in high-income countries where voluntary co-payments are allowed, they are associated with reduced access, especially for people on low incomes. In many countries, co-payments may be charged by a significant proportion of physicians and so cannot be described as voluntary, as access will be denied, and care foregone, in the absence of the patient paying the co-payment.

The third finding of the Rand study – that co-payments affect both necessary and unnecessary care – has been explored by Baicker, Mullainathan, and Schwartzstein (2015). Their conclusion is that co-payment designs are rarely able to distinguish between healthcare interventions (such as prescriptions) that should be encouraged and those which should be discouraged. The moiety might penalise utilisation when it should not and not penalise utilisation when it should. They argue that the moral hazard and co-payment literature naively focuses on the demand curve and fails to take account of mistakes consumers make ('behavioural hazard') in choosing which health services to use. Writing from their perspective as authors based in the United States, they conclude

> Failing to incorporate behavioral hazard into models of health insurance not only generates very wrong answers but very wrong answers with substantial import for millions of people. Much of our health spending is on care that is sensitive to copay changes, and much of that care seems to have an impact on health that differs from that implied by moral hazard alone. Simply assuming that the demand curve reveals the health value of care can generate misleading policy prescriptions. (Baicker, Mullainathan, and Schwartzstein 2015, 1663)

These 'very wrong answers' can have devastating impacts. An increase in pharmaceutical co-payments in Australia was associated with a reduction in use of statins – prescribed to reduce the risk of cardiovascular disease – and an increase in acute coronary syndrome and stroke-related hospitalisations (Seaman et al. 2021). Following a study of people enrolled in the United States' Medicare programme, Chandra and colleagues concluded

> We find that small increases in cost cause patients to cut back on drugs with large benefits, ultimately causing their death. Cutbacks are widespread, but most striking are those seen in patients with the greatest treatable health risks, in whom they are likely to be particularly destructive. (Chandra, Flack, and Obermeyer 2021, 35)

The Tight Funding Argument

Progress towards universal health coverage in low- and middle-income countries is constrained because of their low tax base, large informal sectors, and low average (formal) wages (Bhattacharjya and Sapra 2008). Design of universal coverage in these circumstances often incorporates either compulsory or voluntary co-payments, frequently overtly justified as reducing the risk of moral hazard, but also because it is argued that the proposed government expenditure is all that can be afforded given the tax base. Implicit in this argument is that, to the extent there are disadvantages with individual out-of-pocket payments, these are offset by the disadvantages of attempting to increase taxation to fund any services fully. The 'lack of fiscal room' or 'tight funding' argument should be confronted head on – many low- and middle-income countries have the potential to raise the revenue necessary for universal health coverage (Meheus and McIntyre 2017), and increased government health spending can contribute to economic development (Global Burden of Disease Health Financing Collaborator Network 2019).

But the implicit decision often made is that a unit (dollar) of government expenditure has a different economic value from a unit of private expenditure. That is, in specific circumstances shifting costs onto consumers may be welfare enhancing. The trade-off might involve governments deciding that additional spending in a different sector of the economy may produce bigger gains in social welfare than more spending in the health sector. Indeed, as health is improved through many investments outside the sector, such investments may yield larger health gains than additional health sector expenditure; investing in education, for example, is often posited to lead to improved health outcomes, although the evidence for this is weak (Hamad et al. 2018; Mensch et al. 2019), but, at least in the United States, additional spending on social services in a state – including spending on income assistance – leads to better health outcomes (Bradley et al. 2016).

It may also be that it is seen as easier to have the population pay an extra moiety for healthcare compared to increasing taxes. No general rules can be discerned here – other than that the disadvantages of co-payments need to be kept front and centre – with the context being a significant determinant of appropriate policy design.

Achieving universal health coverage remains a challenge for many low and middle income countries, where there is insufficient tax-based funding to achieve a typical spending target of 5 per cent of Gross Domestic Product on healthcare (McIntyre, Meheus, and Røttingen 2017). However, even in these countries, out-of-pocket payments should be seen as transitional: in some, economic growth could lead to achieving the 5 per cent target and in others, a range of tax initiatives could suffice to meet the target equitably (Elovainio and Evans 2017). Policy should therefore limit reliance on individual contributions, especially for priority services and for the poor (Ottersen et al. 2017, 288), and health financing should be as progressive as possible, as quickly as possible (Meheus and McIntyre 2017).

Even in wealthy economies an argument is sometimes made for increasing private contributions as part of a shift in responsibility for funding healthcare from government to consumers. Again, moral hazard may be front and centre in arguments for these proposals but there may be an implicit value proposition underlying such proposals, that of small government and reducing taxes. Proposals to increase private contributions – except in very rare exceptions – almost always come from centre-right governments ideologically oriented toward small government and the rhetoric of individual choice.

Voluntary co-payments may reduce direct government funding where incomes of physicians and other healthcare workers are established on the assumption of additional income from these informal payments.

Co-payments may also simply be a means for physicians to increase their income in situations of inelastic demand or undersupply, at the expense of equity and access for low-income people.

The tight funding argument can only be valid if it also assumes that relying on private contributions leads to elimination of unnecessary use of care and does not impact adversely on necessary use. As the Rand experiment showed, the evidence is this is not the case.

Where constrained budgets lead to policies for transitional co-payments, then the structure of the co-payment needs to be carefully designed. Typically, co-payments might be levied as fixed amounts or proportional to the total cost of the service, and might also vary with income. There is only a limited literature about co-payment design where equity is an explicit consideration – the objective is generally about savings. But even when equity is the focus, what becomes obvious is that the conception of equity is critical: is the objective of policy to maximise health (Smith 2005)? Or should co-payments be designed to take into account the severity of a patient's illness and the possibility of recovery? The latter approach is based on attempting to avoid double jeopardy 'where on top of the health loss, the patient also faces a substantial monetary loss' (González 2020). Design of co-payment policy is rarely that sophisticated and almost invariably involves crude income (and safety net) thresholds, creating access problems and people missing out on care because of cost. Co-payment policy may be an easier alternative to more sophisticated policies about what should or should not be publicly funded (discussed in Chapter 4). Such policies may be designed with an implicit and erroneous view that tight funding justifies otherwise ethically inappropriate choices (Rumbold et al. 2019).

What has been shown here is that both the moral hazard and tight funding arguments for co-payments are on shaky grounds, and that co-payments lead to inequity and may, by reducing access to needing care, be counter-productive. In the absence of mutualisation, people can be impoverished by catastrophic payments for healthcare, unfortunately a situation that is common in poorer countries (Wagstaff 2009) and in the United States (Dobkin et al. 2018).

Conclusion

An ethic of social justice is an ethic of inclusion: all should have access to care without financial barriers. A Christian ethic would conclude that wealth/money and health/healthcare should be in different spheres

(Walzer 1983, 20) in that extra money should not necessarily lead to one having extra years of life, or better healthcare during any of these years.

Being a neighbour, as the teaching from the parable of the 'Good' Samaritan compels us to be, requires us to take action to address the concerns of all those in need. It calls on us to fall on the side of generosity in our response to needs.

Famous British social theorist Richard Titmuss highlighted that

> Society has to make choices – that is to say, we will have to make choices – between more government or more markets; more freedom for some at the expense of other people's freedom; more justice for some and less freedom for others; and so on. At the heart of many of these choices concerning central question of the politics of the good society – the question of obedience or coercion – lies the conflict between individual equity and social equality. (Titmuss 1974, 131)

Titmuss raises the ugly question of politics: is the quest for social justice too 'political' to be a Christian ethics' cause? Earlier in this chapter I drew on the Magnificat. Justin Welby, Archbishop of Canterbury, also did that in a speech to the British Trades Union Congress:

> Mary's song is revolution in immortal verse. It is describing God, not describing human aspiration. It says justice is who God is. Who God is sets the pattern for who we should be, and what our society should be. That is political, but not party political. The bible is political from one end to the other. But we step into dangerous territory when either left or right claim God as being solely on their side. Jesus was highly political, He told the rich that, they would face woes. He criticised the King of the time as a fox. He spoke harsh words to leaders of the nations when they were uncaring of the needy.
>
> Mary's song, the Magnificat, central to the New Testament, is so revolutionary that anyone who takes it seriously finds it a threat to power and entitlement. (Welby 2018)

So yes, a pursuit of social justice is indeed political – it is about changing policy settings, but it is about pursuit of justice, not political ideology or supporting the policies of one party or another.

The Samaritan parable is an explication of the two Great Commandments. Jesus reversed the Torah's ordering of the two Great Commandments. Although the neighbour-love command occurs earlier in the Torah (Leviticus 19:18), than the commandment to love God (Deuteronomy 6:5), an inclusive true neighbour-love may require filling one's heart with love of God as a precursor:

> Experience dictates that it is very hard to love the unlovely neighbor until the disciple's heart is filled with the love of God, which provides the energy and motivation necessary for the arduous task of loving the neighbor. (Bailey 2008, 287)

Being truly inclusive (and fully compassionate) requires one to have an 'inexhaustible fund of patience' (Zweig 1939, 185), potentially sustained by adherence to the first Great Commandment.

In this chapter, I have argued that contemporary needs are too great to be met by individual responses and that a Christian response to healthcare needs should be informed by an ethic of social justice. This emphasises a social, collective response, funded through progressive taxation and with policies that avoid creating regressive barriers to access such as any use of co-payments, especially for secondary services, including prescriptions. Societies should be aiming to complete all dimensions of the coverage cube because failing to do so may result in long-term inefficiency (deferred or denied visits now may result in greater costs in the future) and will leave in place injustices inconsistent with Jesus' injunction to act like the Samaritan and be a neighbour.

CHAPTER 4

The Call to Responsible Stewardship

> The next day [the Samaritan] took out two denarii gave them to the innkeeper, and said, 'Take care of him; and when I come back, I will repay you whatever more you spend.' (Luke 10:35)

In Chapters 1 to 3, I have argued that the parable of the 'Good' Samaritan and the healing stories of Jesus draw us to compassion as a motivator for healthcare provision, and that we should be driven by a call to justice in healthcare financing. In this chapter, I turn to the vexed question of resource allocation in healthcare: how should we prioritise funding in healthcare and what is the place of efficiency, broadly defined? Should there be a blank cheque for healthcare, with healthcare providers charging or demanding what they like, for whatever services they think might be beneficial? Or should there be limits on what is provided, or, at least, what is publicly funded?

The Samaritan's generosity was probably not unbounded – both because there was a relationship of trust between the innkeeper and him and because of an implicit expectation of reasonableness on the part of the Samaritan.

In the first section of this chapter, I will introduce the economic frame of technical and allocative efficiency, which underpins how economics is used to inform healthcare decision-making and then review ethical issues associated with this contemporary dominant economic frame for priority setting.

The second section of this chapter will develop a Christian ethic of healthcare resource allocation and funding, specifically identifying a Christian rather than a utilitarian basis for resource allocation, arguing that 'responsible stewardship' is an alternative frame that should underpin public resource allocation in healthcare. I will argue, however, that 'responsible stewardship' still involves economic tools for priority setting, but in the context of the other two principles of compassion and social justice.

The Economist's Frame: The Pursuit of Efficiency

In Chapter 1, I introduced the concept of economics as a science of scarcity, a concept developed by British economist Lionel Robbins (Robbins 1932). The theme and message of Robbins' famous work *An essay on the nature and significance of economic science* is that decision-makers in all sectors of the economy face choices in the context of scarcity. Opportunity cost is the core concept in economics, which states that in an environment of scarcity, if money (or another resource) is spent on one purpose, then that resource is not available for another. The cost of the investment in the first purpose is the forgone value that would otherwise have been gained from the second purpose.

In countries where the health system is publicly funded, scarcity has a public financing overlay: tax dollars, pounds, and euros are limited. Public attitudes about appropriate levels of taxation vary across countries and within countries, over time. There are differences between parties of the left and the right about whether to prioritise public or private spending. However, whatever country, whatever time, and whatever ideology, the tax-raising capacities of the government are limited. The 'common pool' of taxes is finite, with demands on the pool having to be weighed one against another, which means that additional public health spending for a new technology comes at the expense of other health spending or spending in another sector, whether this is immediately apparent or not. Collective action – where health service payers and providers come together to plan and manage services – can reinforce solidarity through managing these 'common pool' resources in a collectively accepted way (Ostrom 1990; Sanderson et al. 2020).

A variety of strategies have been implemented to moderate expenditure growth using both global funding caps and improving the benefits of health spending (Mills and Kanavos 2020).

Sometimes spending limits are imposed directly and obviously with policies that the health budget is capped, and the cost of any new technology must be funded by savings from the existing budget envelope. This is how funding of new drugs works in New Zealand, with a 'hard cap' forcing drug manufacturers to offer up savings to make funding room for their new products (Ragupathy et al. 2012; Ragupathy and Jameson 2016; Main, Csanadi, and Ozieranski 2022 (in press)). Sometimes there are formal or informal 'soft caps' (Gusmano et al. 2020), where spending may increase in any one year, but there are reductions that are automatically implemented in subsequent years to bring spending back down (formal soft caps), or there is an informal *modus operandi* where central agencies such as Treasury/Finance demand savings in subsequent years that approximate the increased spending from the prior year (informal soft caps). Within hospitals, continuing budget pressure also operates like a soft cap, forcing a focus on efficiency and elimination of low-value care to accommodate new technologies, although the link between the efficiency actions and the technology introduction may not be direct (Wammes et al. 2020).

The United States, the land of big health spending, paradoxically had a legislated formal soft cap in place for many years for physician spending in its publicly funded Medicare programme. The soft caps were known initially as volume performance standards (Russell 1989a; Rice and Bernstein 1990) and subsequently as the sustainable growth rate (Steinbrook 2015; Hirsch et al. 2016), but physician fee reductions under the plans were more fiction than fact as the provisions were regularly overridden by Congress (Reschovsky, Converse, and Rich 2015).

In an environment of public funding constraints, each individual patient or clinician may argue that they would benefit by just that little bit more – getting around the constraint of waiting times, amenity, or, in some countries, treatment options. But, as Hardin (1968) pointed out, the 'tragedy of the commons' is that if each seeks the additional marginal benefit, then all will be losers. Providers or consumers may also argue that more money for health can be found from the elimination of waste or from another sector, although the resources in the health sector are fully and appropriately employed, that is not so in other sectors (Coast et al. 2002). Within the health sector, advocates for better value for money in healthcare might also advocate a 'look over there' strategy, pointing to potential savings in other specialties rather than their own (Morden et al. 2014). Improved efficiency should always be supported as discussed later in this chapter, and it may be that the marginal benefit of an additional dollar of defence or other spending may be less worthwhile than the additional health spending, but at any given level of health spending there are still trade-offs to be made about where the next dollar of health spending should go, while awaiting any potential redistribution from any other economic sector.

There is a second concept that lies behind the economist's approach to scarcity: a recognition that the value gained by an additional unit of consumption declines with the amount of consumption, termed diminishing marginal returns or diminishing marginal utility. In the economics textbook, a person's seventeenth ice cream on a given day does not bring as much joy as their first or sixteenth on that day. This focus on incremental or marginal benefit compared to incremental or marginal cost has been part of this field since its earliest days (Jiang and Marggraf 2021).

In healthcare, an additional test may not yield as much information as the one before, and generally, more intervention may not yield better outcomes. This phenomenon is known as 'flat of the curve' healthcare, from the graphical presentation with expenditure on the horizontal axis and outcomes, however measured, on the vertical axis: the graph of outcomes against spending increases up to a given level of expenditure and then flattens out.

This concept of the diminishing returns can also apply at the system level: beyond a given level of regional or national health expenditure per head of population, increasing health spending does not lead to significant increases in life expectancy (Self and Grabowski 2003; Fuchs 2004). In OECD (the Organisation for Economic Co-operation and Development) countries – which are all middle to high income – on average a 1 per cent increase in total health spending led to an increase in average life expectancy of approximately 10 days (Joumard et al. 2010), which, although small, may still be cost-effective.

The reality of diminishing returns – for both an individual and society – is why it is naïve to assert that it is not possible to provide best care while still containing costs (Engelhardt Jr 2002, 6): the best is not synonymous with unlimited.

The social licence to manage scarcity through budget caps or other means rests on their being seen to be fair and reasonable (Daniels, Light, and Caplan 1996; Daniels and Sabin 2002). In other environments, rules developed for managing these 'common pool resources' will involve acceptance of limits, and joint accountability – that all hold each other to account for the management of the whole system (Ostrom 2010, 1990). In the health sector this is more likely to be achieved if the system is seen as a communal resource of benefit for all rather than a private resource. The British National Health Service is probably the quintessential community supported system, with Australian and Canadian Medicare not too far behind. The United States system is less well supported. Only 4 per cent of U.K. respondents to an international survey said that their health system needed to be completely rebuilt, with less than ten per cent of Australians and Canadians having that view (Schoen et al. 2013). In contrast more than 25 per cent of United States respondents thought so poorly of their health system that it needed to be completely rebuilt.

There may be many reasons why a health system is seen as broken, including failures of access or quality, but this consequence may also be a failure of legitimacy – that strategies to manage scarcity are not seen as in the public interest, but rather seen as being in the private interest to maximise private profit with patient or communal interest taking a back seat (Jackson 2001b). Public rationing needs to be seen to be fair and reasonable so it avoids the betrayal of trust involved in some forms of corporate cost benefit analysis where safety risks – falling on staff or consumers – are explicitly monetised and accepted in return for additional corporate profits accruing to management or shareholders (Sunstein 2014, 146; 2010).

In tax-funded health systems – in contrast to social insurance systems – the effect of scarcity can be seen in long waiting times for elective procedures and, sometimes, emergency department care. Although waiting times in both areas can be reduced by good funding design and management (Street and Duckett 1996; Duckett and Nijssen-Jordan 2012), long waiting times are an obvious and visible sign that funding is capped. Prioritisation systems aim to ensure that a scarce resource – be it the surgeon's time, hospital beds, or operating room/theatre hours – is allocated so that high-priority patients are given access first (Pomey et al. 2010; Breton et al. 2020; Kalson et al. 2021).

Good health system management should try to ensure that scarce resources are allocated to yield the greatest health benefit: how many beds or operating hours should be allocated to orthopaedics compared to cardiac surgery? To dental care or to social care in the community? The answer to these questions should not rest entirely on political whim. Scarce resources should be allocated to maximise overall health outcomes: in the utilitarian calculus, the greatest good for the greatest number.

Economic Evaluation

It is this recognition of scarcity and opportunity costs that has led to the championing of economic evaluation or 'health technology assessment' as a means of ensuring that any government spending yields the most benefit. For economists that would be paradise. Unfortunately, there are political overlays and the benefits of an additional dollar spent on health may be weighted differently in the political calculus from an additional dollar on roads. Acute health services, such as hospital services, seem to get a higher political priority than less acute services such as rehabilitation; mental health is also often at the bottom of the priority pile, with cancer and children's services closer to the top. Nevertheless, the inevitability of public spending limits provides an ongoing rationale for the use of economic evaluation.

According to Robbins, the essence of choice is about relative valuations. For Robbins:

> The economist studies the disposal of scarce means. He is interested in the way different degrees of scarcity of different goods give rise to different ratios of valuation between them, and ... is interested in the way in which changes in conditions of scarcity, whether coming from changes in ends or changes in means–from the demand side or the supply side–affect these ratios. (Robbins 1932, 15)

Fast forward about ninety years, and Robbins' insights and definition are still relevant, but what has changed is the application and methods. Techniques have been developed about how to allocate resources in an environment of scarcity. The 'ratios of valuations' that Robbins describes has given rise to the subfield of economic evaluation to inform resource allocation; this technique involves assessing the (incremental or marginal) costs of a policy or intervention and weighing those costs against the (incremental or marginal) benefits, with benefits measured either in terms of benefit to 'society' or benefit to the health system (Johannesson et al. 2009).

Cost benefit analysis monetises both costs and benefits; the more common cost-effectiveness analysis quantifies benefits in some other metric such as lives extended. But it is an illusion to imagine that adopting natural units such as lives extended avoids any value or valuation problems (Williams 1993, 36). The underpinning of economic evaluation – even in healthcare – remains utilitarian, aggregating individual utilities into a 'social welfare' function (Charlton and Weale 2021).

The dominant underlying value framework for economic evaluation is 'extra-welfarist', in the sense of seeking a broad maximand, typically 'health', broadly defined, often measured by perceived health status (Booth 2019; Sakowsky 2021). The objective in a particular case might be reduction in pain, in days of feeling low, or self-reported health status on a generic scale aggregated to the treatment population, and cost-effectiveness is assessed on this criterion with hospital treatment ideally assessed against preventive or community-based care.

Robbins also drew attention to the critical distinction between producing goods and services efficiently – what economists describe as technical efficiency – and the economic allocation of resources, what has come to be known as allocative or social efficiency (Bohm 1987). Robbins points out: 'The mass production of particular things irrespective of demand for them, however technically efficient, is not necessarily "economical"' (Robbins 1932, 49).

Allocative efficiency occurs when any reallocation of investments from one use to another cannot improve overall average outcomes; for example, shifting resources from orthopaedics to cardiac surgery does not improve average total benefits to patients. Allocative inefficiency also occurs when resources are devoted to clinically ineffective treatments or unnecessary diagnostic tests (Moynihan, Doust, and Henry 2012; Scott and Duckett 2015; Brett et al. 2017; Brownlee et al. 2017; Chalmers et al. 2018).

An economic evaluation industry has developed, which sets guidelines for how both costs and benefits are to be valued and compared (Drummond et al. 2015; Department of Health. Pharmaceutical Benefits Advisory Committee 2016; Neumann et al. 2017; Kristensen et al. 2019), although there is little guidance on how to consider the implementation of new technologies in economic evaluations (Heggie, Boyd, and Wu 2021). Some health economists have argued for a technique known as programme budgeting and marginal analysis to widen the application of economic evaluation to facilitate explicit consideration of local health trade-offs (Mitton and Donaldson 2001). This approach is perceived as valuable by decision-makers, one criterion for 'success' of the application (Tsourapas and Frew 2011), but this ostensible support generally does not translate into actual use of the technique (Kapiriri and Razavi 2017). The results of economic evaluations are used as a decision-making tool that – either implicitly or explicitly – results in some treatments being publicly funded and therefore widely available, and some not, introducing the 'R' word, rationing (Schmidt 2004).

At its simplest, economic evaluation enables the comparison of different treatment strategies in a single disease: for example, drug A is compared to drug B in terms of improving breast cancer outcomes. But healthcare decision-makers in many countries have extended these within-disease comparisons to between-disease comparisons to compare the improvement in outcomes for a new breast cancer drug against the improvements achieved by other drugs that have been approved for government subsidy, thus evaluating breast cancer outcomes against heart disease outcomes. There are technical and theoretical challenges to such an extension (Bleichrodt and Quiggin 1999), but the underlying argument is whether health funding decisions should be made in order to maximise the benefit in terms of health outcomes across the board for any health spending or whether the health gain achieved from a new intervention is at least as good as its opportunity cost of health gains displaced.

In healthcare, where benefits of interventions include outcomes that extend life and improve the life so extended, this involves 'tragic choices' (Calabresi and Bobbitt 1978) and the extremely complex issue of what (economic) value should be placed on a year of human life, or more accurately, what value should be placed on another 365 days of leading a happy and contented life – this latter involving a measure of subjective well-being.

Choices and controversies abound here. Although the technical write-up often disguises the choices that have been made in equations and formulae, essentially every economic evaluation involves confronting this economic trade-off about how much to invest to gain one extra year of life, and how much should such a year be discounted if it is lived in pain or with a disability. This process creates a metric known as Quality-Adjusted Life Years (QALYs), by discounting ('adjusting') years of life lived by a factor related to the 'quality' or perceived desirability of each year of life (Dolan 2000; Whitehead and Ali 2010; Carlson et al. 2020). QALYs are thus affected by both the duration of life added (adding years to life) and the quality of those added years (adding life to years). The total benefit is then calculated by total QALYs achieved in the number of people affected. Disability-adjusted life years (DALYs) are similarly constructed and, when both quality-adjusted and disability-adjusted life-years are used in economic evaluations, the differences are modest (Feng et al. 2020).

The immediate challenge for QALYs (and DALYs) is in this aggregation – is it ethically reasonable to conceptualise 'capacity to benefit' as a unitary measure combining length and quality of life? Should we view life extension – whether *in extremis* or not – as able to be traded off against life quality? The use of QALYS assumes this is ethically legitimate (Gold, Stevenson, and Fryback 2002), although doing so may not be consistent with society's views on saving identified lives, where society may weight life-saving differently from life extension, as discussed in Chapter 5.

Developing 'quality' or disability adjusters also involves complex and controversial judgements. A person without a disability sees life with a disability differently from someone with that disability, creating the 'disability paradox' (Albrecht and Devlieger 1999; Ubel et al. 2005):

> The Standard View is that disabilities have a very strong negative impact on the quality of life of the individuals who have them. This view is widely held by non-disabled people, both in popular and in academic culture. The Standard View is confronted by … its Anomaly: when asked about the quality of their own lives, disabled people report a quality only slightly lower than that reported by non-disabled people, and much higher than that projected by non-disabled people. (Amundson 2005, 103)

A disabled person is well aware that the impact of their disability is critically determined by social provision; at its most obvious the impact of needing a wheelchair to get around is much less if a wheelchair is available and affordable, if door openings are wide enough to navigate, and if kerbs have ramps. The relevant World Health Organisation classification specifically includes dimensions to assess the interaction with these environmental factors (World Health Organization 2001) and yet disability adjusters (and, by extension, quality adjusters generally) are developed as if the impact of a condition is an individualistic undertaking, independent of the environment within which the person exists, negating all the work of disability activists over decades, and valorising an individual 'medical model' framing over a 'social model' (Amundson 2005).

The reality is that disability is 'complex and multifaceted, with its roots in culture' (Mont 2007, 1662). The corollary is that a unidimensional, individualistic measure, devoid of environmental context, will almost certainly not capture the complex and multifaceted nuances appropriately (Campbell, Nyholm, and Walter 2021). And yet, this is the approach most commonly adopted in economic evaluations. There are now techniques for addressing a parallel weakness of contemporary approaches to economic evaluation: distributional issues in economic evaluations (discussed in Chapter 5). Similarly, economic evaluation could adopt new approaches to use of adjusters, including different adjusters for different purposes or groups (Nord 2005; Mont 2007) as a way of addressing the ethical and policy weakness of contemporary approaches to developing quality and disability adjustments.

Although there are many alternative measurement instruments with different conceptual properties (Olsen and Misajon 2020), quality adjustments are now most commonly measured using an instrument called the EQ-5D – the EuroQol-5 dimension instrument (Szende, Oppe, and Devlin 2007). The five dimensions are mobility; self-care; ability to undertake usual activities; pain/discomfort; and anxiety/depression. Years lived with reduced mobility, for example, are adjusted downwards compared to years lived with full mobility.

Within the economics' value frame, choice in the context of scarcity means giving primacy to the options that maximise the ends, measured in QALYs, relative to the means or costs to achieve those ends. The focus is on the individual benefit, and wider perspectives on value – say to the family or carer – may not be incorporated into the benefit metric as measured by the QALY-gain (Garrison, Kamal-Bahl, and Towse 2017; Bell, Neri, and Steuten 2021; Shafrin et al. 2021; Ryan and Preisz 2022). The QALY gain is the sum of the QALYs of individuals who benefit, or the average QALY gain, thus demonstrating an individualist, utilitarian, and consequentialist calculus.

The use of cost-effectiveness analysis and cost benefit analysis is now all-pervasive in high-income countries shaping what regulatory interventions should be supported to protect life and address broader social concerns, such as environmental regulation. The reach of economic evaluation is so extensive that Posner and Sunstein (2017) suggest the 'regulatory state' is now the 'cost benefit analysis' state.

The work of the regulatory and policy-advising 'econocrats' – the term is from Self (1976) – involves value judgements (Harvard, Werker, and Silva 2020), and assumptions in formulae, about whether the lives of rich and poor should be equally weighted, and whether death from cancer should be valued differently from other deaths, given society may have a greater fear of cancer and its consequences than other illnesses (Sunstein 2014, 2004; Viscusi, Huber, and Bell 2014; Sara Olofsson et al. 2019). QALYs – the metric of choice in economic evaluations – have been challenged on methodological grounds, but have also faced criticisms relating to the ethical basis of the construct including so-called QALY neutrality and implicit discrimination (Rand and Kesselheim 2021).

Normally economic evaluation in healthcare does not involve an explicit calculation that a particular individual will die, nor even that someone will definitively have their life shortened (the case of identified lives is discussed below). Rather, the outcome of economic evaluation in healthcare is the estimate that on average people needing this treatment will have a greater or lesser likelihood of an extra period of life – or extra quality of life – if an intervention is approved or not approved for funding and that if approved, the expected benefit will be within the typical range. It is phrased here as an average benefit across the group, and a likelihood not a certainty. The focus of the economic evaluation is on public resources and overall benefit (Sculpher et al. 2017) and is framed by economists as in the public interest, consistent with a social licence for rationing.

Despite the challenges of the application of economic evaluation to healthcare, discussed below, it is now accepted in many countries as the appropriate metric for judging whether a particular treatment, medication, or preventive strategy is worthy of public funding (Hipgrave et al. 2014; Wiseman et al. 2016; Seixas, Dionne, and Mitton 2021; Seixas et al. 2021). The most notable exception to the use of explicit, economically based, priority setting is the United States (Neumann 2005), with its stronger political emphasis on libertarian philosophies, including in healthcare (Smith 2010, 21), and a lack of a 'common purpose' or shared vision among health system players (Padula and Sculpher 2021), with the interests of insurers and hospitals, for example, being seen as antithetical. However, even there it is creeping into private insurance coverage decisions with the new moniker of 'value-based care' or 'value-based competition' (Porter and Teisberg 2006, 2004), supported by independent assessment services whose advice influences insurers' pricing (Neumann, Ollendorf, and Cohen 2021).

Countries with a Bismarckian tradition of social protection, with a strong emphasis on choice compared to Beveridge-inspired countries, also tend to deemphasise economic evaluation in healthcare priority setting (Torbica, Tarricone, and Drummond 2018).

In publicly funded health systems where economic evaluation is used, healthcare interventions are supported for funding if they cost less than a threshold value for each QALY gained, and not supported if the cost is more than a higher threshold, with a grey area between the two thresholds (George, Harris, and Mitchell 2001; Dakin et al. 2015; Woods et al. 2016; Wang, Gum, and Merlin 2018). The appropriate level of the thresholds (including the upper and lower bounds) will vary between countries, partly related to the country's wealth (Schwarzer et al. 2015; Bertram et al. 2016; Viscusi and Masterman 2017; Cameron, Ubels, and Norström 2018; Leech et al. 2018; Cubi-Molla et al. 2020).

Thresholds – which should be in the public domain, as should be the justification of the chosen threshold (Pekarsky 2015) – should not vary across types of health interventions within countries in the economist's utilitarian frame (Segal, Dalziel, and Mortimer 2010; Schilling, Mortimer, and Dalziel 2016), but may vary for other reasons, for example, to take equity into account, rewarding innovation, or other aspects of societal preferences (Moradpour and Hollis 2021). Allowing thresholds to differ according to payment source – public compared to private payers, for example (Danzon et al. 2018) – would enshrine inequity into the health funding system and should be eschewed.

Analysing cross-country change in aggregate Gross Domestic Product, health expenditure, and life-years retrospectively, Ochalek and Lomas (2020) concluded that an additional adjusted year of life was priced at around one to three times GDP per capita, Daroudi et al. (2021) found lower estimates. These lower and upper bounds might be seen as appropriate 'thresholds' for economic evaluation decisions – although the term threshold may encourage a focus on new technologies rather than reassessing old interventions (Edney et al. 2022) – with the bounds perhaps adjusted downwards in a more resource-constrained and ecologically responsible economic environment (Hensher, Canny et al. 2020; Hensher, Tisdell et al. 2020).

In the United Kingdom and its former colonies, economists at the University of York were the chief proponents of this new religion of economic evaluation (Ashmore, Mulkay, and Pinch 1989), arguing that cost-effectiveness analysis with its utilitarian underpinnings should take precedence over all other bases for evaluation and choice, including political judgements

(Wildavsky 1966), as this would maximise social welfare. For the York economists, this quest also had an ethical basis: 'it is ethical to be efficient (and unethical to be inefficient)' (Culyer 1992, 8), with efficiency here defined as the optimal distribution of healthcare investments as measured using economic evaluations. They were supporters of the United Kingdom's publicly funded National Health Service, and their work was designed to ensure that each pound allocated to healthcare was spent as effectively as possible.

As discussed in Chapter 2, 'need', argued to be a neutral and subjective concept by healthcare planners and advocates alike, is often used in debates about healthcare (Braybrooke 1987). Need can be misused in such arguments, with pathos-based emotional 'shroud waving' used to tear at the heartstrings of the public to support favoured investments. The York economists derided 'need' as an inappropriate concept for resource allocation (Williams 1974) to be supplanted by choices informed by economic evaluation. The York economists went even further, making cost-effectiveness central to even defining 'need': 'Thus health services are needed … only if the outcome is desired and there is no alternative (or more cost-effective) way of realizing (the outcome)' (Culyer 1989, 50–51).

So according to Culyer, recognition of a need necessarily involves some cost-effectiveness calculus. Economic evaluation, cost-effectiveness, and opportunity costs thus 'moved from the wings to centre stage in the rhetoric of decision-making' (Smee 2005, 80). Alan Williams, one of the doyens of health economics and a leader of the York group, posited the centrality and importance of economic evaluation in very general terms:

> An efficient economic system ensures that what people have to sacrifice in order to get something they want is of less value than the thing that they want (and that this difference is as large as possible). (Williams 2001, 251)

The corollary is that an economic system cannot be efficient unless economic evaluation is core to the social priority setting process; it is the way that the opportunity cost of the missed alternatives is brought into the decision calculus. The health economists' argument is that healthcare interventions need to be shown to be cost-effective, as well as clinically effective. In this world view, if an intervention is not cost-effective, there will necessarily be a misallocation of resources; societal welfare will not be maximised, and some other investment will be better for society. Essentially the argument is that any misallocation of resources involves an opportunity cost of foregone benefits.

The economics frame comes into conflict with both clinical autonomy and tailoring clinical interventions to patient preferences. The case for the pre-eminence of economic evaluation was put by another leading York economist, Alan Maynard:

> If evidence-based medicine and the individual ethic are allowed to determine treatment choices, resources will be used inefficiently and unethically … By focusing on the needs of the individual patient, advocates of evidence-based medicine refuse to acknowledge this opportunity lost, or what is given up – i.e., the benefits in terms of the future treatment of other patients. Such an approach is perceived as unethical by those who are concerned with achieving maximum health benefits for the general population from a limited budget. (Maynard 1997, 126–127)

For Maynard and the other York economists, the issues of scarcity and opportunity costs dominated their thinking. Another doyen of the York group, Alan Williams, phrased it this way:

> Many clinicians believe that allowing costs to influence clinical decisions is unethical. They are mistaken in this belief, because it cannot be ethical to ignore the adverse consequences upon others of the decisions you make, which is what 'costs' represent … So if someone says to me that they must have something *no matter what it costs*, I take them to mean that they must have it *no matter what sacrifices have to be made*. And it is always easier to make such statements if the costs (or sacrifices) are going to be borne by somebody else! (Williams 1992, 7, emphasis in original)

Even when balancing individual needs in the context of wider scarcity, the York economists favoured considering cost-effectiveness and challenged the place of clinical autonomy:

> Social values must, in a publicly financed system, be balanced with clinical values to determine which patients will and will not get treatment. Neither the clinician nor the economist should dominate decisions about who will live in what degree of pain and discomfort and who, in extremis, will die. Such choices are informed by the evidence base of cost-effectiveness, and determined by independent professional judgments. (Maynard 1997, 128)

But not all health economists accepted this nuanced view:

> I want to highlight the uncomfortable fact that, as practised, medical ethics, particularly in the form of clinical freedom, tends to breed inefficiency. Indeed, it seems that it sometimes provides a convenient escape mechanism for the romantic member of the medical profession neither to pursue efficiency nor to attempt any rationalisation at all of the potential for pursuing efficiency in health care. (Mooney 1986, 89)

This criticism of medical ethics was – even at the time – unfair and failed to consider how ethics and efficiency might be pursued jointly, incorporated naturally into clinical decision-making (Levinson, Born, and Wolfson 2018; Varela 2018; Grimshaw et al. 2020). Further, as I will show later, one of the challenges of cost-effectiveness analysis is that in some decisions, especially involving rare diseases, there are identifiable lives at stake, compared to statistical lives in the abstract, and the mindless application of economic evaluation might be inconsistent with social preferences and valuations of outcomes and is certainly inconsistent with the Christian ethic of stewardship of resources.

Technical Efficiency

The focus of health economics on economic evaluation was to some extent at the expense of the less theoretically appealing and more mundane issue of technical efficiency. Technical efficiency, defined as the (optimal) ratio of inputs to outputs, relies on measurement of outputs. (Allocative efficiency is essentially optimising the ratio of outputs to outcomes or ends.)

In his review of the scope of health economics, York economist Alan Williams identified technical efficiency as important (Williams 1997a) as would be expected since allocative efficiency cannot be achieved in the absence of technical efficiency; that is, societal welfare will not be maximised if a more technically efficient process could be implemented to achieve the agreed ends or outcomes. Ironically, in healthcare the principal work on technical efficiency was initiated outside the purview of the York economists in the United States, the most expensive health system in the world.

Measuring outputs in healthcare is a non-trivial task. The intellectual breakthrough in terms of hospital output measurement was achieved by a team at Yale University led by an academic industrial engineer Bob Fetter and nurse academic John Thompson who conceptualised the output of hospital care as treated patients (Fetter, Brand, and Gamache 1991; White 2003). The issue was how to distinguish between different types of patients, which Fetter and Thompson did through the development of a categorisation scheme for inpatient care known as Diagnosis Related Groups (DRGs) (Fetter et al. 1980). Contemporary DRG classifications have hundreds of categories, distinguishing patients with Chronic Obstructive Airways Disease from those who had appendicectomies, and within those groups, by the extent of their comorbidity.

DRGs were initially developed to *describe* hospital in-patient activity, but it was a logical step to move from description to paying hospitals on the basis of DRGs, initially in the United States (Russell 1989b), and subsequently in many publicly funded health systems (Kimberly, de Pouvourville, and D'Aunno 2008; Busse et al. 2011), in this case with the Yale group being the chief proponents.

Activity-based funding, as the process became known, involves describing the activity of a hospital – normally using DRGs for inpatient ('admitted') activity – and the payer funding the hospital based on its activity. Under this payment system, the payment for each treated patient is independent of the hospital's own costs, with the payment normally set at a target price or the average across all hospitals. Introduction of activity-based funding thus creates an incentive for efficiency, with more expensive hospitals funded at less than their historic levels.

Although there is still some criticism of the pursuit of technical efficiency in healthcare (Stein 2001), paying healthcare organisations on the basis of their activity is now the dominant payment method for healthcare organisations. Activity-based funding is discussed further in Chapter 5.

The Challenges of Economic Evaluation

The York (and other) economists make a strong case for economic evaluation in healthcare. Indeed, it is difficult to argue against the logic that society is better off if no more worthwhile investments to improve QALYs can be found within a budget cap. It is logically and rhetorically seen to be sensible to spend where there is the greatest capacity to benefit – which QALYs measure – without regard as to who is benefitting, or whether the benefit is life extending or life improving, providing the measurement is fair, as is the QALY claim (Rand and Kesselheim 2021).

The alternative to a system where priorities are set using economic evaluation is also difficult to develop. Assuming that scarcity is an economic reality rather than politically (Jackson 2001a) or socially constructed (Hughes and Light 2002), what alternative metrics for priority setting for public funding can be articulated? In fact, no alternative has been developed or gained acceptance, with the consequence that rejecting economic evaluation for priority setting is likely to be associated with health costs consuming a larger proportion of the total economy, at the cost of meeting other social, or indeed, individual, goals.

Application of cost-effectiveness within the health sector, however, creates an engine for health expenditure growth, albeit with that expenditure growth having a concomitant increase in benefits (Donaldson et al. 2008; Lomas et al. 2018). Rarely is there any explicit analysis of the opportunity costs of this increase in spending compared to spending in another sector of the economy that has not embraced economic evaluation, or other parts of the health sector. Economic evaluations are often commissioned by proponents of a new product as part of the process of creating a government- or other payer-subsidised market and possibly for that reason, there are fewer economic evaluations of public health relative to somatic interventions (Cyr et al. 2021), potentially contributing to underinvestment in this sector.

Although there is some variation in thresholds and decisions internationally (Nanavaty et al. 2015), recent empirical analyses suggest that the cost-effectiveness thresholds up to which new drugs might be approved by funding agencies are too high, compared to what the public might see as reasonable, resulting in decisions that inappropriately favour new technologies by underestimating what is foregone by these new investments (Claxton et al. 2015; Edney et al. 2018; Karnon, Edney, and Afzali 2018; Edney, Haji Ali Afzali, and Karnon 2019; Siverskog and Henriksson 2019; van Baal et al. 2019; McDougall et al. 2020), and this despite the fact that thresholds and associated estimates of the value of an additional (quality-adjusted) life year in the health sector are generally lower than in other sectors (Cubi-Molla et al. 2021). Post-approval review processes are often weak, and the promised benefits shown in early studies may not eventuate when an intervention is used in ordinary clinical situations (Cipriani et al. 2020).

In Australia, recommendations for new drugs that involved a large incremental cost to the budget formerly had to be considered by Cabinet. However, the cries from stakeholders that these drugs are 'cost-effective' meant that it became politically impossible to maintain this extra gate – after cost-effectiveness has been demonstrated – even when expenditure was large. The extra gate was, in fact, illogical:

> To say that an alternative is cost-effective but not affordable must mean that the [implicit or explicit] 'threshold' used to judge cost-effectiveness does not reflect the scale and value of the opportunity costs. (Lomas et al. 2018, 274)

Despite decades of development (Williams 1995; Spencer et al. 2022), cost-effectiveness analysis is not without its controversies (Smith 2010), even from within the economic frame (Gray and Wilkinson 2016; Sen 2000), including the appropriate valuation of a year of life, what to do about future medical costs (de Vries, van Baal, and Brouwer 2019), whether benefits in the near future should be valued the same as benefits in a few years' time (Craig et al. 2018), and what are the appropriate thresholds for what is deemed cost-effective and what is not.

Important decisions are made on the basis of economic evaluations, with differences in incremental cost-effectiveness ratios presented with a degree of precision that contributes to an 'illusion of validity' (Kahneman 2011) and an assumption that the whole process is 'value free' (Harvard, Werker, and Silva 2020). The illusion of validity and the consequential subjective confidence in the results of economic evaluations are at odds with economic evaluation's foundation, which may be built on the shifting sands of spurious accuracy. Recent studies have confirmed this spurious accuracy showing that a shift from using the EQ-5D with a three-level scale for each dimension as the principal outcome measure to one with a five-level scale may change decisions from an intervention being deemed cost-effective to the reverse (Hernandez Alava et al. 2018; Pennington et al. 2019). The source of funding of economic evaluations also influences the results: studies funded by pharmaceutical companies are more likely to show the product is cost-effective than those funded from other sources (Friedberg et al. 1999; Neumann et al. 2000; Lundh et al. 2012). Methods for recognising uncertainty around estimates are still being developed (Soares, Sculpher, and Claxton 2020).

In real-life policymaking, there is rarely a single metric that is used in decision-making: there may be a budget cap, costs of implementing change, differences in decision-makers' risk tolerance, and concern about the uncertainty of estimates, which all conspire to dilute the mindless application of economic evaluation. However, the econocrat's argument is that these factors can be taken account in an economically rational way (Hauck, Thomas, and Smith 2016; Sendi 2021), and that by so doing, societal welfare is enhanced.

There are also critical, controversial value choices in the application of cost-effectiveness analysis, including the issue of whether someone can be 'better off dead' (Dewitt and Torrance 2020; Sampson, Parkin, and Devlin 2020; Schneider 2022). Following a review of some of the weaknesses of economic evaluation, and the assumptions incorporated in cost-effectiveness studies and valuations of QALYs, Nord (1999, 73) went so far as to conclude:

> I contend that to rank projects in terms of cost-per-QALY as often as not may tend to distort resource allocation decisions rather than to inform and aid them.

Nord's criticism is in part based on how QALY weights are often calculated: aggregations of the answers from individuals about what health states they might value or be willing to pay for, the latter basis arising from Cold War strategising (Schelling 1968; Banzhaf 2014; Enthoven 2019). Such aggregations are unstable and probably inequitable (Dolan et al. 2008; Rice 2015; Kniesner 2019); indeed, Nobel Laureate Amartya Sen has suggested that

> When all the requirements of ubiquitous market-centred evaluation have been incorporated into the procedures of cost-benefit analysis, it is not so much a discipline as a daydream. (Sen 2000, 952)

The alternative favoured by Nord and others (Ubel et al. 1996; Shiell, Hawe, and Seymour 1997; Anand 2001) is that QALY weights for public resource allocation should be developed based on what people think is appropriate for *public investments*, helping to convert the individual utilitarian approach to a communitarian one (Etzioni 1988, 1999; Mooney 2001).

A more fundamental issue is how to incorporate the reality that 'the public' is not homogeneous and so there is heterogeneity of values (Baker et al. 2021) and whether the whole approach to measurement of benefit should differ for different populations. For example, Indigenous populations conceive of health differently from non-Indigenous people (Angell et al. 2016; Butler et al. 2019; Willing et al. 2020), and so it would be logical for the approach to measuring benefits for programmes focusing on Indigenous populations to be constructed differently; failure to do so would be inequitable and probably inefficient because of inappropriate priority setting.

Economic evaluation for policy compares the outcomes of an intervention for a group of people with the outcomes from an alternative intervention (on either the same or a different group of people), and thus involves comparing lives in the abstract – 'statistical lives'. The quantification involved in cost-effectiveness analysis also disguises inherent value choices in measuring QALYs, including deemphasising equity. Both issues create critical challenges for the use of cost-effectiveness analysis.

Statistical Lives and the Rule of Rescue

Aristotle long ago recognised three bases of rhetorical argument: ethos, logos, and pathos. Economic evaluation is based on logos, the logical choice to be made; it excludes the emotive sway of pathos. QALYs are about groups of people – people in the abstract – and the outcomes of care for them are measured in (discounted) statistical lives (Hammitt and Treich 2007).

Ethicists distinguish the general situation where we describe benefit in unidentified statistical lives from those situations where an individual, or a small group of individuals, is able to be identified as benefiting from a specific intervention (Emanuel 2002). In those latter situations general rules of priority setting are often overridden with the 'Rule of Rescue': that a supererogatory intervention may be evoked to save an identified individual

(Jonsen 1986; Hadorn 1991, 1996; McKie and Richardson 2003; Lipsitch, Evans, and Cotton-Barratt 2017), and this response to identified lives over statistical lives might be a deeply programmed part of our evolutionary biology (Moore 1996).

Economic evaluation is normally based on groups and ignores issues of specific cases and unique circumstances. It is not only the situation of the trapped miner or a lone sailor to which the Rule of Rescue applies: cost-effectiveness measurement may also be challenged in its application to small, reasonably identifiable groups of people with, for example, rare cancers or rare genomic anomalies (Drummond et al. 2007; Onakpoya et al. 2015; Rodriguez-Martin et al. 2018). The abstract calculus of theory may be challenged when it collides with political realities:

> When budget decisions are made in real life, nobody is behind a veil of ignorance. It is inevitable that people, making judgements concerning others, let themselves be influenced by emotions stirred by the specific characteristics of the allocation options presented (e.g., that the disease in question occurred in one's own family). It is not to be expected that the preferences following from these emotions should entirely coincide with long-term preferences expressed in cool, neutral circumstances behind a veil of ignorance. (Nord 1999, 10)

Nord is here questioning whether even decisions at the group level, when people are not identifiable, can be uninfluenced by individual experiences and emotions. Establishing 'neutral' criteria behind a Rawlsian 'veil of ignorance' (Rawls 1999), and applying them in practice, becomes more difficult when there are clearly identifiable individuals who are affected by the general rule, and especially so when issues of life and death are at stake. Clinicians and the general public might be impacted adversely – experiencing 'denial or deprivation disutility' – if confronted with making harsh, explicit, rationing decisions (Coast 1997, 2001).

This is the problem that is confronted in the clinic on a regular basis. The up-to-date clinician knows of a new treatment which has been 'shown to work' in overseas trials and if this treatment is not currently approved for use or publicly funded locally what does the clinician do? Some clinicians will accept the rationality of government priority setting, some will not (Coast 2000; Feiring and Wang 2018; Pace et al. 2021). Definitions of what 'shown to work' means will vary across clinicians – is an early-stage descriptive study enough to claim a treatment works, or is a randomised trial required? Or a randomised trial replicated a few times? What about side effects? Over what timeframe should they be evaluated to apply the label 'shown to work'? When some treatments are not funded, some clinicians will face a tragic choice – for them, the statistical lives of the econocrat have become personalised into the patient they are treating and to whom they are explaining treatment options.

The Internet has also changed the role of clinicians as gatekeepers. Patients can and do search on-line for information about 'patients like me' (Frost and Massagli 2008). Patients can source information themselves about treatment options, form their own views about the benefits and risks of treatment in their specific situation, and justify their concerns about their illness (Stevenson et al. 2021). In some cases, this will be based on a good understanding of probabilities of the outcomes, in some cases not. As discussed in Chapter 2, compassionate care involves recognising and valuing patients' choices: the patient is the only one who can weigh the importance of different outcomes at play, both in terms of the potential clinical outcome and the side effects of the treatment. In evaluating treatment options, one of the clinician's roles is to inform patients and their carers about the probability or likelihood of each of these potential outcomes and potential side effects, including potential adverse events.

The challenge for clinicians, health services, and health systems is when the assessment of what is the average outcome as measured for a group of patients may not be relevant to the individual patient. The average may be a poor measure of the distribution of outcomes – there may be a group of outliers that pull the average in one direction or another, the average may sit in a very wide distribution, or the average may have been calculated on a small number of patients so is inherently unstable.

Application of standard economic evaluation is challenged in all these scenarios. Individual patients – or small groups of patients – can claim to be different and seek to be treated differently. The homogeneous group becomes heterogeneous, and the decision rules based on average statistical lives do not survive confrontation with the personalised life in the clinician's office (Lessard, Contandriopoulos, and Beaulieu 2010; Brousselle and Lessard 2011).

Technological change is also challenging the 'average across the group' approach of yesteryear. New treatments are becoming more personalised: the intervention targets and works only in people with these genomic characteristics and does not otherwise. The number of people may be small, and the difference for them is great. The handful of people who benefit is easily identifiable and the benefits to them easily recounted. Gene therapies – where benefits accrue over a lifetime and across economic sectors (i.e. outside the health sector) – are often expensive but deliver benefits that are multiples of comparators (Goswami et al. 2019; Elverum and

Whitman 2020). These are challenging conventional approaches to economic evaluation (Firth et al. 2021).

Decisions in these circumstances – where treatment eligibility requires identification of the patient's genomic make-up – can slip quickly into looking more like Rule of Rescue than standard economic evaluation.

The Rule of Rescue – a pathos-based allocation when confronted by the individual case – is antithetical to the normal conception of a systematic economic evaluation approach as it overrides the priority setting criteria and thresholds of the 'rational' approach. In the context of a fixed health budget, and the economist's frame, it means that identified lives are inappropriately valued more highly than non-identified lives, and, as the York economists argue, were the Rule of Rescue to be applied, more statistical (quality-adjusted) lives would be lost than identified lives saved.

Hope (2001, 182), in arguing against the legitimacy of allowing the Rule of Rescue to justify interventions with costs above established thresholds, suggests that those opposed to the Rule of Rescue are not callous and lacking in compassion, rather

> The callousness (of those supporting the Rule of Rescue) lies in the relative indifference to death and suffering simply because the specific individuals concerned cannot be identified. There is a lack of imagination in those preferring rescue rather than a lack of sympathy in those (who don't).

However, 'not everyone thinks like an economist' (Fein 2010, 161) and the economist's championing of 'rational' decision-making does not take place in a neutral environment. Economic rationality is also challenged on the basis of self-interest. Public spending on healthcare is the income of employees and contractors to healthcare organisations, including pharmaceutical and other suppliers (Reinhardt 2012). It is therefore in the interest of suppliers, especially pharmaceutical suppliers, to weaken the logos-based arguments in favour of pathos-based arguments highlighting specific cases of individuals whose lives will be foreshortened or made a misery in the absence of public support for the company's patented prescription (Booth, Aggarwal, and Sullivan 2022). Patient advocacy organisations are funded by pharmaceutical companies to join such campaigns (Batt 2017; Mattingly and Simoni-Wastila 2017; McCoy et al. 2017; Moynihan and Bero 2017; Rose et al. 2017), converting the role of consumer from expert informant to advocate (Ghinea, Lipworth, and Kerridge 2020), and there is selective media support for special consideration for drugs used for some diseases, especially cancer, despite their lack of cost-effectiveness (Lewison et al. 2018), increasing pressure for public spending on drugs, which may confer little benefit on patients.

But the advocates for applying the Rule of Rescue can also advance logos-based arguments. There are technical reasons why it may be difficult to undertake valid cost-effectiveness studies in the circumstances where the Rule of Rescue might apply. Measurement of cost-effectiveness relies on studies with sufficient statistical power to show a statistically significant difference, and this may not be feasible in health conditions that occur rarely (Ghinea, Little, and Lipworth 2017; Mattingly and Simoni-Wastila 2017). In the absence of good evaluation studies policymakers need to consider the type of mistake that may be preferred:

- treatment might be funded which is ineffective; or, the alternative error,
- funding is not provided for treatments that are effective and so people miss out on a cost-effective intervention because of the inability to identify it as such.

The Rule of Rescue leads to weighing cost-ineffective access and ignoring the opportunity cost of the Rule of Rescue investment over the goal of limiting the potential waste of money on those cost-ineffective treatments. The place of the Rule of Rescue in funding in a Christian ethic of resource allocation is discussed in Chapter 5.

A challenge for economic evaluation, and somewhat related to the issue of Rule of Rescue, is a situation where people have only a short time to live; should decision-making prioritise people in those situations? That is, should there be an end-of-life premium?

The evidence about whether, and to what extent, the public supports a premium for those with only a short time to live in the absence of treatment as a legitimate basis for overriding normal cost-effectiveness criteria is quite mixed. A recent review identified eleven studies that did not find an end-of-life premium, eight studies that did find public support for such a premium, and four studies that were inconclusive (Shah, Tsuchiya, and Wailoo 2018). Even where an end-of-life premium is found, its incremental value may be modest (Gu et al. 2015; Pennington et al. 2015; McCabe et al. 2016; Shah 2016; Olofsson et al. 2018). A study by Hansen and Kjær (2019) suggests that the public preferences quality of life gain over life extension and so measures such as QALYs, which conflate the two, may not be sufficiently nuanced to elicit the public views.

Qualitative studies suggest there is not a single public view of rescue, rather views are quite heterogeneous (McHugh et al. 2015; Wouters et al. 2017; Gyrd-Hansen 2018; McHugh et al. 2018). McHugh and colleagues, for example, identified three distinct clusters of views:

- population perspective: value for money, no special cases;
- life is precious: valuing life extension and patient choice; and
- valuing wider benefits and opportunity cost: the quality of life and death (McHugh et al. 2018, 67).

About half the respondents in this study adopted the second viewpoint, essentially endorsing the legitimacy of a Rule of Rescue premium, with just over one third adopting the first viewpoint, which would preclude such a premium, and about 10 per cent the third viewpoint. This diversity should not be a surprise – especially when discussing end-of-life interventions – and highlights a common weakness in preference-elicitation studies, which aggregate the heterogeneous views into a single aggregate measure (Baker et al. 2021).

Despite this equivocal public support for an end-of-life premium, and, indeed a weak ethical justification for one (Cookson 2013), the United Kingdom's National Institute of Health and Care Excellence has accepted an 'end-of-life' premium for more than a decade (McCabe et al. 2016), albeit 'not always consistently conducted or transparently reported' (Bovenberg, Penton, and Buyukkaramikli 2021, 697). *Prima facie*, this divergence between public views and policy guidance 'challenges' the current policy of an end-of-life premium (McHugh et al. 2020, 8), but it might equally be a methodological challenge – that the views expressed in the abstract in the context of discrete choice experiments or other methods of eliciting the public's views (de Bekker-Grob, Ryan, and Gerard 2012; Soekhai et al. 2019; Bahrampour et al. 2020) may not survive the first encounter with actual identifiable, rather than hypothetical, statistical, lives.

I will return again to the issue of the public's views about an end-of-life premium in Chapter 5 where I discuss the tension between compassion and stewardship.

Valuation of QALYs

The starting point for the valuation of lives in QALYs is supposed to be 'person neutral': an assumption of 'QALY egalitarianism' (Culyer 1991) or 'distributive neutrality' that

> the healthcare system should aim at maximising health benefits with the resources that are available, irrespective of how these benefits are distributed across people. (Nord 1999, 23)

Implicit in the use of QALYs are two disturbing assumptions. Firstly, there may be an implicit age bias. Interventions that target older people will naturally have a lower potential for life-years to be gained than interventions that target younger people. Secondly, social justice and equity in the distribution of benefits is almost universally ignored.

The Age Bias

Some measurement approaches cap expected life-years gained at age 70 (Brenner 2017; Taksler and Rothberg 2017), the most notable example being the original measure of 'Potential Years of Life Lost' used for international comparisons of health systems, such as those using data from the OECD health data repository.

The concept of Potential Years of Life Lost stems from a Canadian paper, which proposed it as a method of priority setting in that country. Although a life expectancy of 70 has a biblical resonance (Psalms 90:10), the authors had a more pragmatic justification:

> In choosing a cut-off age above 70 one should consider that the determination of the underlying cause of death becomes difficult, particularly for very old people. On the other hand age 65, proposed by several authors, appears rather young, since a great proportion of people are still productive at this age. (Romeder and McWhinnie 1977, 147)

At the time the paper was written Canadian life expectancy was around 74, but it is now around 82 suggesting that if a single age threshold is to be used it should be revisited, perhaps to 80.

More recent estimates of potential years of life lost use a dynamic life table approach where, rather than a single life expectancy, years of life lost is calculated based on life expectancy for the relevant age group so a death of a person aged 95 would accrue 3.6 years of potential years of life lost derived from the relevant life table (GBD 2016 Causes of Death Collaborators 2017, Appendix Table 18).

The implicit age bias has been justified in terms of the 'fair innings' argument: 'the feeling that everyone is entitled to some 'normal' span of health, usually expressed in terms of life-years, for example, 'three score years and ten' (Williams (1997b, 119); see also Culyer and Maynard (1997, Chapter 21). This 'fair innings' argument is expressed in terms of living a 'fair share' of life, which may have little to do with a 'fair share' of health resources, and risks introducing an explicit bias of denying resources to older people inappropriately, when they could benefit (Hazra, Gulliford, and Rudisill 2017, 213–214). However, as we saw in the discussion of the Rule of Rescue, public opinion seems to accept that there are limits to life, and to the extent there is a case for *additional* weightings for interventions at the end of life, they are very modest. A systematic review that examined studies of public opinion about the appropriateness of age weightings (as part of a wider review), concluded that if anything (and there are methodological difficulties, notably the conflation of age and proximity to death), the direction of opinion is that investments in younger people should be weighted more favourably than investments in older people (Gu et al. 2015).

Equity

Economic evaluation does not set out to be equitable: it is about efficiency – it asks which alternative is better, but it does not 'encourage us to divide the alternatives into two distinct classes, those that involve serious ethical wrongdoing and those that do not' (Nussbaum 2000, 1032). The general position adopted in economics is that issues of equity – and the creation of inequity could certainly be a 'serious wrongdoing' in Nussbaum's language – and the distribution of benefits should not enter the economic evaluation calculus, but rather equity should be dealt with through income redistribution policies (Zajac 2001, Chapter 7). As the pursuit of equity in healthcare is often seen as being a separate objective, it is no surprise that systematic reviews of economic evaluations show distributional issues completely neglected (Sassi, Archard, and Le Grand 2001).

The reason for this neglect is perversely 'QALY egalitarianism', that economic evaluation does not

> commit us to the equal distribution of healthcare resources. On the contrary, the QALY method requires us to put resources where they will produce the most QALYs for each dollar of the health budget – and this might mean that some individuals and groups will get more resources than others, and some individuals and groups may get none. The QALY approach is egalitarian in the sense that, if all else is equal, a QALY gain to one person is of the same value as a QALY gain to anyone else, not in the sense that it advocates the equal distribution of resources regardless of benefit. (McKie et al. 1998, 41)

So, it is no surprise that

> The neglect of equity concerns is ubiquitous across all economic evaluations in the health sector, in both clinical medicine and public health. (Cookson, Drummond, and Weatherly 2009, 232)

The result of regarding equity as a separate objective is that economic evaluations ignore equity, contrary to the views of the public: the public is 'inequality averse' (Costa-Font and Cowell 2019) and, consequentially, there is public support for some form of consideration of equity. The value of health improvement in low socio-economic status groups was often seen by respondents as an order of magnitude greater than an incremental improvement in higher socio-economic status groups (Lal, Moodie et al. 2018; Lal, Siahpush et al. 2018). However, equity preference may be contingent on how equitable allocation of care occurs (Ubel 2000). Although health economists recognise the importance of equity, and advocate for its inclusion in considerations of healthcare priority setting (Kahneman, Knetsch, and Thaler 1986; Fuchs 1998; Cohen and Ubel 2001; Dolan and Olsen 2002; Danis and Patrick 2002; Dukhanin et al. 2018), this recognition and advocacy has not translated into policy action.

In their study of decision-making criteria, Guindo et al. (2012, 9) reported that 'equity and fairness' was the most frequently reported, but that it 'is difficult to operationalize in decision-making and priority-setting processes in a pragmatic manner'. Ghijben et al. (2018), following a systematic review, concluded that decision-makers espoused use of equity in health technology assessment (stated preference studies), but this was not followed through into decision-making (revealed preference studies). 'Frameworks' that include equity as one of a number of criteria, but do not precisely define how it should be included in priority setting, effectively relegate it to being an afterthought or footnote (Krahn et al. 2018).

Proposals for inclusion of equity considerations have been around for some time, ranging from formally drawing decision-makers' attention to equity impacts of options to equity-weighting of benefits (Evans and Brown 2003; Cookson, Drummond, and Weatherly 2009; Love-Koh et al. 2019; Avanceña and Prosser 2021;). Decision-making bodies, such as the United Kingdom's National Institute for Health and Care Excellence (NICE), have been 'extremely reluctant' to incorporate equity into their decisions explicitly, but appear to have incorporated equity considerations implicitly (Shah et al. 2012). Importantly, the most recent checklist for publication of economic evaluations recommends that study results show 'how impacts are distributed across different individuals or adjustments made to reflect priority populations' (Husereau et al. 2022), and this may make result in these implicit approaches becoming more explicit in the future.

Asaria, Griffin, and Cookson (2015) demonstrate the use of distributional cost-effectiveness analysis in a comparison of reminder strategies for bowel cancer screening. Although a universal reminder may be better on a simple cost-effectiveness criterion, a targeted strategy yields a more equitable, but still cost-effective, outcome, thus highlighting the importance of considering 'inequality aversion' in priority setting.

The public's preference is reinforced by the Christian emphasis on social justice, which suggests that resource allocation and stewardship informed by a Christian ethic would incorporate equity weighting into decision-making, transforming the decision criterion from simply maximising efficiency to maximising equity-weighted benefit (Cookson, Culyer, and Norheim 2020), an issue discussed in more detail in Chapter 5.

Economic Evaluation as a 'Reasonable' Process

Its use as part of decisions about what is to be funded from the public purse enshrines economic evaluation as part of the democratic process (Broome 2000; Schneider 2021), and thus rests on a social licence: ethicist Norman Daniels and his colleagues have argued that any system of rationing – which the application of economic evaluation that I have described here is – needs to meet certain ethical criteria (Daniels, Light, and Caplan 1996; Daniels and Sabin 1997). Their framework, known as accountability for reasonableness, requires transparency of the decision-making process, that decisions are based on relevant criteria, and those decisions are revised in the light of new evidence.

As I have shown above there are controversies within health economics about how to deal with particular situations including when and whether the Rule of Rescue should apply, and whether equity weightings should be used. Application of the accountability for reasonableness framework suggests that there should be transparency of these choices (Butler 1999, 108–114) and these decisions should not be shrouded behind a veil of apparently ethically neutral technocratic choices.

The implications of different value-assumptions should be highlighted as part of sensitivity analyses in economic evaluations (Luyten and van Hoek 2021), but structural reform of decision-making processes may be needed too. The principal health technology assessment agency in the United Kingdom – the National Institute for Health and Care Excellence (NICE) – has opened up its processes and implicit choices through a structured form of community participation (Shah et al. 2012) and greater public engagement and public deliberative processes have also been proposed in Canada (Bentley et al. 2019). Implementation of more structured public involvement in decisions about medication subsidies in Canada highlighted the challenge of incorporating different perceptions of legitimacy: 'scientific legitimacy' – that is, the traditional, mechanistic application of economic evaluation – and 'democratic legitimacy', which involves structured ways of listening to patient and public voices and experiences (Boothe 2021).

Engaging with the consumer voice is a distinct phase of the decision-making process (Kleinhout-Vliek, de Bont, and Boer 2021). Mere structural change – such as adding a token consumer to committees – will not shift the way listing, prioritising, or rationing decisions are made, nor will any change shift thinking overnight. But strengthening public engagement in decision-making needs to be a necessary element for use of economic evaluation, although it alone will not address all the shortcomings of the black box of economic evaluation in practice.

The criterion in the accountability for reasonableness framework relating to review highlights the importance of disinvestment decisions (Garner and Littlejohns 2011; Haas et al. 2012; Airoldi 2013; Day, Norman, and Suzanne 2016; Hofmann 2020, 2021). The health sector does this poorly, partly because of policy inertia and cognitive and affective biases, partly because of pressure from interest groups and providers who benefit from the contemporary approval, and partly because the evidence standard to remove a subsidy – often that there is no benefit – is higher than the standard to add a subsidy, which is often simply that there is an incremental benefit that is greater than the incremental cost.

Biblical Views of Scarcity

Much biblical teaching is about how *individuals* should live their lives, including in terms of their economic relations (Barrera 2013). However, *general* principles of resource allocation and economic ethics at the societal level can be discerned from the Scriptures. A Christian ethic of healthcare resource allocation has the same starting point as economics – scarcity. Robbins recognised this in his *Essay*, alluding to the Garden of Eden story as the initiation of scarcity:

> We have been turned out of Paradise. We have neither eternal life nor unlimited means of gratification. (Robbins 1932, 15)

God created a world of abundance; however, outside the Garden of Eden that abundance is conditional (Barrera 2005, 26–27) and scarcity has become a reality. Cooper-White (2009) contrasts theologies of prosperity, often preached by Pentecostal churches (Maddox 2013), scarcity, and abundance. But for Cooper-White, a theology of abundance is still one where

> Every individual and each faithful community that embodies a theology of abundance will refuse to place themselves in a competitive posture against others to garner scarce resources; rather they will seek opportunities for collaboration and cooperation on all sides. (Cooper-White 2009, 204)

A theology of abundance involves responsible stewardship, recognising the earth's limits and cycles of growth and decay. Jesus' promise in John 10:10, 'I came that they may have life, and have it abundantly', is not a justification to eschew any attempt to manage the earth's limits, but rather a promise one will have an abundant joy in life (Miller 2012; Deane-Drummond and Rossing 2013; Hrynkow 2017). A theology of abundance can in contemporary reality only be a theology of partial or conditional abundance, one which recognises the brokenness of the world outside the Garden of Eden, which means needs cannot always be met, and that stewards must care for available resources.

Demands for healthcare are not infinite (Frankel 1991), but, as argued earlier in this chapter, extra spending on healthcare – whether by governments or individuals – has the potential to squeeze out expenditure on other worthy goals. This forces consideration of stewardship of health spending.

Scarcity in the Hebrew Scriptures

Gordon (1989) traces biblical conceptions of the scarcity problem and its solutions across both the Hebrew Scriptures and the New Testament. The five approaches to 'solving' scarcity he identified in the Hebrew Scriptures are

- the *Solution by Faith*. Abram is directed by God to leave 'his father's house' to go to another land where he will be blest (Genesis 12:1–4);
- the *Solution by Wisdom*. Jacob becomes wealthy through skill and guile (Genesis 30:32–42). A second example is the more problematic one of Joseph who uses foresight in the face of famine first to buy, on behalf of the Pharaoh, all the grain in Egypt, then all the livestock (in exchange for grain), and then all the land (in exchange for livestock). Joseph thus acquires all the land of Egypt for the Pharaoh, but it is returned for use to the people, only now with a 20 per cent tax;
- the *Solution by Observance*. Following settlement in Canaan, new codes of law were established, which governed relationships, including economic relationships. Gordon (1989:12–13) summarises the Solution by Observance as based on

  > the promise that the community or the individual adhering to its statutes will not know deprivation … If the conquerors of Canaan obey the law, they will experience population growth, capital expansion, favourable seasons, abundant output, political security, and international domination. On the other hand, failure to keep the law will result in economic disaster, plague, political subservience and slavery to foreigners. (Deuteronomy: 28:1–46)

- the *Solution by Mediation*. This was developed in the context of the Babylonian exile: Israel will flourish if its people take on the role of mediator between YHWH and other nations; and
- the *Apocalyptic 'Solution'*. Gordon's fifth solution from the Hebrew Scriptures is that scarcity ends in the context of the end times.

These 'solutions' are of two kinds: Firstly, consistent with much other teaching in the Hebrew Scriptures, is the idea that faith and reliance on YHWH is what Israel must do. The solutions by faith, observance, and mediation, and the Apocalyptic Solution are all variants of this. Although YHWH had promised a land flowing with milk and honey, the avoidance of scarcity was clearly 'conditional and not absolute' (Barrera 2007, 82): it relied on being faithful to the Covenantal relationship.

Secondly, there are practical guidance and lessons. Here the Solution by Wisdom has two examples: one of skill and guile (Jacob) and one of foresight (Joseph). In the first case, the problem of scarcity is shifted from Jacob to his uncle, Laban, by Jacob's cunning. In the other, foresight is used to smooth out the problem of scarcity over time.

Unfortunately, none of the 'solutions' proposed in the Hebrew Scriptures to scarcity really address how to make competing judgements about alternative uses – the scarcity problem.

Matthean Approach to Scarcity and Resource Allocation

Gordon (1989, Chapter V) labels the New Testament solution to scarcity the *Solution by Seeking the Kingdom*. Here he cites the Sermon on the Mount as the main formulation:

> Therefore do not worry, saying, 'What will we eat?' or 'What will we drink?' or 'What will we wear?' For it is the Gentiles who strive for all these things; and indeed your heavenly Father knows that you need all these things. But strive first for the kingdom of God and his righteousness, and all these things will be given to you as well.
>
> So do not worry about tomorrow, for tomorrow will bring worries of its own. Today's trouble is enough for today. (Matthew 6:31–34)

Jesus' response to the problem of scarcity – what people will eat, drink, and wear – is somewhat enigmatic, deferring those scarcity issues as being second order to seeking the Kingdom of God, and seeking God's righteousness. The Sermon on the Mount is thus simply a starting point for exploring what a Christian theology of scarcity might look like.

The Matthean formulation has many similarities to the Solution by Faith, albeit rephrased into Matthean Kingdom of God discourse. The clue in the Sermon on the Mount involves discerning the relevance of Seeking the Kingdom of God and God's righteousness. Disentangling what this might mean in practice for economic resource allocation decisions is helped by updating the androcentric, geography-based (Sölle 1990, 139; Wenell 2017) 'Kingdom' language of Matthew, to a reference to the Realm of God, or better, the Rule of God or God's ruling style (Crossan 2012, 119). This helps, but it is clear that adhering to the rule of God involves 'a mixed array of precepts and counsels' (Barrera 2007, 88).

Righteousness is a specific and distinct concern of the writer of Matthew, especially in the Sermon on the Mount: the term righteousness occurs seven times in Matthew, more frequently than in any other part of the New Testament (Hagner 1998; Viljoen 2013). However, the Realm of God should not be seen as a separate concept from seeking God's righteousness. They are synonyms: the rule (Kingdom) of God occurs if and only if God's righteousness abounds and is lived. Jesus did not invent the concept of God's righteousness, it comes with a long tradition in the Hebrew Scriptures and teachings (Weinfeld 1995), generally coupled with justice (e.g. Jeremiah 22:3; Amos 5:24), and Matthew was probably drawing on this tradition to invoke this older concept of 'ethical righteousness' (Hagner 1998, 367).

Earlier in the Sermon on the Mount, the Matthean Jesus cites approvingly 'those who hunger and thirst for righteousness' (Matthew 5:6). Describing a hunger for righteousness is strong language, but adding thirst provides a further emphasis, given the importance of water in the lands of Israel historically (Kugel 2008, 236), an importance that continues as a source of conflict (Zeitoun 2008; Brooks, Trottier, and Giordano 2020).

The Matthean version of the Beatitudes contrasts with the Lukan version (Luke 6:21a) by its spiritualised language (Bowe 2017, 155). Luke, who probably knew Matthew's account (Goodacre 2001; Malan 2014), stripped away the concepts of righteousness as what is sought, and thirst, sharpening the injunction to focus on justice and poverty (Mealand 1980). Ireland (1992, 195) attempts to re-spiritualise Luke, suggesting that 'all the material on riches and poverty in Luke-Acts is religious. What matters most is one's attitude toward God'. Although I don't agree with Ireland's thesis, his conclusion that 'How one uses material possessions is indicative of one's ultimate loyalties' (Ireland 1992, 217) is consistent with the theology of stewardship that I am advancing here.

Righteousness in Matthew 5:6 and especially later in Matthew 6:33, where it is coupled with the rule of God, can best be interpreted as being about the 'desire and aim to live in accordance with the will of God' (Viljoen 2013, 5). Seeking God's righteousness, then, is a summary for adhering to all of Jesus' other teachings, including about justice, care, and compassion; the link to the pursuit of justice is made explicit in the Douay-Rheims translation of Matthew 5:6 as 'Blessed are they that hunger and thirst after justice: for they shall have their fill'.

Righteousness, especially as seen in the Sermon on the Mount, is about communal identity and communal values: it is a social value that refers to communities and relationships (Viljoen 2013). It is thus about how relationships to community should be lived. Jesus' concern for justice and seeking God's righteousness provides an emphasis on community and inclusion. It can reasonably be considered to encompass a concern for the common wealth and stewardship.

Gordon (1989) cites the Sermon on the Mount as the principal New Testament source on the question of scarcity and characterises the solution as directing us to seeking the rule of God and God's righteousness. An alternative reading, especially of verse 34, is a rejection of the very concept of scarcity – Jesus enjoining the listeners to the Sermon on the Mount not to worry about scarcity tomorrow, for tomorrow will worry about its own things: 'Let the day's own trouble be sufficient for the day' (Revised Standard Version).

The implication here is that if one seeks, or works towards achieving, God's righteousness, then one's needs for food, drink, and clothing will be provided, both now and into the future. However, this will only be possible if under the rule of God resources are available, distributed fairly, and managed appropriately. 'Seeking God's righteousness' therefore requires us to live according to a Christian ethic of resource allocation. That is, living or seeking the rule of God and God's righteousness involves appropriate stewardship of God's resources.

In the first creation story (in terms of ordering in the Torah) the 'ādām was given responsibility to be the guardian of earth's resources, translated in the King James Version as being given dominion over other living creatures (Genesis 1:28). More recent exegesis invokes the concept of stewardship (Harrison 1999; Bergant 2013; Francis 2015), an interpretation more consistent with the language in the second creation story of the 'ādām being placed in 'the garden of Eden to till it and tend it' (Genesis 2:15; Jewish Study Bible translation).

Oikonomia: What Is Stewardship?

The Greek word for steward commonly used in the New Testament is *oikonomos*, often transliterated as 'household manager' (Oosthuizen and Lategan 2015), and is also the root of the word economics; Aland et al. (1994, 124) translate the Greek as steward, manager, treasurer (of a city), or trustee. The related word *oikonomia* refers to stewardship, although perhaps 'a stewardship' may be a better translation of the concept. The Greek may be translated as 'management of a household, task, work, responsibility, and (divine) plan' (Aland et al. 1994, 124).

There appears to be a distinction in biblical usage of the terms *oikonomos* and *oikonomia* (see Table 4.1).

Oikonomos appears to be used neutrally and can refer to good and bad stewards: good in Luke 12, 1 Corinthians 4, and Titus; bad in Luke 16; neutral in Romans and Galatians. *Oikonomia,* on the other hand, is only used frequently in the Pauline corpus with a positive, often spiritual overlay (1 Corinthians 9, Ephesians, Colossians, 1 Timothy). Paul also tends to describe his role as involving a stewardship (Story 1976). The biblical view of stewardship is therefore

> grounded in the nature of God as creator and redeemer, as protector of the oppressed, and as just administrator of creation itself. (Foster 1995, 15)

The etymology of *oikonomia* and its connotations at the time Jesus have important differences from how we think of economics today.

Leshem (2016, 231) cites a first century BCE source to describe rational management or *oikonomia:*

> the one who conducts himself in this rational manner, with fruits and profits of it shall be used for his earnings and enough for the prosperity of his body and food for those in his household, and he should leave some on top of this to help his relatives and acquaintances. And a small measure of it to women and the poor people of his polis and he should save some so as to be helped in dire times and it is worthy of him not to ask for more than this and he asked more than this he is subjected to a bad thing.

So in that time, rational management is seen not only to be about the household, but also about ensuring a small surplus for distribution to the poor and about not consuming to excess (Gotsis and Merianos 2012). In contrast to Robbins (1932), who saw economics as not being about values and ethics, at the time Jesus was speaking, and as the New Testament was being written, *oikonomia* (and stewardship) were inherently and inextricably linked with meaning, purpose, and values. Singer (1958, 42) suggests the suffix, nomos, had a connotation of 'to care for (the flock), to apportion, to allocate and to provide for'. This again points to a value-based use of the term.

By 300–100 BCE, *oikonomia* was generally used in the context of what we might call estate management rather than household management, and the same principles were seen to apply to administration of a nation as to a household (Reumann 1957, 207, 501–507). In this same period *oikonomia* began to take on a wider meaning about rational management including management in politics and medicine (Reumann 1957, 320; Leshem 2016, 228).

Table 4.1 *Use of* oikonomos *and* oikonomia *in the New Testament*

Verses	New Revised Standard Version translation
Luke 12:42	And the Lord said, 'Who then is the faithful and prudent manager (οἰκονόμος) whom his master will put in charge of his slaves, to give them their allowance of food at the proper time?'
Luke 16:1–4	1 Then Jesus said to the disciples, 'There was a rich man who had a manager (οἰκονόμον), and charges were brought to him that this man was squandering his property. 2 So he summoned him and said to him, "What is this that I hear about you? Give me an accounting of your management (οἰκονομίας), because you cannot be my manager (you are unable to manage οἰκονομεῖν) any longer." 3 Then the manager (οἰκονόμος) said to himself, "What will I do, now that my master is taking the position (the management οἰκονομίαν) away from me? I am not strong enough to dig, and I am ashamed to beg. 4 I have decided what to do so that, when I am dismissed as manager (οἰκονομίας), people may welcome me into their homes."'
Luke 16:8	And his master commended the dishonest manager (οἰκονόμον) because he had acted shrewdly; for the children of this age are more shrewd in dealing with their own generation than are the children of light.
Romans 16:23	Gaius, who is host to me and to the whole church, greets you. Erastus, the city treasurer (οἰκονόμος), and our brother Quartus, greet you.
1 Corinthians 4:1–2	[1]Think of us in this way, as servants of Christ and stewards (οἰκονόμους) of God's mysteries. [2] Moreover, it is required of stewards (οἰκονόμοις) that they be found trustworthy
1 Corinthians 9:17	For if I do this of my own will, I have a reward; but if not of my own will, I am entrusted with a commission (οἰκονομίαν)
Galatians 4:2	but they remain under guardians and trustees (οἰκονόμους) until the date set by the father.
Ephesians 1:10	as a plan (οἰκονομίαν) for the fullness of time, to gather up all things in him, things in heaven and things on earth
Ephesians 3:2	for surely you have already heard of the commission (οἰκονομίαν) of God's grace that was given me for you,
Ephesians 3:9	and to make everyone see what is the plan (οἰκονομία) of the mystery hidden for ages in God who created all things;
Colossians 1:25	I became its servant according to God's commission (οἰκονομίαν) that was given to me for you, to make the word of God fully known
1 Timothy 1:4	and not to occupy themselves with myths and endless genealogies that promote speculations rather than the divine training (οἰκονομίαν) that is known by faith.
Titus 1:7	For a bishop, as God's steward (οἰκονόμον), must be blameless; he must not be arrogant or quick-tempered or addicted to wine or violent or greedy for gain
1 Peter 4:10	Like good stewards (οἰκονόμοι) of the manifold grace of God, serve one another with whatever gift each of you has received.

Rational management was integral to the life of both the head of a household and by inference, the head's agent:

> In the writings of the ancient Greeks, the life of the head of household – the *oikodesptes* (*sic*, should be *oikodespotēs*) – … was conducted in three dimensions: the spiritual realm of philosophy, the heroic realm of politics, and the economic realm. The role of the economic dimension was to secure the means necessary for existence and to generate a surplus that sustained the two other dimensions that were deemed worthy of man. This could be done in two ways: either by increasing production or by moderating consumption. (Leshem 2016, 229)

Oikonomia thus contemplated at its essence both appropriate management of resources and that the purpose of rational management was to support broader goals, with the connotation that it is about the 'flourishing of the community' (Francis 1993, 136). This intertwining of *oikonomia*, and stewards as delegate for the *oikodespotēs*, and the purpose for which rational management takes place, occurs in a number of texts. Foster (1995, 15) refers to this 'spiritual vein' of *oikonomos* as occurring in 1 Corinthian 4:1; 1 Peter 4:10; and Titus 1:7. Oosthuizen and Lategan (2015, 556) use the same examples to refer to the '*practical* as well as *spiritual meaning*' of *oikonomia* (emphasis in original). Hays goes further in drawing attention to the broader ethical concept of stewardship rather than a wealth accumulation or wealth preservation role: 'Luke always refers to stewards in their capacities as giving away the goods of the Master (whether licitly or not)' (Hays 2012, 50).

Three Parables on Stewardship

Stewards and how stewardship ought to be exercised are highlighted in two parables: the parable of the watchful steward and the parable of the unjust steward. A third parable, of the talents, also has some stewardship connotations. As with all the parables, they are enigmatic and need to be interpreted carefully.

The Watchful Steward, the Overseer, or the Faithful and Unfaithful Stewards (Luke 12:35–48; Matthew 24:45–51)

This parable, the least enigmatic of the three, is about preparedness. It is one of a group of 'servant parables' that 'concern a master-servant relationship and a time or moment of reckoning' (Crossan 1992, 94). In this parable the expected outcome occurs. The bulk of the story is the forewarning that one must be prepared – living God's righteousness – at all times, not just, for example, on Sundays. The complexity comes in the last few verses about differential punishment for those who know what is expected and do not deliver compared to those who don't know and also don't deliver. The Matthean version is perhaps clearer: Blessed is that slave whom his master will find at work when he arrives (Matthew 24:46).

Although often interpreted in eschatological terms, the parable should also be interpreted in the context of Luke's wealth ethics, consistent with the value-base inherent in Luke's teachings:

> the imagery and language of the Parable of the Unfaithful Stewards is typical of the rhetoric of Lukan wealth ethics, and indeed, coheres with and complements Luke's teachings on possessions elsewhere in the Gospel. Thus, this parable encourages the ethical disbursal of money: wealth is to be used to meet the needs of those unable to provide for themselves (perhaps even for their daily needs), and not to be squandered on selfish indulgence and excess. (Hays 2012, 52)

A further message here is that stewardship is ongoing and requires continuous attention; it is not a 'set and forget' exercise. As argued earlier, economic evaluation is an ongoing task and as new technologies are developed, they need evaluation.

The Unjust Steward or the Shrewd Manager (Luke 16:1–15)

This is another one of the servant parables or 'parables of reckoning' (Crossan 1992, 114), with the parable ending at verse 7, 8, or 9 (Crossan 1992, 106), with explanatory teaching after that. In this parable, the expectation of the reckoning is reversed. This reversal is probably what led to it being described as 'notoriously one of the most difficult parables to interpret' (Morris 2008, 262), a view also shared by Goodrich (2012).

It is no surprise then that interpretations of this are quite mixed and include claims that the steward is buying favour from those who owe money by reducing the steward's own commission (Soards 2010, 1860). In this interpretation, the steward is doing nothing dishonest and in fact, is being prudent about preparing for his own future and hence wins commendation from the master. This interpretation has been challenged, though, as the steward's commission may have been a fabrication to get around contemporary laws against lending money at interest (Morris 2008, 263; Wright 2014, 193), a matter that will be discussed in the context of the parable of the talents.

Crossan (2012) identifies this parable as a typical 'challenge parable', those that are meant to be debated, shock, and possibly even to mean the reverse of a simple reading (Crossan 2012, Chapter 6). In the brief rendition we have seen in Luke, we do not know how Jesus used the parable. Did he tell the story (verses 1–9) and then immediately continue with his interpretation and associated teaching (10–13)? Or did he pause and let the crowd debate and discuss the story?

But, however used, an important lesson here is the parable's emphasis on trustworthiness of stewards:

> The key to it all is in the opening verses: it's about faithfulness. Money is not in possession, it's a trust: God entrusts property to people and expects it to be used to his glory and the welfare of his children, not for private glory or clamour. (Wright 2014, 196)

Goodrich (2012) situates the parable in the context of voluntary debt remission – which conveyed reciprocal benefits on the debtor and the lender (Goodrich 2012, 565) – and suggests in that context the steward can be seen as acting fairly and faithfully. Dormandy (2002) proposes yet another focus of the parable. Rather than the parable being about the steward and his actions, Dormandy argues it is about the 'rich man', and indeed suggests that the parable should be called the parable of 'the rich man converted':

> ... within the Lukan context, which contains such an emphasis on what rich people should do with wealth, it is reasonable to infer that the rich man ends up by beginning to realise that his attitude to wealth must change: he is being converted to a more just lifestyle by the actions of his own 'wasteful' steward. (Dormandy 2002, 520)

A superficial reading gives a reversal of the expected outcome of the reckoning. Crossan's approach is to argue that this is to stimulate discussion. Dormandy, in contrast, suggests that the appropriate focus is on the rich man and his actions: he is the one that reversed his position and caused the difficulty with the typical interpretation. A common thread in all the interpretations is one of appropriate stewardship and use of resources.

The Talents (Luke 19:12–27; Matthew 25:14–30)

The parable of the talents is another parable of reckoning, with graded responses by the nobleman. The parable can be interpreted as teaching about using one's 'talents' and being rewarded for that. Morris (2008, 293) takes this view. It makes more sense in my view to see it as another 'challenge parable', which Jesus intends to be debated and discussed.

As with the parable of the unjust steward, the first century Jewish context is a strong tradition in the Hebrew Scriptures against lending money at interest (Gordon 1982). The only mention of 'interest' in the New Testament is in this parable. Crossan (2012) portrays the challenge:

> it is surely strange, then, to presume that the first two slaves are positive and the final one negative example – for a first century Jewish audience faithful to covenant and tradition. In other words is the audience being provoked to agree or disagree with the master's actions? To agree or disagree with which slaves' actions? And thereby to think for or against the multiplication of money known as interest?. I suggest therefore that, on the immediate level, the intention of Jesus was to create audience debate between the Roman pro-interest tradition within the Empire and the Jewish anti-interest tradition within the Torah. (Crossan 2012, 104–105)

If it is accepted as a challenge parable, it provides a springboard for discussion about the extent to which people should stand with 'the needy or the greedy' (Crossan 2012, 106). In the context of teaching about stewardship, it forces reflection about whether investment decisions are consistent with seeking God's righteousness, and what the ethical purpose of these investments is.

The Parables Overall

The overall flavour of these parables is the value-basis of stewardship: the linking of stewardship and the appropriate use of resources. These parables force us firstly to recognise that a stewardship involves being attentive and 'watchful'. Secondly, investment choices involve ethical choices and there will be a reckoning of the choices that have been made. The parables are all consistent with my main argument, that value choices are critical, and that the role of stewardship is to be one of rational management of resources, and to be fair in that process.

Stewardship Is a Fundamental Principle for a Christian Ethic of Healthcare Funding

At the time the Bible was being written, the future was seen as being in God's hands with little thought to shaping the future in any management or policy sense (Bernstein 1996, 19), statistical analysis was hampered by use of Roman numerals, and there was thus no economic calculus of what good stewardship of the future would look like.

Moreover, stewardship and *oikonomia* as used at the time of the New Testament writers were not value neutral terms:

> The ancient Greeks saw economic behaviour as rational when it was frugal in its use of means towards what they deemed as worthwhile ends. (Leshem 2016, 232)

These same themes are evident in the Pauline epistles, which preach economic self-sufficiency and that when a surplus exists, it should be distributed to the poor (Gotsis and Dodd 2002), and in the early Christian leaders such as Clement who also preached self-sufficiency (Finn 2013, 77). Stewards had the responsibility of effecting this and so stewardship was about rational management which had two distinct elements:

- being prudent in the use of resources, eschewing greed and over consumption; and
- being concerned about social justice and those, outside the immediate household, who were in need.

The second of these elements links to the discussion of social justice in the previous chapter and will not be discussed here. The other element can provide the basis for a Christian ethic of resource allocation, based on responsible stewardship. Importantly, harking back to the Sermons on the Plain and on the Mount, proper stewardship today, and pursuing the rule of God today, not only is concerned with scarcity and ensuring adequacy of resources today, but it also helps to ensure that resources are available for tomorrow. In that sense it provides for intergenerational equity – that any funding decisions made today are cognisant of the needs of tomorrow and a prudent use of today's resources in the context of future needs, and so consider a 'time margin' as well as a resource margin (Gustafson 1977).

The three parables discussed above provide further context for a stewardship of prudence: the parables of the watchful steward and the talents direct us to the ethical distribution of money; and the parable of the unjust steward again points to faithfulness in managing resources. Stewards are to be judged on the management of resources, both in the short and in the long term.

What Is Prudence and Avoidance of Over-Consumption?

Although the possibility that extra treatment may not be valuable has been around since the time of Hippocrates (Reiser 1980; Jecker 1991; Kerridge, Mitchell, and McPhee 1996), it has been brought into starker focus in the last quarter of the twentieth century with technological advances in healthcare. With increased life expectancy, more interventions are legitimately being undertaken on older people, leading to the so-called bio-medicalisation of ageing (Kaufman, Shim, and Russ 2004). Intensive care units apparently perform miracles daily where people who in earlier decades might have died survive. The contribution of healthcare as a driver for the increase in life expectancy changed over the last century but was never the overwhelming cause of the increase in life expectancy (Kaplan and Milstein 2019; Buxbaum et al. 2020). More tellingly, in recent decades overall improved survival benefits of newly approved drugs in Europe is generally modest (Davis et al. 2017) and the cost of each increment in average life expectancy is increasing (Catillon, Cutler, and Getzen 2018), both suggesting high-income nations are clearly in an era of flat of the curve medicine.

The drivers of the increase in life expectancy include public health interventions, and improvements in the living standards. So, prudence in healthcare funding means that healthcare decision-makers must recognise that the improvement of the population's health status may come from policy action outside the health sector, such as addressing the social determinants of health including improving education and employment, and so healthcare spending decisions need to be weighed against these alternative choices.

There is a long tradition of Christian social thought, which advocates prudence in consumption and sharing 'superfluous income' for the benefit of others (Barrera 2007, 106; 2011, 159). Much New Testament teaching suggests that there are dangers in the love of money and that 'the road to salvation would be eased for [rich] people if they gave away all their riches' (Dodd and Gotsis 2000, 28). Our relationship with God can be evaluated in terms of 'how well one treats one's neighbour' (Barrera 2007, 158), as Matthew 25:45 makes clear. Lukan teaching also shows that 'to dissipate wealth is to sin against God' (Kim 1993, 248).

Prudence in consumption might also be traced back to the Decalogue, where the Tenth Commandment injunction against coveting other's property (and family) is part of the set of injunctions about dealing with others generally. Unlike the other Commandments which are about words and deeds, the injunction against coveting is much stronger, about thoughts (Baker 2005).

The Tenth Commandment can also be clearly traced into the New Testament (Kanagaraj 2001). The Tenth Commandment implicitly condemns greed, where one covets resources (and people) that are not one's own. In the context of healthcare resource allocation, this message might also be about condemning overconsumption, pursuing unnecessary healthcare consumption, and seeking to spend more on healthcare than the economy can sustain. Prudence in consumption and the theology of limits is an accepted part of Roman Catholic moral theology where it plays out in debates about ordinary versus extraordinary and proportionate versus disproportionate care (McCartney 1980; Engelhardt Jr 2002, 6; Taboada 2002; Kelly 2019).

Economic concepts can legitimately inform a Christian ethic of prudence in consumption. Specifically, overconsumption occurs when there is limited value from the consumption of an additional unit. This can be translated back to economic evaluation language as when the marginal or incremental benefit of consumption is less than the marginal or incremental cost. But how might a Christian approach to the use of economic evaluation address the weaknesses in cost-effectiveness identified earlier (statistical lives, age bias, and ignoring equity)? And is discounting lives consistent with other Christian teaching?

Any Christian ethic of resource allocation must start with recognition of the limits of the earth's resources, and that the reality of scarcity, choice, and opportunity cost is confronted because of a broken post-Eden world. There is now an extensive theological literature on resource limits (Gustafson 1977; Scharper 1998, Chapters 14–16; Horrell 2015; Pedersen 2015; Williams 2015), which draws us to consider not only how we live our comfortable lives in high-income countries, but also our need to consider how our resource consumption impacts on countries not so fortunate as our own. Our neighbour, as the Samaritan story teaches us, may come from, and reside in, a place further from our comfort zone than we thought possible (Levine 2015).

Some have argued that if only we were to be wiser in our use of healthcare resources, we would be easily able to meet all needs (Brook and Lohr 1986, 1991; Weil 1989; Ayres 1992). There are two elements to this claim: firstly, the current use of resources is allocatively inefficient, in that we are not getting the best outcomes for given inputs, and secondly, there is substantial technical inefficiency within the health system.

The allocative inefficiency argument is that vast resources are committed to clinically ineffective treatments and eliminating them would solve the problem of scarcity: as Brook and Lohr (1986) succinctly summarised the issue in the title of their paper 'Will we need to ration effective healthcare?'. These arguments are mostly made by authors from the United States, the country that spends almost twice as much per head or as a share of gross domestic product as any other country (Papanicolas, Woskie, and Jha 2018). The United States' level of excess may be unique, and there is certainly evidence of quite different use of resources between, say, the United States and the United Kingdom in treatment of a number of conditions (Aaron and Schwartz 1982; Figueroa et al. 2021) and also within the United States (Wennberg, Freeman, and Culp 1987; Gawande 2009b).

There are three reasons why the 'only effective care' strategy will not obviate the need for priority setting.

Firstly, although 'effective care' is framed as clinically effective care, that is care for which there is a net benefit to the patient, the critical issue for resource allocation is whether these net benefits to patients are affordable. Many new drugs provide only limited benefits to patients (Davis et al. 2017; Vivot et al. 2017; Wieseler, McGauran, and Kaiser 2019; Rodwin et al. 2021), and yet some come at high cost. Tax funding is not unlimited and at the margin one will always have to make a trade-off about value. If taxes were higher, the funding threshold might relax, and drugs that cost $200,000 per QALY will be funded rather than limiting funding to those which cost less than $100,000 a year.

Secondly, there is little public support for increasing the threshold infinitely and so at any level of spending there will always be decisions to be made about whether additional spending is worthwhile. Even in countries such as Australia, with a much lower health spending than the United States, the same arguments about a high proportion of spending being wasteful are made. These often rely on United States data as justification without any check on the source data's veracity (Rosenbaum 2017), nor any modification for Australia's circumstances (Strategic review of health and medical research (Chair: Simon McKeon) 2013; Braithwaite, Glasziou, and Westbrook 2020), but the point they make is the same: some proportion of existing healthcare is wasteful and ineffective. The 'effective care' argument will only defer the issue of addressing choices and trade-offs, not avoid them. Pursuit of effective care should be a central part of policy but even such most aggressive policies will not mean that rationing can be totally avoided.

Thirdly, as healthcare technology advances, newer technologies will become available for introduction and their worth will need to be evaluated, at the very least to ensure that these new technologies are cost-effective. As pointed out earlier in this chapter, the opportunity costs of clinically ineffective care are certainly easy to observe where there is a hard budget cap, but also exist where there is a 'soft cap'.

Although some argue that the alternative to rationing is simply to argue for more spending (Rawles 1989), the reality is public and private finance is limited, and the only issue is where that limit occurs. Informed public debate is thus not about whether there is to be some form of rationing and limitation, but rather how that is to occur, whether limits apply to both private and public spending, and how tightly resources in the health sector are to be rationed, that is when is additional spending justifiable and when is it not?

The issue with technical inefficiency is somewhat similar. Certainly, improved technical efficiency ought to be a fundamental part of responsible stewardship, and technical efficiency ought to be the first strategy pursued in addressing scarcity, but eventually it is unlikely that technical efficiency strategies alone will obviate the need for some form of priority setting.

In summary, if we accept limits imposed by scarcity, then we must accept trade-offs and choices, and this requires some consideration of benefits and costs, albeit with some modification to address the weaknesses of the contemporary economistic approaches. A theology of limits suggests that a Christian ethic of healthcare funding must incorporate a principle of stewardship and prudence in the use of resources.

Stewardship and the Dignity of Humanity

One of the fundamental tenets of Christian faith is the dignity of humanity: that humans have been created in the image of God and so all life is to be valued. This raises the issue of to what extent is this belief consistent with ranking interventions?

Not all countries adopt a ranking approach: the United States rejects explicit rationing of public funding. Whether the anti-rationing position is causative or not, the United States spends about twice as much on its health system as other countries in the Anglosphere (Organisation for Economic Cooperation and Development 2019a). Despite the rhetoric, rationing in the United States is unfortunately built into the design of the system – the poor and people of colour have systematically worse access and outcomes (Dickman, Himmelstein, and Woolhandler 2017; Hero, Zaslavsky, and Blendon 2017). The excess spending is associated with terrible inequity in access – even after the Obama reforms – and very poor health outcomes overall, with poorer life expectancy than other comparable countries (Organisation for Economic Cooperation and Development 2019a). Certainly, the United States' experience is not one of prudence, and/or avoidance of overconsumption.

Although we must recognise that there are very clear risks to letting money be our main way of measuring value (Goodchild 2009; Welby 2017), priority setting in healthcare, or 'rationing' to use harsh language, involves comparisons of the value of investments in cancer compared to heart disease, and investments in prevention of cancers compared to treatment. This necessarily involves estimating the value of the benefits gained from these interventions, however measured. Because the investments are monetised, we end up putting a value, in monetary terms, for the benefits of the investments.

Philosopher Michael Sandel has challenged us to consider whether there are some decisions that should be excluded from the market role. He advanced two objections:

> The fairness objection asked about the quality that market choices may reflect; the corruption objection asked about the attitude and norms that market relations may damage or dissolve. (Sandel 2012, 110)

Sandel expands on the corruption objection arguing that markets 'promote a degrading, objectifying view of the human person, as a collection of spare parts'.

Harcourt (1994, 211) also points out that markets, without specific interventions, do not work in a 'socially desirable manner' (see also Harcourt (1992)). Supporting economic evaluation is not the same as supporting marketisation of every aspect of healthcare, but the same warnings need to be heeded. I will discuss in Chapter 5 how a Christian ethic of resource allocation can adapt contemporary approaches to economic evaluation to incorporate equity considerations. Sandel's corruption objection – which was articulated in the context of markets for organs – also needs to be addressed.

It might at first appear logical to argue from a Christian perspective that human lives cannot be traded or valued one against another, their exchange is 'blocked' (Walzer 1983; Andre 1992) or 'taboo' (Tetlock 2000) and that they are indeed incommensurable. However, Broome (1999) has challenged the logic of incommensurability. Once we have recognised that there are limits, and once we have decided that improved health status is our objective or end, we logically must accept at least some means needs to be pursued toward that end:

> Deciding on an end gives you no reason to take a means to it, but in a different way it does commit you to taking a means. Deciding on an end is itself deciding to take some means to it .... To put it another way: intending an end is intending some means to it. So the movement from end to means is not mediated through reasons but through intention. (Broome 1999, 160–161)

That is, a theology of limits necessarily involves – at least in healthcare – addressing the theology of what a Christian ethic of resource allocation might involve, and what elements of standard economic evaluation might need to be incorporated and what excluded.

Discounting Lives

Fundamental to the use of economic evaluation as currently practised is that some lives, or more accurately, conditions of living – say with reduced mobility – are valued more highly than others. Explicit in the QALY metric is that some incremental life-years are less valuable than others: the value of some life-years is adjusted down because they are lived with reduced mobility, increased pain, or increased anxiety. Standardised weights – which appear common across cultures (Salomon et al. 2012) – have been developed for years lived with different combinations of scores on the common quality-of-life measurement instruments such as the EQ-5D (Kind, Hardman, and Macran 1999; Viney et al. 2011). This comes perilously close to starting to objectify the human person as Sandel's corruption objection forewarns.

This would, *prima facie*, seem inconsistent with the recognition, which occurs in many different phrasings in the Scriptures, that all are equal before God. However, adjusting for different conditions of living is not the same as discounting lives or, more accurately, incremental life-years, and does not involve valuing the human less, but rather recognises that an intervention has a better outcome if it leads to better mobility, less anxiety, less pain, and so on. This better outcome would then be reflected in a higher QALY. The human who has less mobility remains equal in God's sight, but the average outcomes of an intervention would be regarded as better with better mobility.

Nord (2005) has called out the sloppiness of language that has contributed to confusion about what QALYs (and DALYs) are and what they measure. He has helpfully distinguished three concepts:

- the worth of a person, or the value of a person's life;
- the impact on a person's well-being of a condition; and
- the desirability of some conditions of life, and conversely, the undesirability of other conditions.

Weights to be used in economic evaluation can be conceptualised as either being about (subjective) well-being or about the desirability of avoiding a particular condition (Nord 2005, 139). In neither case do weights (and economic evaluations) involve an assessment of the worth of a human.

Innumerable studies lie behind the weights used in economic evaluation studies, and there is public acceptance that different outcomes can be valued differently in a compassionate society. This argument does not require us to reject the 'sanctity of life doctrine' – 'it is absolutely prohibited … to base decisions relating to the prolongation or shortening of human life on considerations of its quality or kind' (Kuhse 1987, 171) – but rather accepts the intrinsic value of life in aggregate and, that different outcomes of care can be more or less beneficial or desirable, and that QALYs can be used as a metric to reflect that.

Let us consider two interventions, one where all the people treated had an extra five years of life with outcomes at the top of any quality-of-life scale, the other with an extra 10 years of life but at half the quality-of-life scale. An economic evaluation would normally rank these two interventions equally (assuming equal costs and that the quality-of-life rankings are valid). If adjustment for the condition of living is seen as illegitimate, the second alternative would be ranked twice as valuable as the first. Ignoring the conditions of living achieved is not consistent with public expectations. In my view it is also not consistent with a Christian ethic of resource allocation.

Christian compassion (and indeed humanistic compassion) calls us to ameliorate pain and suffering. If we have a choice, we will want to help someone move up the quality-of-life scale to lesser pain, similarly, on depression/anxiety, and mobility. This individualised compassion has parallels to a societal view. Society should value healthcare interventions that have lower average pain as an outcome over higher average pain. This does not mean that people with higher levels of pain are less valued, rather that society values the reduction of their pain.

Nord (1999) has proposed a non-utilitarian approach to replace QALYs as a way of ranking outcomes. This communitarian rather than individualistic approach to weight setting has merit and should be used as an alternative way of framing an outcome metric, allowing weights used in QALY calculations better to reflect the views of the collective for priority setting (Denburg et al. 2020; Schneider 2021). In the meantime, the values underpinning the black box of QALY weightings should be opened up, with more transparency and greater clarity of any uncertainties in economic evaluations (Grimm et al. 2020; Sculpher and Palmer 2020; Soares, Sculpher, and Claxton 2020; Rand and Kesselheim 2021).

I introduced Daniel's framework of accountability for reasonableness earlier. The elements of that framework sit well with the Christian ethic of resource allocation. When rationing decisions are to be made, they should reflect a clear ethical basis consistent with Christian values. Setting relative weights to be used in calculating discounts for QALYs based on willingness to pay or other utilitarian principles seems inconsistent with that.

Most international experience with involving consumers is still poorly conceptualised and structured (Sarri et al. 2021). Ghinea et al. described consumer engagement as

> still sporadic, inconsistent, and lacking in transparency, and there remains considerable uncertainty among stakeholders about how efforts to engage consumers in [health technology assessment] should be designed, implemented, and evaluated. (Ghinea, Lipworth, and Kerridge 2020, 88)

Although the United Kingdom has had a guideline for incorporating consumer views into its process for priority setting more than a decade, it is under challenge (Littlejohns et al. 2019). Consumers, and consumer participants in decision-making, are heterogeneous. Rajan and colleagues have identified three types of 'publics':

- 'Unaffected' (or 'pure') public: assumed to be unfamiliar with the issues;
- 'Affected' public: those with relevant personal experience; and
- 'Partisan' public: those with a special partisan interest, technical expertise or professional identity (Rajan et al. 2022, 10; Koch and Rajan 2021, 73).

Ghinea, Lipworth, and Kerridge (2020) introduce a similarly helpful distinction between consumers as expert informants and consumers as advocates. In the former role, consumers can supplement dry quantitative measures both by bringing the human to the statistical and giving meaning to what the 'quality adjustment' to their real life means. In the latter case, consumers go beyond a neutral, information-giving role to advocate for funding of a particular intervention, influencing the outcome (Charlton 2022 (in press)), and potentially introducing inequity into the decision-making process.

Nevertheless, structured engagement with the views of consumers as expert informants would bring economic evaluation processes closer to a system where society collectively can articulate priorities in decision-making. A Christian ethic of resource allocation should prioritise such processes, in addition to the other criteria in the accountability for reasonableness framework.

From the very early days of the application of cost-effectiveness analysis to healthcare there has been recognition that QALY weights and their equivalents have a value base:

> The first general point that has to be made is that every effectiveness measure implies some value judgement. These frequently go unrecognised, because the effectiveness measure has come to be so widely used that it is conventionally accepted as the appropriate technical way of doing things. (Williams 1992, 9)

The implicit challenge that Williams highlights is to make those unrecognised value bases explicit. Despite the ubiquitous acceptance of QALYs, their construction involves choices that can still be challenged, to ensure they reflect values that communities – of citizens and consumers – accept should be incorporated in priority-setting processes.

The Place of Technical Efficiency

The theology of limits calls us to abhor waste. Addressing technical inefficiency – one of the many types of waste in healthcare (Bentley et al. 2008; Berwick and Hackbarth 2012; Black 2017; Organisation for Economic Cooperation and Development 2017) – should be a key part of responsible stewardship (Cafferky 2013). Technical efficiency is not the same as simple-minded cost-cutting, nor is it cost shifting from one funding source to another; it is not shifting costs to families and patients, and nor is it privatisation. What technical efficiency is about is ensuring that each type of healthcare service is provided at the least cost, subject to the standard economist assumption of *ceteris paribus*, other things being equal, such as, crucially, the quality of care.

Conclusion

Oikonomia as used at the time of Jesus had a clear ethical value base. This appears to have all but disappeared from the practice of economics today which appears implicitly to deemphasise justice. A Christian ethics of resource allocation should be founded on Christian values, rather than utilitarian principles, and emphasise responsible and ethical stewardship, clawing back the historic ethical connotations of stewardship and its objective of releasing funds to assist the poor. As the relevant parables show, stewards have an obligation to manage resources wisely.

I have argued that stewardship has two distinct elements:

- being prudent in the use of resources and eschewing greed and over consumption; and
- being concerned about social justice and those, outside the immediate household, who were in need.

This means that a Christian approach to resource allocation needs to accept that resources are limited and that extra spending on healthcare should be scrutinised and assessed against alternative priorities. In turn, this calls for the use of economic evaluation, as a tool for doing this. However, contemporary approaches to economic evaluation fall short of the Christian ideal.

The critical difference though, between the utilitarian underpinning of resource allocation decisions, and a Christian ethical basis, is that stewardship in a Christian ethic of healthcare funding sits alongside the two other principles of compassion and social justice.

Table 4.2 *Responsible stewardship and its implications*

Elements of responsible stewardship	Healthcare policies based on responsible stewardship
Being prudent in the use of resources Eschewing greed and over consumption	Pursuit of technical efficiency • Use of economic evaluation in priority setting, so that services where the benefits do not outweigh the costs are not supported (subject to the exception below) • Ensuring that social value judgements are incorporated into the economic evaluation system and that the system meets standards of reasonableness. • Recognise the Rule of Rescue to allow some leeway in decisions in situations where the number of people affected is small (discussed further and operationalised in the next chapter)
Being concerned about social justice and those, outside the immediate household, who were in need	Incorporate an explicit requirement to consider the equity implications of rankings and the distributional consequences (discussed in the next chapter).

A Christian ethic of resource allocation, based on responsible stewardship as developed in this chapter, should be characterised as shown in Table 4.2.

A Christian ethic of healthcare funding is framed within a theology of limits and an ethic of prudence. It accepts that unlimited spending is not just, and that healthcare may need to be rationed to ensure equitable and efficient use of scarce resources.

Although I have been somewhat critical of economic evaluation and the York economists who have led its application to healthcare, I accept its underlying principles. As one of the York economists argued:

> Resort to numbers is not an abdication of moral responsibility, nor an attempt to conceal the moral issues involved. On the contrary, it is a means of avoiding the impasse which much moral argument reaches, when platitudinous generalisations about striking a balance, or finding an acceptable compromise, or weighing conflicting views one against another, block further thought and progress. (Williams 2001, 255)

It is possible to reframe economic evaluation so the 'moral arguments' are addressed and incorporated appropriately in resource allocation policies. Responsible stewardship, so operationalised, thus involves a modification of contemporary economic approaches to resource allocation but still recognises the centrality of scarcity.

A Christian ethic of resource allocation calls us to be rational stewards of healthcare resources, paraphrasing Benedict XVI (2009, para. 37), it recognises that every healthcare resource allocation decision has a moral consequence. In publicly funded health systems, it calls us to ensure that taxpayer dollars are invested wisely, in the context of ensuring social justice and promoting compassionate care.

CHAPTER 5

A Christian Ethic of Healthcare Funding

> A man was going down from Jerusalem to Jericho, and fell into the hands of robbers, who stripped him, beat him, and went away, leaving him half dead. (Luke 10:30)

In Chapters 1–4, I argued that a Christian ethic of healthcare funding should be motivated by and show compassion, be just in access, and be guided by a theology of limits and prudence, evidencing responsible stewardship. A Christian ethic of healthcare funding is not one of choosing which of compassion, social justice, and stewardship to prioritise and which to ignore: the Samaritan showed all three. The healthcare funding challenge is how to hold all three in tension, and how to reconcile all three.

In this chapter, I start by discussing the tensions involved in pursuing all three objectives and then come down a level, moving from principles to the specific, discussing how the three principles might apply when paying organisations and professionals for public health and healthcare.

The Compassion-Social Justice Tension

Compassion as the motivator may occasionally come into conflict with social justice in the context of stewardship – resources are limited, and choices need to be made. But normally, compassion will point in the same direction as justice, and we will show compassion to all, inclusively. I have argued compassion should be an attribute of communities, and it is hard to see a compassionate community not pursuing social justice.

However, as I noted in Chapter 3, individuals and societies may suffer compassion fatigue, and this may force choices about which groups will receive attention. The nicer, cleaner groups – more like us – will be prioritised. The antidote to this is reflection, remembering again the story of the sorting of the sheep and the goats (Matthew 25:31–46), and the preferential option for the poor. Compassion – the visceral need to act – should be directed to address not only individual, present needs but also the broader social and economic factors that might have caused the immediate needs to occur.

Health needs are unevenly but not randomly distributed, and a focus on need and the factors that give rise to the need will almost inevitably be pro-poor. The risk is that if social justice is not explicitly considered, resource allocation may be skewed, an issue discussed in the following text.

The Compassion-Stewardship Tension

I have argued in Chapter 4 that economic evaluation is consistent with a Christian ethic of resource allocation and, indeed, prudence in consumption and good stewardship requires such priority setting. But the challenges for economic evaluation outlined in that chapter are particularly relevant for a Christian ethic of healthcare funding. Specifically, how to reconcile a principle of compassion and one of stewardship? This is most obviously an issue when we – decision-makers and the public alike (Sinclair et al. 2008) – see the plight of individuals and feel compassion for them, yet meeting their need would not, *prima facie*, be consistent with economically rational priority setting criteria: that is, what is the place for the Rule of Rescue in a Christian ethic of healthcare funding?

Even though public opinion surveys seem to put only a modest value on the Rule of Rescue or an identified life premium, a Christian ethic of resource allocation should challenge that. We are told by the priestly writer in the first creation story that humans were created in the image of God (Genesis 1:26–27), a concept sometimes referred to as *imago dei*. The theology of these verses has been extensively debated but the consensus is that 'image' is not to be reduced into a simple matter of physical appearance (Barr 1968). 'Image' probably connotes power or decision-making roles, immediately followed by the reference to having dominion over fish and animals, and certainly humans are unique and distinguished from the other inhabitants of the living creation (Bird 2011). Sawyer (1974, 424) suggests that an alternative translation better captures the nuances of the Hebrew:

> So God created the man with a resemblance to Himself
> With a resemblance to divine beings he created him

In Christian theology, Christ is the very image of God, as many New Testament references attest (Kilner 2015). *Imago dei* has also provided the fundamental underpinning of Christian bioethical teaching (Lustig 2017; Pilkington 2017). Much of Roman Catholic doctrine on bioethical issues and, indeed, broader social issues is explicitly based on the dignity of humanity. The first chapter of the principal document to emerge from the Second Vatican Council, for example, is entitled 'The dignity of the human person' (Paul VI 1965) and a major instruction on bioethics commences:

> The dignity of a person must be recognized in every human being from conception to natural death. This fundamental principle expresses a great 'yes' to human life and must be at the center of ethical reflection on biomedical research, which has an ever greater importance in today's world. (Congregation for the Doctrine of the Faith 2008, para. 1)

Imago dei leads us to value all human life. We are also taught in the quite complex theological dialogue between Abraham and YHWH in Genesis 18 (Macdonald 2004; Zvi 1992) that God recognises the value of small numbers of people.

However, one does not have to be a Christian to value human life, whether because one sees God in the face of fellow humans or because of simple humanity. Valuing human life calls out a compassionate response – a response which is stronger the more one can identify with the person or people affected either because they are like us in location or wealth (Berlant 2004) or because they have names and are identifiable (Kogut and Ritov 2005; Slovic 2010). A compassionate response, regardless of its limitations in breadth of acceptance, is something to be welcomed, not derided, diminished, and denied as being inconsistent with economic rationality.

This leads to an argument about how compassion should be considered in responsible stewardship. The identified lives issue applies not only to the unique individual but also to small groups of beneficiaries, possibly identifiable with genomic tests. Here it is not only the argument from compassion that is relevant but also the risks of statistical or research errors that increase the likelihood that the research results used to inform cost-effectiveness analysis may be spurious. The challenge then becomes how to reconcile the broader concerns for the dignity of all human lives with setting priorities that might exclude people from life-improving or life-extending treatment.

Stewardship has a key place in a Christian ethic of healthcare funding because it is about addressing prudence in consumption: that in aggregate the common good requires that our healthcare investments are worth it. Economic evaluation is about prioritising in the economic realm, but this realm operates within a broader context and needs to consider how economic evaluation might still 'maximise respect for the equal dignity of persons' (Beckley 2011, 360).

When the beneficiary is identifiable, we need to leave the economic realm and enter the world of personhood where each person is valued uniquely and inalienably. We no longer are considering averages but are now considering individuals each of infinite (non-monetary) value, and the aggregation arithmetic is confounded and irrelevant. The only way to reconcile respect for human dignity and economic evaluation's world of aggregates is to specify the limits of the economic realm.

I have already alluded to the 'illusion of validity' of economic evaluation (Kahneman 2011). It would therefore seem inappropriate to rigidly rule in or out potential healthcare interventions in circumstances where the Rule of Rescue might come into play. Nevertheless, it is appropriate to set some limits about the circumstances in which ordinary 'rational' criteria are overridden. Responsible stewardship should identify such criteria where the Rule of Rescue is appropriate, including small numbers or where the benefit is large despite large costs.

Small Numbers

Different rules may apply when there is a small number of people affected. This is partly because our compassion is evoked, especially when children are involved, and individuals, professionals, and communities are loathe to be accused of 'playing god' (Chadwick 1989; Incandela 1996; Coady 2009). But there are also technical reasons to eschew economic evaluation when small numbers are involved: that small sample sizes have greater statistical margins of error, and so the findings of economic evaluations may not reflect the true underlying cost-effectiveness of an intervention. In addition, 'heterogenous patient pathways, limited clinical experience, and often no accepted standard of care, makes it more difficult to generate the same standard of evidence in rare and ultra-rare conditions as in more common conditions' (Henderson et al. 2021, 4).

Many countries – especially high-income countries – have developed special policies for rare, 'ultra-rare', or 'orphan' diseases (Pant and Visintini 2018; Chan et al. 2020). The threshold for defining 'small' or rare is a matter of judgement and ranges between 2 and 80 per 100,000 population (Pant and Visintini 2018). Although the prevalence of each 'rare' disease may be very low, with improvements in genomic technology, more such diseases are being identified and the overall prevalence may be 3.5–5.9 per cent of the population (Nguengang-Wakap et al. 2020).

Unless the costs of an intervention are exceedingly large – the issue of fair prices is discussed below – applying different rules for efficacious treatments in small cohorts with a tight definition of 'rare' will generally cause only a small increment in total health expenditure. A critical issue will be identifying how one defines the cohort and this will increasingly be through genomic testing.

But even when small numbers are involved, the theology of limits still has a part to play, and large spending for experimental treatments – or treatments with a low probability of success in life extension – should not be part of responsible stewardship. Societies will need to debate and develop thresholds for supererogatory interventions, potentially related to the size of the economy and average lifetime disposable income (Emanuel 2019).

Where the Benefit Is Large Despite Large Costs

Cost-effectiveness analysis would typically reject interventions with a high cost for each QALY (on average). With developments in genomics, it is now possible to identify with precision people who might benefit from an intervention and have dramatic effects. The tension between stewardship and compassion must prioritise compassion over mechanistic application of economic evaluation. Well-designed and ethically sound systems of differential access – including access to an intervention/drug not yet approved to be sold and to interventions not yet approved for public funding – should be introduced in an ethically responsible way (Hanna et al. 2018; Pace et al. 2018; Löblová et al. 2019).

However, consistent with the reality of 'no blank cheque for the health system', decision-makers still need to be wary of prices charged for the intervention. The proposed price for each intervention might be high, as patent owners seek to maximise returns from their investments, including recouping payments an order of magnitude greater than the cost of their investment (Tay-Teo, Ilbawi, and Hill 2019). Responsible stewardship would first seek to attack this rent-seeking behaviour by attempting to negotiate a just price (Barrera 2007, 100–103) reflective of benefit (Vokinger et al. 2020). This might involve innovative drug payment regimes such as risk-sharing where drug companies only get paid when a patient responds to treatment, so that payments reflect the benefit observed in practice, rather than benefits claimed in submissions for approval of the treatment (Neumann et al. 2011; Garrison et al. 2013; Navarria et al. 2015; Ghinea, Lipworth, and Kerridge 2016; Department of Health and Human Services. Centers for Medicare & Medicaid Services 2020; Lauenroth et al. 2020; Lopez et al. 2020; Bohm et al. 2022), or other innovative pricing or financing approaches (Hanna et al. 2018; Dabbous et al. 2022), or simply tougher and more sophisticated negotiations with drug manufacturers for access to a subsidies (Main, Csanadi, and Ozieranski 2022 (in press)).

Drug prices vary significantly across countries, with prices highest in the United States (Salas-Vega, Shearer, and Mossialos 2020), which essentially eschews tough negotiations with drug manufacturers (Trujillo et al. 2020). Emanuel (2019) has proposed a specific measure of what is a 'just price', suggesting prices for the United States above 11 per cent of average lifetime disposable income are excessive and unjust; many current drug prices exceed that threshold.

Rent seeking by pharmaceutical companies needs to be addressed directly. Their intellectual property is, in fact, a legal artefact, granting the patent owner a monopoly for a defined period to compensate for the costs of development of the drug (Kapczynski and Kesselheim 2016). The extent to which patents promote innovation and are appropriately structured is debatable (Boldrin and Levine 2013), and so the net benefit of the pharmaceutical patents as a way of encouraging innovation has been called into question (Gøtzsche 2018; Baker 2021; Neumann, Ollendorf, and Cohen 2021). The COVID-19 pandemic has brought the benefits of patents into sharp focus with vaccine developers making large profits from vaccine roll-out in wealthy countries (Malpani and Maitland 2021) while seeking to maintain patent coverage in the face of very low vaccination rates in low-income countries. This has led to calls for relaxing patent protection in low-income countries, supported by the United States' government (Iacobucci 2021). Patents are not, of course, the only barrier to low rates of vaccination (Le and Samson 2021), albeit without affordable vaccines the other barriers are moot.

In order to ensure dynamic efficiency in healthcare, there may need to be a rethinking of how innovation is encouraged and paid for (Hensher, Tisdell et al. 2020): just pricing for pharmaceuticals must incorporate a fair payment for innovation, but such payments must also recognise adequately the opportunity costs of investments and health sector payments for the innovation (Woods et al. 2021). Traditionally, innovation is encouraged and rewarded through patents, which guarantee an income stream for the patent holder. Prizes have been proposed as an alternative reward structure to overcome the potential for price gouging that patents provide and to delink reward for innovation from product pricing (Gandjour and Chernyak 2011; Pan et al. 2017; Hong, Kesselheim, and Sarpatwari 2019).

The benefits of the social license granted through patents may need to be constrained to prevent price gouging, regulating prices of patented medicines to align with some measure of their value as measured using economic evaluation (Schaffer et al. 2018; Gurwitz and Pearson 2019; Humphries and Xie 2019). This approach could be supplemented by considering a drug monopoly as any other essential service monopoly, such as water supply, and have a regulated rate of return (Laffont and Tirole 1993; Drummond and Towse 2019) similar to other drugs or to that prevailing in other industries (Ledley et al. 2020), taking into account the risks associated with the investment in drug development (Berdud, Drummond, and Towse 2020).

Whether or not fair pricing can be negotiated, where dramatic benefits can be shown (good quality of life for years compared to poor quality of life for weeks), there is a legitimate argument to allow a higher approval threshold, where the number of people who might benefit is small and identifiable. This Rule of Rescue approach should not be specific to a particular diagnosis such as cancer (Chamberlain et al. 2019; Chim et al. 2019), and should be neutral as between medications and other types of healthcare interventions (Saing et al. 2019).

Age Bias

Former Archbishop of Canterbury, Rowan Williams, has identified ageing as a spiritual issue (Williams 2015, 246), and discrimination against older people is both unlawful in most high-income countries (Macnicol 2006; Freedland and Vickers 2016) and unethical. However, as argued earlier, responsible stewardship must recognise limits. The death of anyone often leads to sadness for those left behind, but death is inevitable. Although we talk colloquially of healthcare interventions 'saving lives', they do not; they extend lives. Sometimes life extension is measured in decades, but sometimes it is only in days, weeks, or months.

Despite all the advances in health technology and treatment in recent decades, the life expectancy for a woman aged 75 in 2012 in Australia was only five years longer than her counterpart in 1952 (13 vs 8 years; Australian Bureau of Statistics (2014)). The same pattern of small change in life expectancy is true in all high-income countries and is projected to continue into the future: female life expectancy at birth in high-income countries is expected to increase from 83.5 years in 2017 to 86.1 years in 2100 (Vollset et al. 2020, Appendix 2 – Table 1). There is also some evidence that maximum life expectancy – as evidenced by the longevity of the oldest person alive at any time – has not changed over the last decade (Dong, Milholland, and Vijg 2016; Einmahl, Einmahl, and de Haan 2019; James 2020), although whether this will be a stable finding into the future is disputed (de Beer, Bardoutsos, and Janssen 2017; Barbi et al. 2018).

Although a Christian ethic of resource allocation should value all people, older people should not be singled out to have additional weight attached to their extra years of life compared to anyone else in the population, or to have a new allocation metric related to percentage improvement in longevity (Shuster 2019). This will mean that interventions principally targeted at older people will be less likely to meet cost-effectiveness thresholds compared to interventions aimed at younger people – an average 10-year improvement in quality-adjusted life expectancy will be easier to achieve in people aged 35 than in people aged 85 (Palmer et al. 2021), even without the additional weighting sometimes now accorded to interventions which have longer term – say greater than 30 years – benefits (Charlton 2022 (in press)).

Nor should an additional year of life for an older person be weighted less than that of a younger person (Lancsar et al. 2020): with equal values for each additional life year, healthcare interventions targeted at older people are already less likely to achieve cost-effectiveness thresholds, and so an additional discount would make interventions at older ages even harder to attract public funding.

I argue that the absence of pro-age loadings is not an age bias but age neutrality – an extra year of life should be valued equally, neither discounted nor weighted positively at any age, so interventions that cost less than the threshold per QALY should be endorsed for public funding whether the intervention is targeted at 35- or 85-year-olds.

Care at the End of Life

Care at the end of life requires ascertaining and valuing the preferences of the dying person but as was discussed in Chapter 2, this does not mean that 'disputed care' needs to be provided. The frame for provision of care should be a focus on the individual, with compassion, not rationing or economics, driving an individual's treatment.

However, end of life care takes place within a social context of families and carers, hospitals or palliative care services, and a wider society (Kluge 2007; Misak, White, and Truog 2014). A significant proportion of health expenditure is spent on people in the last years of their life but this is not a surprise, as people closer to death are also sicker (Wammes et al. 2018). In any event, this higher expenditure cannot be easily predicted in an individual case (Einav et al. 2018). The policy issue is whether the health system is responding appropriately to people's needs and whether there is too much intervention occurring that is providing too little benefit to the patient.

Anesi et al. (2019) have called out what they see as 'irresponsible use' of healthcare, specifically in intensive care units, which is driven by a combination of system and individual factors. According to research by Anesi et al., in the United States, a surfeit of resources leads to excessive use, and the United States public's aggressive opposition to anything remotely like rationing encourages this.

Alongside these developments, there has been an increase in expectations of patient autonomy but without a serious effort to develop the skills of health professionals to work with patients to help them understand their choices and their implications. It is not good clinical practice to provide patients with a bewildering array of options and expect them to comprehend complex statistical concepts of risk and likelihood, which baffle many economists (Kay and King 2020), and clinical concepts about potential outcomes. Healthcare has changed over time, not only in technological capacity but also in the way it is practised:

> (There has been a) shift from medicine rooted in paternalism to medicine as guided centrally by the principle of patient autonomy. Under the new approach of extreme autonomy, physicians gave patients, families, and surrogates options in which none were presented before, and then asked what these patients wanted. Simultaneous to this approach, the capabilities for critical care, including life-support therapies such as mechanical ventilation and cardiopulmonary resuscitation, greatly expanded, and allowed more to be interpreted as better in the absence of evidence to the contrary (and sometimes even in the face of such evidence). Perhaps most influentially, the American medical community placed immense medical decision-making authority in the hands of patients, families, and surrogates who are not medically trained, and did so without any appropriate context. These patients and families were told medical risks and benefits, concepts even many trained physicians have difficulty interpreting, but not how different treatment choices might align with patients' values or what they viewed as acceptable and unacceptable clinical courses, recovery trajectories, and qualities of life. Taken together, this approach was a setup for a massive expansion in the delivery of aggressive care. The family of a sick patient, who is not getting better, or getting worse, and for whom the physician thinks the outlook is not good, was given the options to make them comfortable, perhaps continue with current (ineffective) therapy, or go to the ICU for aggressive care or to do everything. Without proper context, there is no decision: more is better, if the alternative is death. (Anesi et al. 2019, 608)

The language here is somewhat excessive, including 'extreme autonomy', but the point being made is an important one: the compassionate dialogue that needs to take place between a treating team and a patient and their family is an extremely complex one. If this is the first time there has been a discussion about the patient's intention at the end of life, the compassionate dialogue is much harder. But as Anesi et al. argue, the role of the treating team is not a simple one of laying out 'the facts', but a critical part of clinical communication in listening carefully and being sensitive about the nuances of what is said or not being said. Anesi et al. coined the term 'facilitated autonomy' to describe the role. Writing as they do in a country that does not have a social justice underpinning of healthcare, it is no surprise that they also warn of the risk that this role could easily slip into discriminatory behaviour, offering fewer options to poorer people than the wealthy.

This balance of how a patient's social context influences treatment options is a complex and fraught one. There are not going to be hard and fast rules that apply across every clinical situation, but a Christian ethic of healthcare funding and resource allocation should continue to emphasise the importance of listening to the patient and their caregivers and helping them to explore the options for them, but with a particular obligation to be realistic about prognosis and treatments.

This does not mean that there is no place for economic evaluation in end-of-life care (Hunter 2016; Johnston 2016; Coast et al. 2021), but rather that compassion has an important place. Standard economic evaluation metrics such as QALYs do not work well at the end of life – especially in children facing death where a QALY gain is not the most important factor in decision making (Hinde et al. 2021) – and more appropriate measures of benefit, such as focusing on a person's capabilities, need to be used (Coast et al. 2016; Sampson 2016).

In summary, the compassion-stewardship tension resolves with a balance towards compassion incorporating explicit acceptance of the Rule of Rescue in economic evaluation. All the examples involve areas where simplistic application of economic evaluation in decision making might be in conflict with community values, including the Rule of Rescue. They all highlight the importance of public and patient engagement in deliberative processes as identified in Chapter 4.

The Social Justice-Stewardship Tension

The third tension to be addressed is between social justice and stewardship. The contemporary application of economic evaluation, where it effectively ignores equity, is not consistent with responsible stewardship. I have demonstrated in Chapter 3 that social justice is a core concern of biblical teaching, and this must be incorporated into priority setting.

Distributive Justice

If a decision-maker were considering two projects, equally ranked in terms of cost per QALY, but one where the benefits were skewed towards the poor and one to the rich, responsible stewardship, founded in social justice and a preferential option for the poor, would favour selecting the pro-poor option. The challenge arises when there is an equity-efficiency trade-off. What if the project where benefit accrued disproportionately to the rich was marginally but statistically significantly better in terms of the cost per QALY metric? Conventional economic evaluation, ignoring as it does the equity dimension, would decide in favour of the pro-rich project.

Contemporary approaches to economic evaluation – especially by public funding agencies – tend to emphasise simple QALY maximisation. But there is no reason there should be a single maximand. Charlton and Weale argue that the United Kingdom's health economic evaluation assessment agency, the National Institute for Health and Care Excellence (NICE), should

> break free from the intellectual shackles of QALY maximisation. As the dominant social value judgement in NICE's approach, any departure from this goal is counted by some as a dilution of the pure milk of the health economics gospel; other considerations may modify, but they cannot compete on equal terms. (Charlton and Weale 2021, 6)

In contrast to a singular focus on QALY maximisation, a Christian ethic of resource allocation should require explicit consideration of the distribution of benefits of projects. The cost per QALY should not be deified as a magic number, which is the sole determinant of an intervention's relative priority. Decision-makers should recognise the uncertainty surrounding cost per QALY estimates (Häyry 2002; Griffin 2020; Sculpher and Palmer 2020; Soares, Sculpher, and Claxton 2020), and accept that pro-poor projects can be supported at a more expensive cost per QALY than less equitable projects, or, in one framing, what should be maximised is equity-weighted benefit. Sunstein (2013) makes a similar point in arguing that distributional considerations might over-ride cost-benefit analysis' rankings in the context of considering statistical vs identifiable lives. QALY weights could also be adjusted to incorporate an equity-weighting directly (Carlson et al. 2020).

Consideration of equity can easily be incorporated into existing ranking approaches, which recognise a grey zone in project approvals by highlighting the sensitivity to both the incremental cost-effectiveness criterion and the equity impact (Griffin et al. 2019). Cookson et al. review several approaches as to how equity analysis can be incorporated into economic valuation. They conclude

> we see a role for equity-weighting sensitivity analysis as an aid to deliberation in the context of specific decisions in light of information on who gains and loses … [Equity-weighting analysis] … can be used as an aid to deliberation

> in the context of specific decision via sensitivity analysis of different equity parameters to help decision-makers and stakeholders explore the implications of alternative value judgements about equity. (Cookson et al. 2017, 211)

The failure of economic evaluation as it is practised to consider distributional issues explicitly is a major weakness and not consistent with a Christian ethic of healthcare funding. Equity considerations should be incorporated into decisions for approving new drugs, vaccines, or treatments for public funding using appropriate techniques (Cookson et al. 2020; Bell, Neri, and Steuten 2021; Ward et al. 2022). Submissions for public funding should be required to incorporate distributional analysis – as now recommended as best practice in reporting economic evaluations (Husereau et al. 2022) – including, where possible, information about the incremental cost-effectiveness ratios for different population groups.

The preferential option for the poor has specific application here: new interventions that are pro-poor – or that have a progressive distributional impact on other equity criteria – should be approved at the upper end of any approval range in terms of cost for incremental benefit.

The World Health Organisation has highlighted the importance of distributive justice in its three-stage approach for the move to universal health coverage, which:

- categorises services into priority classes. Relevant criteria include those related to cost-effectiveness, priority to the worse off, and financial risk protection.
- first expands coverage for high-priority services to everyone. This includes eliminating out-of-pocket payments while increasing mandatory, progressive prepayment with pooling of funds.
- while doing so, ensures that disadvantaged groups are not left behind. These will often include low-income groups and rural populations (World Health Organization 2014; Norheim 2015).

The start of the universal health coverage process relates to the stewardship criterion, identifying what is to be covered, and ensuring that covered services are cost-effective. The second two elements of the strategy are about equity: expanding coverage for everybody without out-of-pocket payments for high-priority services and addressing the most disadvantaged.

Co-payments

As discussed in Chapter 3, co-payments impact adversely on the poor, and the argument in favour of co-payments based on 'moral hazard' is on shaky grounds. Chandra and colleagues phrase their conclusion particularly starkly:

> One conclusion remains clear: patient cost-sharing introduces large and deadly distortions into the cost-benefit calculus. (Chandra, Flack, and Obermeyer 2021, 38)

There are four main clusters of strategies to reduce co-payments including oversight and stewardship (e.g. better monitoring of private payments), improved coverage, reforms to service delivery, and increased investment (Jalali, Bikineh, and Delavari 2021). All should be pursued.

Because of their adverse impact on the most disadvantaged, and the ambiguous at best impact of moral hazard, co-payments should have a limited role in healthcare funding design informed by a Christian ethic. Ideally, there would be no out-of-pocket payments in wealthy economies, and to the extent out-of-pocket payments are necessary to support the phasing in of universal health coverage in developing countries, they should be phased out when feasible (McIntyre 2007). The international evidence suggests this is a common pattern – what Fan and Savedoff (2014) refer to as the 'health financing transition' – that as countries spend more on healthcare, the share contributed by out-of-pocket payments declines.

Use of Private Money

In Chapter 4, I argued that healthcare resources are limited, and indeed, not all investments in healthcare are worthwhile. But what if I have my own money to spend? Should I not be able to spend it as I choose? But this immediately draws our attention to who is the I in this question? The answer is obvious and confronting: this is only a question for those with the wealth to participate in a private market and so immediately raises issues of equity.

Private payments are a feature of all health systems and come in a variety of guises.

A prominent feature of the health system in many low- and middle-income countries are so-called *informal payments* – payments to providers that fall outside the purview of the state and are often under-the-counter cash payments (Lewis 2007; Cherecheş et al. 2013; Stepurko, Pavlova, and Groot 2017). These might be required to get any access to care because of resource shortages (Gaal and McKee 2004; Gaal et al. 2006), expedited access, or access to what might be perceived as better quality care (Cohen 2012). They occur for a host of reasons, including topping up official salaries, which are perceived as inadequate and may be an endemic part of the local culture (Gaal and McKee 2004; Cohen 2018, 2012). In some cases there may be an element of coercion (Chereches et al. 2013), but in others there may be an expression of gratitude, although even here the gratuity may be expected or required (Gaál 2006; Moldovan and Van de Walle 2013). Whether couched as gratitude or not, coercive payments act as an additional rationing device and have all the undesirable features of formal out-of-pocket payments described above.

A second type of private payment is common in all high-income countries and that is private payment for services that *complement* the publicly funded system, that is they provide coverage for services that are not covered in the public benefit schedule. In most countries, cosmetic procedures – surgery for purely aesthetic reasons – fall outside the public programme and are fully privately funded. Dental services are not covered in some countries, nor are some medications, especially 'over-the-counter' medications.

A third type of private payment is for services in the public benefit package. Private payments may be a mandatory component of the public benefit package, with the disadvantages of out-of-pocket payments previously discussed. Private payment is particularly inappropriate for public health interventions – such as immunisation – which convey wider social benefits (Shafrin et al. 2021). Here, as well as being unjust, private payment undermines social solidarity and potentially undermines responsible stewardship if people cannot afford to be part of a public health programme.

Policies on vaccines against the SARS-CoV-2 virus – which causes COVID – provide a case in point. A small Chilean study showed that people would pay for vaccination, albeit with the anticipated equity effects: people on lower incomes or unemployed were less willing to pay (García and Cerda 2020). Nevertheless, COVID vaccination was almost universally seen as a right, with vaccination quickly included in public benefit packages or mandated to be covered by private insurers (Keith 2020), perhaps because of a strong expectation by the public that this was just – and part of a commitment to the 'common good' (Yunus, Donaldson, and Perron 2020), or because of perceived benefits of herd immunity (National Academies of Sciences Engineering and Medicine 2020).

In some countries, such as Australia, private health insurance provides full or partial coverage for the same services that are included in the public benefit package. In this case private payment may be claimed to act as a *substitute* for public funding: that is, if it were not for the private payment, these services would be fully funded from the public purse. The marketing of substitute insurance might emphasise faster access to care, bypassing public-sector priority setting, different thresholds for admission – that is treatments might be provided with private funding that have lower benefit to risk ratios and so might not be eligible for public funding – or better amenity.

A key argument for private funding is a libertarian one: people should have a freedom to spend their own money as they wish. Färdow, Broström, and Johansson (2019, 518) somewhat pejoratively refer to this argument as a hedonistic one:

> people typically *feel good about* being able to choose and, conversely, *feel frustrated when they are* being barred from a choice between alternatives that could have been offered to them. [emphasis in the original]

However, there are very few occasions when only private money is at stake: arguably the resources devoted to 'aesthetic medicine' – the surgeon's time, the beds, and operating rooms/theatres staffed by nursing and other personnel – could have been used for other purposes and so cosmetic access impinges on general access, creating an opportunity cost to the use of private money. Similarly, the educational preparation of those involved in providing these services may have been subsidised by the state so there is an inherent, albeit small, implicit government subsidy.

The place of private funding can be evaluated in the light of its impact on compassion, social justice, and stewardship.

Compassion might, *prima facie*, support unfettered use of private funding for any of the three types of private funding referred to above, especially private funding that is a complement to the public benefit package. Even if thresholds for admission are different between public and private funding, maybe it should be up to the consumer, if they have the ability, to assess their own willingness to pay for services which are of marginal benefit. The compassion argument assumes no coercion and that the consumer has full information to make that decision.

Coercive informal payments fail on every criterion: they are not compassionate, inhibit access and so are not just, and by operating outside a regulatory framework, they almost certainly undermine stewardship as well.

Private payment of complementary services, even though there is an opportunity cost and a small implicit subsidy, does not undermine the public benefit package (Krohmal and Emanuel 2007, 2009). If one assumes the public benefit package has been established fairly, necessary services should be covered in the package and so the adverse impact of private payments on social justice might be limited. In situations where the public benefit package is unreasonably narrowly defined, private payments will impact on social justice and the health status of the most disadvantaged.

The public policy response should be to expand the public benefit package to incorporate necessary services, that is, the critical question for policymakers should not start with what is an individual's responsibility (Tinghőg, Carlsson, and Lyttkens 2010), but rather what should be a social responsibility (Stabile 2015).

The case of *substitute* services is also clear: private payment undermines both social justice and stewardship.

Private payments exist because of the disjunction or asymmetry between the established institutional processes in the health system and informal norms, values, and cultures (Williams and Horodnic 2017; Horodnic and Williams 2018). There is a significant difference in the role of private payment for substitute services in Canada and the United Kingdom on the one hand, and Australia on the other. There is little private payment in the first two countries, and indeed in Canada private payment for substitute services is strictly limited and, in most provinces, prohibited. A recent legal challenge to this prohibition was rejected (Flood, Thomas, and White 2020; Flood 2021).

The informal norms, values, and cultures in Canada and the United Kingdom and the formal policies about Canadian Medicare and the U.K. National Health Service are closely aligned. The public systems in both countries are strongly supported – there is an expectation in both countries of equitable access, with preferential access or requirements to pay out-of-pocket being neither part of the informal nor the formal systems. In both countries the public system was initially disputed but was quickly accepted by the medical profession and consumers (Houston 2002).

In contrast, in Australia private payment for substitute services is widespread and even encouraged, especially by conservative (Liberal) governments (Duckett and Nemet 2019). Australia's Medicare system was only introduced after vociferous and bruising fights (Scotton and Macdonald 1993; Boxall and Gillespie 2013). It was originally introduced in 1974 and then dismantled shortly thereafter. It was reintroduced in 1984 and the Liberal Opposition continued to oppose it in election after election, promising to dismantle it, for the next decade.

Even though the medical fee schedule in Australia was based on the prevailing 'most common fees', a significant number of medical practitioners view the fee schedule as illegitimate and charge above the schedule fee. Although charging a higher fee might connote higher quality, there is no Australian evidence of an association between out-of-pocket payments and quality, and the limited United States evidence suggests an inverse relationship between provider price and quality (Whaley 2018). Contrary to naïve economic theory, competition in the primary medical care market appears to reduce quality but have no meaningful impact on price (Johar, Jones, and Savage 2014).

In Australia there is a significant difference between the informal values, norms, and cultures, especially of the medical profession and the formal health system provision under Medicare. This leads to a culture of significant out-of-pocket payments, and private health insurance, for services in the public benefits package.

The ethics of private payments for substitute services involves the consideration of the balance of stewardship and social justice. The existence of private payments inevitably involves the creation of a two-tier health system, although the French-Canadian expression *à deux vitesses*, may be a more accurate given what is often purchased is faster access. A two-tier or two-speed health system is antithetical to social justice. It also undermines commitment to solidarity and weakens support for the stewardship function of the health system (Weale and Clark 2010). Preferential access for those who can afford it weakens support for a *universal* health system and undermines the legitimacy of public priority setting.

The intersection of a parallel private health system saps resources from the public system (Hurley 2020; Cheng, Joyce, and Scott 2013; Cheng, Kalb, and Scott 2013) and, contrary to the argument of advocates, does not reduce waiting times for those in the public sector (Duckett 2005, 2018b). A Christian ethical position should be that adopted in Canada: that parallel systems of public and private payment are more likely to harm than help public systems (Tuohy, Flood, and Stabile 2004) and should not be supported, albeit with the recognition that this choice leads to increased public spending, or reduced private earnings, or both.

The Broader View of Social Justice and Stewardship – Beyond Health

Priority setting and stewardship are not only issues for healthcare, but are also tasks for, and responsibilities of, every sector of the economy. A Christian ethic of healthcare funding should be cognisant of the impact of healthcare on other sectors and how decisions in healthcare contribute to, or harm, other sectors.

Health services and the social care sector exhibit 'reciprocal interdependence', the most complex form of interdependency (Thompson 1967) – better rehabilitation services might reduce demand for social care, especially residential aged care, and better social care might prevent some hospitalisations (Bradley et al. 2016). As a 24/7 endeavour, the health sector consumes significant energy resources and is a major contributor to a country's energy consumption, which, depending on how it is sourced, might contribute to global warming (Eckelman and Sherman 2018; Sherman, MacNeill, and Thiel 2019; Duckett, Mackey, and Stobart 2020; Hensher, Tisdell et al. 2020; Pencheon and Wight 2020; Sherman et al. 2020), which in turn might have an adverse impact on human health (Rocque et al. 2021), including increasing the risk of pandemics (Carlson et al. 2022 (in press)). The issue of responsible stewardship of environmental resources is critically important as the burgeoning literature on eco-theology (Deane-Drummond 2017; Hrynkow 2017), pronouncements from church leaders (Francis 2015; Zink 2017; Bartholomew, Francis, and Justin of Canterbury 2021), and local 'green' action (Nche 2020; Mash 2021) attest.

Both these examples – of the social care-healthcare link and the health sector's environmental footprint – involve externalities, where the health sector can impact, potentially adversely, on another sector. Health sector negative externalities should be fully considered in priority setting as part of responsible stewardship in the health sector. In the case of environmental impacts, the health sector might be held to a higher standard than other sectors because it is one of the few sectors where its poor environmental record impacts directly and adversely on its future demand/workload.

Another form of negative externality is that the health sector might be seen as having a higher political priority than spending in another sector and so meeting health sector needs might 'crowd out' spending on other projects that might rank higher on non-political criteria. Just as humility should be a core underlying value in healthcare (Gill 2006), the healthcare decision-maker should be humble in their advocacy to avoid the downsides of crowding out.

More broadly, a core task of government is priority setting across sectors. In an economist's ideal, allocatively efficient world, the marginal benefit of an extra dollar of expenditure in one sector would be the same as in every other sector. This requires a fungible measure of benefit so that the gain in quality-adjusted life years from a healthcare investment can be judged against the benefit of investing in extra schooling, enhanced public security, or pensions.

We are a long way from that ideal. It is obviously possible to identify broad government social goals and assign programmes with like objectives into those clusters, for example, the OECD 11-item list: income and wealth, housing, work and job quality, health, knowledge and skills, environmental quality, subjective well-being, safety, work-life balance, social connections, and civic engagement (Organisation for Economic

Cooperation and Development 2021). However, this still leaves open the question about how to prioritise each of the clusters.

One approach – as recommended in the United Kingdom's Treasury Green Book for investment appraisal (United Kingdom. Her Majesty's Treasury 2018) – is to monetise the metrics. But this approach is fraught (Hurst 2019), requiring heroic assumptions to shoehorn everything into a money metric. How does one credibly ensure that the monetisation of outputs of projects aimed at improving 'social connections' is in any way commensurate with the monetary values of outputs designed to address 'environmental quality', for example? Although the Treasury and Finance officials' spreadsheet will have cells populated by numbers with impressive precision, able to be sorted in rank order, any ordering will be spurious with the ranking dependent on the relativities put into the ranking model and the implicit value choices of those who drive the modelling.

Monetisation will often resolve into how each sector contributes to Gross Domestic Product, incorporating all the failures of that measure, such as devaluing women's work – both in the home and in the workforce – failure to take into account environmentally damaging externalities, overvaluing risky financial transactions, and assigning zero value to anything not traded (Waring 1988, 1999, 2003, 2018; Coyle 2014; Stiglitz, Fitoussi, and Durand 2018; DeRock 2021; Prügl 2021; Mügge 2022). Such an approach cannot be reconciled with a Christian approach to resource allocation. The measurement of Gross Domestic Product must certainly be improved, with a greater emphasis placed on distributional issues as promoted by the Organisation for Economic Co-operation and Development(Stiglitz, Fitoussi, and Durand 2018).

An alternative approach is to create a new overarching measure of social welfare. The Himalayan kingdom of Bhutan is the most prominent example of this with its use of rankings based on a measure of Gross National Happiness (Musikanski 2014; Burger Araujo Santos and Dorji 2021). This measure has nine domains (standard of living, good governance, environment and access to nature, community, culture, access to education and learning, psychological health, physical health, and time balance), with scoring against twenty-six factors, with a maximum of four points on each factor.

Importantly, the Bhutanese approach is not simply a modern reaction to the weaknesses of Gross Domestic Product as the measuring stick of social progress. Almost three centuries ago the Bhutanese legal framework – which has its basis in Mahayana Buddhism – incorporated references to 'happiness' goals (Givel 2015). A lineage can be traced from those ancient ethical principles into the modern-day social calculus, contributing to the perceived legitimacy of the approach.

Another challenge to the standard budget processes is occurring in New Zealand, which implemented a 'well-being budget' in 2019 (Mintrom 2019; New Zealand Treasury 2019; Sharma 2021). This goes beyond presentational change – allocation of investments to grouped social goals – but rather involves a different budget process, with the published budget being the output. The well-being budget process is described in the official documents as involving:

> 1. Breaking down agency silos and working across government to assess, develop, and implement policies that promote well-being;
> 2. Focusing on outcomes that meet the needs of present generations at the same time as thinking about the long-term impacts for future generations; and
> 3. Tracking our progress with broader measures of success, including the health of our finances, natural resources, people, and communities. (New Zealand Treasury 2019, 5)

Even recognising that the budget documents are garnished with self-serving hyperbole, the process appears to have the elements of an appropriate whole-of-government model, which incorporates an iterative approach that recognises interactions, interdependencies, and contributions of different portfolios to common goals.

Although the New Zealand 'well-being budget' appears close to what a budget setting process based on compassion, social justice, and responsible stewardship should look like, it is too early to tell whether the New Zealand model will provide a robust example of a new approach to budgeting, and whether it can be adopted in larger jurisdictions with different cultures.

Both the Bhutanese and the New Zealand approaches are founded on consensus, acceptance of common goals, and relegating the interests of the silos to second place. In the Bhutanese case, it also involves being overt about relative weightings for the contributing measures. This transparency characterises a less formal approach to improving cross- or multi-sector priority setting, namely highlighting anomalies, quantifying where possible.

A number of different sectors have objectives about reducing deaths, for example, in the transport sector a goal of reducing road fatalities. However, the value of a statistical life used as thresholds vary significantly across sectors (Cubi-Molla et al. 2020; Cubi-Molla, Buxton, and Devlin 2021; Cubi-Molla et al. 2021) suggesting opportunities to improve allocative efficiency.

So even where a common metric does exist, it is often not used as a key basis of decision-making. A further challenge for multi-sector decision making is the reality that, in the absence of credible common measures, budget decisions rely on judgement, and particularly, the politics of the budgetary process (Wildavsky 1988). This political overlay is inevitable, and perhaps even an appropriate part of a democratic political system. Some sixty years ago, famous American political scientist, Aaron Wildavsky, identified the limits of normative budget processes, noting that

> No progress has been made [on developing normative budget processes] for the excellent reason that the task, as posed, is impossible to fulfill … [it] is utopian in the fullest sense of that word. (Wildavsky 1961)

Pace the Bhutanese and New Zealand experiences, budgeting and priority setting is the quintessential political process about who gets what and when (Lasswell 1936), so advocates of responsible stewardship may have to content themselves with seeking to assist political decision-makers by making the impacts and distributional consequences of their decisions clear (Tran, Zimmerman, and Fielding 2017), including the longer term and intergenerational consequences (Jacobs 2011). Paraphrasing American jurist Louis Brandeis (Brandeis 1914): Transparency is justly commended as a remedy to ensure responsible stewardship in multi-sector allocation decisions.

So even if there is no magic right amount that should be spent on healthcare compared to other sectors, transparency of metrics can inform whether health spending has approximated the Goldilocks position – not too much and not too little. Charlesworth and Bloor (2018, 3) suggest

> we can examine inputs (by comparing spending with other countries), processes (by examining waiting times, which might indicate demand exceeding provision), and outcomes (by analysing life expectancy over time, although this is complicated by wider determinants of health).

But they go on to conclude that

> Technical indicators of expectations, capacity, need, and demand for (health care) can inform expenditure decisions, but (the) amount of spending remains largely a matter of politics.

A Christian ethics of healthcare funding would add that the amount of spending should also be a matter of ethics and values, and consideration of the stewardship-social justice (and compassion) tension.

Holding the Tensions in Balance in Public Health and Prevention

The ethics of public health are somewhat different from the Beauchamp and Childress (2013) clinic-oriented traditional biomedical ethics – the focus of choices in public health is at the population level, with trade-offs often between different population groups – with the traditional ethical criteria being replaced by broader concerns, including of equity, liberty, and justice (Baylis, Kenny, and Sherwin 2008; Kahn and Mastroianni 2009; Faden, Bernstein, and Shebaya 2020; Scovronick et al. 2020).

Compassion calls for societies to prioritise appropriate preventive interventions. The alternative – not investing in prevention appropriately – is an abrogation of the core protection function of society and morally repugnant. But not all prevention is cost-effective (Russell 1986, 2007; McDaid, Sassi, and Merkur 2015), and so is it still morally repugnant not to prevent, whatever the cost?

Screening programmes may not be cost-effective because of 'false positives', where the test may identify that a person is at risk when in fact they are not. A screening intervention may therefore lead to unnecessary anxiety by a person identified as at risk, and to a stream of further investigations, both of which add to costs but not benefits (Russell 1994). Here there is no real conflict – uncertainty, increasing the anxiety of an individual because of false positives, is not compassionate.

The World Health Organisation's criteria for screening programmes recognised this trade-off of costs and benefits with a criterion for programmes including the need for 'economic balance of the cost of case-finding in relation to total expenditure on medical care' (Wilson, Jungner, and Organization 1968, 35) and suggested that the cost-benefit threshold should be similar to that used for other health programmes. A more recent Delphi process to develop screening program criteria also supported an emphasis on cost-effectiveness of screening programmes (Dobrow et al. 2018).

This same criterion – that preventive interventions should be just as cost-effective as any other intervention – is reasonable on stewardship grounds and, because the nature of prevention is that one is dealing with large populations, does not conflict with the Rule of Rescue. The tension with social justice is discussed below.

Where cost-effective interventions are available, both compassion and stewardship would call for implementation of preventive policies. This position is in contrast to that of Calman (2009, e8) who suggested 'Do nothing or simply monitor the current situation', as the first step on a public health intervention ladder, was the one that required the least justification. However, a non-decision is equally a decision (Bachrach and Baratz 1963), and inaction, a sin of omission, should require at least as much justification as any other decision.

Legitimate Rules or Illegitimate Impacts on Freedom?

In general, public health interventions aimed at changing taxes, laws, and regulations, often targeting the commercial determinants of health, are the most cost-effective public health and prevention interventions (Vos et al. 2010; Masters et al. 2017). The same is true for health promotion interventions: those aiming at changing structures and preconditions are more effective than health promotion efforts aimed at individual behaviour change (Swerissen and Crisp 2004). These cause no conflict with compassion, although some claim that they impinge inappropriately on liberty (Buchanan 2008; Faden, Bernstein, and Shebaya 2020), often citing philosopher John Stuart Mill's famous 'Liberty Principle':

> That the only purpose for which power can be rightfully exercised over any member of a civilized community, against his will, is to prevent harm to others. His own good, either physical or moral, is not a sufficient warrant. (Mill's 1859 essay, *On Liberty*, as reprinted in Mill (1977, 223))

The argument here is that people are, and should be, completely autonomous in their health decisions and behaviours, and distorting their choices to protect them from making 'bad choices', for example, smoking or consuming sugary drinks, is not a legitimate exercise of the role of state power. Rather than 'nudges' and taxes, health promotion strategies informed by the Liberty Principle focus on 'individual responsibility' (Brown, Maslen, and Savulescu 2019). Mill argued the individual responsibility line explicitly: 'Each is the proper guardian of his own health, whether bodily, or mental or spiritual' (Mill 1977, 226) and that 'over himself, over his own body and mind, the individual is sovereign' (Mill 1977, 224).

But the reality today is that individual choices are influenced by a range of factors, including advertising, peer pressure, availability of alternatives, and an individual's ability to weigh benefits and costs, including those which become apparent only sometime in the future. Further, health is in part generationally and genomically determined (Wolfe, Evans, and Seeman 2012; Balasooriya, Bandara, and Rohde 2021), and so not totally in one's own control, even with the best intentions. The consequences of genomic conditions are also mediated by one's environment (Bann 2021).

However, Mill recognised the importance of society and its role:

> To individuality should belong the part of life in which it is chiefly the individual that is interested; to society, the part which chiefly interests society. (Mill 1977, 276)

Mill accepted that 'everyone who receives the protection of society owes a return for the benefit' (Mill 1977, 276), and recognised a broad role for society including that children should be educated, even against their parents' wishes, as this was for the overall benefit of society (Mill 1977, 301–302).

A key economic concept, externalities, is relevant here: an externality occurs when some of the costs or benefits of an economic trade falls on someone other than the two trading parties. A polluting factory, for example, imposes costs on others who are neither involved in the production nor the consumption. Immunisation also involves an externality – being immunised both protects the immunised person and also contributes to protecting others. Although controversial, there is some evidence of externalities in income distribution – more equal societies are healthier (Wilkinson and Pickett 2010; Pickett and Wilkinson 2015; Kragten and Rözer 2017; Barnett 2020). The existence of externalities is a stewardship-based reason for supporting some public health initiatives and is another reason why immunisation is normally available without charge.

In a society where costs of ill-health are shared, the issue of negative or pecuniary externalities becomes important (Greenwald and Stiglitz 1986; Laffont 1989). These externalities can be created by individual decisions: one person's consumption of sugary drinks requires an increase in another's taxes to pay the health system costs generated by that consumption. Addressing that externality fits within the parameters of Mill's Liberty Principle as an appropriate use of state power, and is consistent with obligations of solidarity (Davies and Savulescu 2019).

Many public health interventions that might, on a naïve reading, be derided as an exercise of 'nanny state' powers – the state telling us what is in our best interest (Wiley, Berman, and Blanke 2013; Le Grand and New 2015; Magnusson and Griffiths 2015) – may instead be reframed as simply addressing externalities and market distortions (Duckett, Swerissen, and Wiltshire 2016; Lloyd and MacLaren 2019). This is particularly important for healthcare funding, as taxes on unhealthy products are increasingly being used successfully as instruments of health policy (Eykelenboom et al. 2019; Vecchio and Cavallo 2019; World Health Organization 2019; Dodd et al. 2020; Mounsey et al. 2020).

The Place of Justice in Public Health and Prevention

Public health interventions are frequently directed at the whole population – shifting and reducing the mean of the distribution of illness. The effect of this is often that the better educated and those with more social capital will follow the health messages and those under stress will not (Hernández-Quevedo and Weatherly 2015). What was designed as a positive measure for all ends up exacerbating inequality.

A Christian ethic calls us to focus on social justice in public health interventions – addressing distributional effects of messaging and targeting the most disadvantaged for additional resources and support. Public health interventions should involve shifting both the mean of the distribution (Rose 1985) and the statistical tails. Generic messaging is cheap, visible to all, and shows that the government is doing something – part of the 'political spectacle' (Edelman 1988). Messaging specific at-risk populations is difficult and more expensive. In these circumstances mainstream media may need to be supplemented by local, even face-to-face, messaging.

Public health and prevention already focus on the causes of health and disease, and so include strategies to reduce the spread of disease through personal preventive activities such as immunisation. But public health and prevention policy should also address the prior question, what are the causes of causes (Braveman, Egerter, and Williams 2011; Braveman and Gottlieb 2014; Marmot 2018)? It will lead us to put the proximate causes – often cast as individual decisions such as individual choices about food, alcohol, or drugs – into the context of an obesogenic environment, stress at work, or social isolation. These distal causes include those that lead to 'deaths of despair' – deaths from suicide, drugs, or alcohol (Case and Deaton 2020) – and the social factors that create stress and alienation. It asks us to question why some people are at risk of risks – why are some people exposed to certain risk (or protective) factors and others not (Link and Phelan 2005)?

Addressing the causes of causes will require overturning those social and economic factors such as unemployment, poor education, and racism, which shift the incidence of health to those most disadvantaged (Commission on Social Determinants of Health 2008; Raphael 2009), and those made vulnerable by social choices about the economy and the environment that create unemployment and poor living conditions. It is here that the social justice overlay inherent in a Christian ethic of healthcare funding comes to the fore, where the last are first in any policy consideration. A Christian approach to funding of public health and prevention should highlight the need for concern about the distributional effects of public health interventions and in design of policies.

Acting on social and economic determinants of health will involve working with broader coalitions outside the health sector – to advocate for and implement programmes that create jobs, ensure adequate and safe housing, overcome barriers to participation in schools and the community, and build community resilience. In government, it will involve cross sectoral collaborations of health and economic portfolios, health and social security, health and housing, and so on (McDaid and Wismar 2015), aiming to reduce the adverse impacts of the social and economic determinants on health and their consequential impact on healthcare in terms of hospital admissions for 'economy-sensitive conditions' (Colvin et al. 2020).

Stivers (2011) identified a hierarchy of Christian responses to homelessness as:

- 'Rescue and recovery', essentially a response that ameliorates the situation for the individual and sees the problem of homelessness as caused by individual behaviour, which can be addressed;
- 'Low-income home ownership', one step from an individual response, but still is about providing individual services to individuals, albeit now providing a home;
- 'Prophetic disruption assessment and response', moving towards empowerment of the homeless, and advocating a more compassionate society; and
- 'Constructive organising', building a social movement to end homelessness.

This same hierarchy might apply to prevention and public health strategies. A proximate response is the *care* response, to fix the presenting symptoms. At the next level are the personal preventive strategies – counselling, medication, or surgery to reduce obesity. But effective prevention must also engage at the two higher levels, addressing the causes of causes, empowering communities to act, and taking relevant, preventive public policy action. This involves economic policies to promote inclusive growth, taxing, and regulatory policies to affect the commercial determinants of health, and policies to address social and economic determinants of health such as social housing.

A social justice focus on causes and social, economic, and commercial determinants of health stands in stark contrast to a focus on individual responsibility in health promotion, public health, and prevention. A focus on personal choices deflects back to the individual responsibility for their own health, and deflects away from government and society responsibility to address these causes of causes (Levy 2019). Individuals of course have a responsibility to care for themselves, but it is the responsibility of society to make that easier rather than harder (Brown, Maslen, and Savulescu 2019).

Charitable and policy responses informed by a Christian ethic should ensure they balance immediate ameliorative strategies with action to ensure that the Jericho Road is a safe one, and that travellers are not exposed to risk time and time again, and that some travellers are not more likely to be at risk than others. As the Samaritan enlisted the aid of the innkeeper, so Christian organisations should be involved in broad movements to change the fundamentals, to deflect the determinants so they have less impact on individuals in need. Funding of prevention initiatives should support and encourage this broader focus.

But a social justice and community-level focus might also still recognise that there is a role in talking to individuals about their specific situation and guiding and strengthening them to address it. Although finger-wagging and victim-blaming by society is often an easy way out – avoiding societal action to address social, economic, and commercial determinants of health – this does not mean that individual responses are never to be discussed. It is still legitimate for people who are with the person in the gutter to stand alongside them in fighting broader determinants, but simultaneously taking action individually.

Jackson and her colleagues – writing from their experience in a local community health centre in Australia – advanced the concept of 'developmental casework'

> developmental case work has, as an explicit goal, the development of the individual receiving such support, and the creation of links between individual service users … By working with individuals and families on everyday survival issues, workers stay in touch with the reality of the lives of those they seek to empower. (Jackson, Mitchell, and Wright 1989, 68)

Their point is that action against broader determinants takes place on a continuum, starting with the individual afflicted by those determinants. This may involve individual counselling about obesity and their food intake, but the problem arises if action stops there and eschews any wider, preventive action: 'rescue and recovery' is not a valid endpoint.

But this form of action has more legitimacy if the counsellor/adviser looks more like the person in need, that they have been alongside them in the gutter, and they are standing as close to them in work or mission as possible. Wilson (2012) refers to this as the 'proximity principle' involving both reducing physical distance – by living in community – and working to reduce relational distance, by being an authentic part of the community (Grinnell 2021).

Holding the Tensions in Balance in Payment Policy

Payment policy is about how healthcare funding flows from those who collect taxes or premiums (governments or health insurers) to providers – doctors, hospitals, rehabilitation facilities – for care of patients and to provide preventive programmes. The ideal health system will keep the public healthy and restore people to health as efficiently as possible when they fall sick. Payment policy may be designed to encourage providers to meet these twin objectives or more commonly just the latter.

There are a limited range of options for healthcare payment, with different incentives and complexity (Quinn 2015). Total health expenditure in a community is a function of the number of people, their illnesses, and the costs of treating those illnesses. This identity can be divided in different ways to assign responsibility for managing (or not managing) the variables to either the payer or the provider/funded organisation (Miller 2009).

A classic graphical presentation arrays the payment options on a horizontal spectrum, with the vertical axis notionally portrays the level of risk borne by payers and providers (Averill et al. 2010; Frakt and Mayes 2012). The spectrum focuses on whether the payer or the provider bears the risk for specific types of inefficiency.

At one end of the spectrum is capitation payment – the funded organisation/provider gets paid a fixed amount to provide all the necessary care for a person (and their family) for a given period, typically a year. In this payment model, the funded organisation/provider bears all the risk of variations in use of care, including the exogenous epidemiological risks of incidence of disease and all the endogenous risk of variations in efficiency of service provision, including how the patient is managed clinically and in the technical efficiency of services used.

In the capitation model the payer bears neither the epidemiological nor the technical efficiency risk but does carry the risk of setting the capitation rate in a way that minimises the risk of gaming by funded organisations. By assigning management of the epidemiological risk to the funded organisation/provider, those organisations have an incentive for prevention.

At the other end of the spectrum may be cost-based reimbursement, where the payer bears all the utilisation and efficiency risk, with the provider carrying neither risk. Cost-based reimbursement is now only rarely part of any healthcare system, a recent exception being where other payment methods were over-ridden during the SARS-CoV-2 (COVID) pandemic (Quentin et al. 2020).

Fee-for-service is another typical end point of the spectrum, and, although derided as 'perhaps the single biggest obstacle to improving healthcare delivery' (Porter and Kaplan 2016, 88) is a very common payment method for physicians in many countries (Robinson 2001; Zuvekas and Cohen 2016). Under fee-for-service, responsibility for variation in use of care, including disease incidence, falls on the payer. The provider's risk is the efficiency one: that their costs are less than the fees received. Both capitation payment and fee-for-service approaches are discussed in more detail later.

There are different intermediate points on the spectrum, representing different degrees of bundling of activities: services can be aggregated daily or over other time periods, or into 'episodes' with the episode being more or less narrowly defined; for example, bundling hospital and doctor/physician payments; or bundling acute hospital and rehabilitation, or acute admissions and pre- and post-care. The broader the bundling, the more the payment option approaches capitation, the narrower the bundling, the more it has attributes of fee-for-service.

Concomitantly, the broader the bundling, the more the risk of utilisation and efficiency falls on, and thus must be managed by, the funded organisation or provider; the narrower the bundling, the more the utilisation and efficiency risk falls on the payer. In the graphical presentation the provider and payer risk curves slope in opposite directions – providers have the highest risk with capitation and the lowest with fee-for-service, the payer's risk curve is the opposite. The risk curves intersect at a happy medium, with the intersection falling at one of the bundling options.

What is significant about this common analytical frame is that only two key interests are highlighted: the payer and the provider. The consumer interest is not even on the map.

The concept of responsible stewardship, as developed in the previous chapter, supports a concern with efficiency *and* overall utilisation; the elements of the traditional payer-provider risk allocation are important. However, efficiency or stewardship within a Christian ethic of healthcare funding sits alongside, and is in tension with, both social justice and compassion.

I argued in Chapter 1 that we need to place ourselves in the position of the traveller in the gutter in the Samaritan story. The interests of the consumer cannot be ignored: a Christian ethic of healthcare funding augments the two-dimensional focus of payer versus provider risk into a three-dimensional space where the impact of the various options on the consumer or patient is part of the calculus.

Consumer interests are not homogeneous, as different consumers will experience the healthcare system differently because of their gender, race, age, location, identity, and illness among a myriad of factors. However, there are some common concerns for all consumers, albeit weighted differently by different consumers because of their circumstances, with those common concerns including the expectation of being treated with dignity, the ability to exercise choice, timeliness of care, and potential out-of-pocket payments (Duckett and Ward 2008).

Each of the options for payment has certain consumer risks to be considered alongside the payer and provider efficiency and epidemiological risks.

The Sources of Consumer Risks

The standard economic market model is one of consumer sovereignty: the consumer weighs up products on offer and exercises choice. Choice is theorised to be exercised independently and the ability to make choices is available equally to all (Gabe, Harley, and Calnan 2015). The explicit assumption of the market model is that the consumer has the information required to make such a choice. Unfortunately, that is not the market reality in healthcare. In the prototypical market it is assumed that the consumer can assess their own needs or wants and can judge all relevant attributes of the product they are buying. Neither is true in healthcare.

Information Asymmetry

The interaction between the patient and their physician or other provider is a complex one. It involves two people, 'one of whom is suffering … and the other of whom knows, knows how, and offers his assistance' (Ricoeur 2007, 213).

The health professional brings years of training and experience into the relationship, the consumer their lived experience of their own illness and their history. There is an imbalance or asymmetry in the information of the two parties: the professional may have seen dozens or even hundreds of people with similar symptoms and might have learned about the patterns of symptoms as part of their training. The consumer expects professionals to bring their knowledge into the treatment interaction, and so this information asymmetry is inherent in healthcare.

The patient-professional relationship is also one of trust: the patient needs to assume that the professional will act in the best interest of them as a patient, as their honest agent. Referrals and tests ordered are accepted on this basis. However, the patient's expectation is not always realised in practice. The professional is an imperfect agent (McGuire 2000) and may order more tests than warranted because of their risk aversion, fear of litigation, or a monetary incentive. The professional might also order more tests because of specific concerns of the patient.

If a professional has time on their hands – insufficient demand to fill up their appointment schedule – they may encourage the patient to come back for another appointment, from an overabundance of caution, or because of the income that will be generated if they are remunerated on a fee-for-service basis, or a mix of both. The additional appointment could easily be justified, but the incremental benefit may be substantially less than the cost of the visit. Additional visits generated by physicians in these circumstances are referred to in the literature as physician-induced, and the phenomenon as supplier-induced demand (Evans 1974, 2016b; Wennberg, Barnes, and Zubkoff 1982; Bickerdyke et al. 2002; Mohammadshahi et al. 2019; Callison, Kaestner, and Ward 2021).

Supplier induced demand can lead to problems of overdiagnosis – illnesses diagnosed inappropriately when no treatment is necessary – and over-ordering of tests, which also increases the risk of overdiagnosis (Welch, Schwartz, and Woloshin 2011; Moynihan, Doust, and Henry 2012; Justman 2015; Korenstein et al. 2018; Shaffer and Scherer 2018; Brownlee and Korenstein 2021; Korenstein et al. 2021). Both can impact adversely on the patient.

Information asymmetry also has implications for co-payment policy. As the Rand experiment showed, consumers react to co-payments by reducing both effective and ineffective care – 'potentially valuable care e.g., preventive services and potentially wasteful care e.g., imaging services' (Brot-Goldberg et al. 2017) – an unsurprising response because a consumer cannot be expected to have the knowledge to make the same judgements as a professional about what is valuable or not; people also make mistakes in their valuation of the benefits of healthcare, what Baicker, Mullainathan, and Schwartzstein (2015) refer to as behavioural hazard.

Access to the Internet has reduced information asymmetry to some extent, but not all websites purvey up-to-date evidence-based information (Daraz et al. 2019; Valizadeh-Haghi et al. 2021), nor are all patients internet users. Further the Internet cannot undertake the same physical examinations as a professional so even a well-informed consumer will still not have the same knowledge as their provider. Consumers value on-line sources of information but as a complement, not an alternative to a medical practitioner (Farnood, Johnston, and Mair 2020; Stevenson et al. 2021).

Incomplete Information and Product Definition

The economist's ideal market involves the complete specification of a product being purchased: the consumer knows the price in advance and can assess all relevant aspects of the product – colour, weight, speed, etc. This is not the case in healthcare where important aspects of the 'product' may not be known in advance – for example, whether this specific patient will be treated with dignity – and may not be knowable, for example, aspects of quality may not be measurable using contemporary techniques. Even when quality is measurable, the information may not be specific to this provider, or, where it is measured, the results may not be disclosed to the consumer or the provider.

In the healthcare market, the patient may therefore be called on to make a choice with inadequate or incomplete information, most commonly incomplete information about quality. Nobel prizes in economics have been awarded because of contributions to this vexed problem of how to deal with inadequate and incomplete information.

Oliver Williamson, awarded the prize in 2009, studied the attributes of transactions and the situations when it made sense for firms/organisations to purchase supplies in a market, and when it made sense for the firm to produce the needed supply internally, a choice characterised as markets or hierarchies (Williamson 1986, 1975, 2002). The relevant factors included how specific the product was to the firm, and how well the product could be specified.

Oliver Hart, awarded the prize in 2016, contributed to the understanding of 'incomplete contracts' – situations where the contract between purchaser and provider could not specify all the relevant elements, including the situation where the quality of the product cannot be fully specified (Hart 2003; Hart and Moore 1999, 2007). Again, in these circumstances, the conditions for a market to yield the best outcome for the purchaser may not apply as they cannot be fully sure of what they are purchasing.

In an ordinary market there is an assumption that the product is of a standard quality. One risk of poor product specification in healthcare is that the provider can redefine aspects of the product to respond to efficiency or other pressures. For example, in response to pressure to manage length of stay, a hospital might redefine when a patient is ready to be discharged and lead to discharging patients too early, 'quicker and sicker' discharge (Kosecoff et al. 1990), thus shifting costs onto carers at home, most commonly women, or increasing readmission risk. A Swedish study of ambulance privatisation showed that private ambulances cost less than public provision in terms of cost per hour. However, probably because the contracts' poorly specified quality (e.g. competence of staff to be employed), the three year mortality rate was higher for people seen by a private compared to a public ambulance (Knutsson and Tyrefors 2022 (in press)).

The theoretical advances of Williamson and Hart are probably insufficiently applied to real-world contract and market design, and so policymakers should be sceptical about how healthcare markets function and assume the healthcare market is awash with market failure, a case of *caveat emptor*, or perhaps, more accurately, *cave mercatus*.

The Types of Payment

There are a variety of payment options for healthcare and an extensive literature that summarises their strengths and weaknesses (Jegers et al. 2002; Miller 2009; Quinn 2015; Heider and Mang 2020) and in this section I will consider three: capitation, episode payments, and fee-for-service. Although not strictly speaking payment methods, I will also consider global budgets and 'value-based *payments*' and the quest to pay for consumer-relevant outcomes.

Capitation or 'Population-Based' Payment

Payment to look after a patient holistically for a reasonable time period creates an incentive on the funded organisation to keep an eye on prevention, and also an eye on ensuring a whole episode of illness is managed efficiently (Miller 2009). Known as capitation, it is a payment for each person's healthcare needs for the coverage period.

The payer makes a risk-adjusted payment – a payment that varies according to the age, gender, and other relevant social factors of the person covered (Ellis, Martins, and Rose 2018) – to the organisation. All the risk of utilisation and efficiency of provision falls on the funded organisation, including the risk of provision of unnecessary or 'low-value' care (James and Poulsen 2016). This method of payment is widely used in United States, originally associated with 'health maintenance organisations', the title alluding to the prevention objective, but it is also common in Europe.

Capitation or population payments can be made to organisations with a defined geographic catchment with all residents automatically assigned to the organisation, or alternatively, people can opt into the capitated organisation in a competitive marketplace. The former model is more common in public systems, with the term 'population funding' used; and the latter in systems with a strong private orientation such as the United States, where it is more commonly referred to as capitation. In either case, the payer needs to develop a risk-adjusted formula, a non-trivial task that has spawned a vast literature (Ellis et al. 1996; Van de Ven et al. 2007; Van de Ven 2011; Iezzoni 2013; Juhnke, Bethge, and Mühlbacher 2016).

The most common capitation period in the competitive model is one year, and at the end of each year people can elect to change providers; this is designed to mitigate the risk that the provider will skimp on service provision or provide a narrow range of potential providers limiting consumer choice (Mazurenko, Taylor, and Menachemi 2022), risking exits if they do. Of course, the providers may want some people to exit – especially high-cost consumers for whom they are inadequately compensated under the risk-adjusted formula.

Area-based capitation in publicly funded systems is slightly more complex as it not only has to address fairness in terms of who is covered by the capitated organisation, but consideration must be given as to fairness for what: is the capitated organisation to be compensated so people covered can have equal access to care for equal need (horizontal equity), or the stronger conception of unequal access to achieve equal health outcomes (vertical equity)? The different conceptions of need will lead to different distributions of resources and the relative emphasis on the different objectives may shift over time (Asthana and Gibson 2020).

Consumer risks with capitation payment include under-provision: providers may manage their costs by not providing sufficient care (Rich et al. 2013), and/or making it difficult for consumers to access care by limiting the outlets where care covered by the package or plan may be obtained (Porter and Kaplan 2016; Mazurenko, Taylor, and Menachemi 2022).

Unscrupulous plan providers might also attempt to game the payment arrangements in competitive markets by using additional information on potential clients to ensure their enrolment profile is, on average, healthier within each risk stratification of the payment model, a process known as risk selection or cream skimming (Fioretti and Wang 2019), or to inflate diagnoses artificially where they affect risk stratification (Porter and Kaplan 2016; Geruso and Layton 2020; Chernew et al. 2021).

Models where all patients who live in a geographic area are assigned to a provider cannot use plan switching as a risk mitigation strategy, and if out of area services are also constrained, then the consumer risk from under provision can only be managed with effective consumer complaint mechanisms ('voice') or linked to political action (Hirschman 1970).

Episode Payments

The most common type of episode payment is for hospital care. As discussed in the previous chapter, the DRGs classification system was developed in the United States by Fetter and Thompson (Fetter, Brand, and Gamache

1991) and involved bundling services provided within a hospital stay into a single category, where the category is defined based on the diagnosis of the patient and any procedures performed. Services for which separate fees might have previously been paid – days of stay, tests performed, medications provided – are all bundled into a single category, the treated patient. Classifications have now been developed for other aspects of healthcare such as mental healthcare (Jacobs et al. 2019; Tran et al. 2019), emergency departments (Zaerpour et al. 2020), and palliative care (Guo et al. 2018).

When used in payment, normally there is no additional payment to the hospital for a longer length of stay or additional tests, and so the hospital has an incentive to manage all the inputs into care. There have been few rigorous evaluations of implementations of activity-based funding (Valentelyte, Keegan, and Sørensen 2021), but nevertheless DRGs are now widely used for payment for hospital inpatient care (Kimberly, de Pouvourville, and D'Aunno 2008; Busse et al. 2011).

A downside for consumers is that, as mentioned above, if a hospital has strong incentives for efficiency, it may respond perversely by changing the definition of when treatment has concluded and thus shift costs to the consumer or their family with early discharge. Pressure for speedy discharge may also affect the time that staff have to care for patients. If separate payments are made for rehabilitation, then there is a further incentive on the hospital responsible for the acute phase of treatment to 'unbundle' care into an acute episode and a rehabilitation episode, each attracting separate payments. Such post-acute services increase in many implementations of activity-based funding (Palmer et al. 2014).

Payers have responded to this unbundling by proposing re-bundling episodes of care into larger bundles, in this example, bundling the acute and the rehabilitation components of a single episode of treatment. Broader bundles facilitate continuity of care and manage the appropriate site of care, be it an acute ward or a rehabilitation unit. Broader bundling, to achieve both improved continuity and efficiency, is behind a number of contemporary reform strategies (Embuldeniya, Gutberg, and Wodchis 2021), including 'accountable care organisations' in the United States (Michael Wilson et al. 2020), which may also bundle hospital and physician costs (Porter and Kaplan 2016).

A downside for consumers of broader bundling is a reduction in choice – for example, consumers can no longer choose whether to go to a specific rehabilitation provider – and care bundling may reduce the likelihood of the acute organisation to refer to separate, specialist, providers in the interest of maintaining the full payment for the total episode.

Because providers are paid for each hospital admission, activity-based funding, unless managed with activity caps, creates an incentive for more hospital admissions. Unlike capitation or population funding, the hospital funded for activity has no incentive to reduce admissions and no financial incentive to invest in prevention. A common response to this criticism is to attempt to shift healthcare funding 'from volume to value', a strategy discussed further below.

Episode bundling can also be used outside hospital settings. It is possible, although unusual, to bundle care in the community into, say, a single payment for managing a patient with diabetes or mental illness. These implementations exhibit some of the characteristics and downsides of capitation models unless there is good outcome measurement as part of the implementation (Volmink et al. 2014).

Fee-for-Service Payment

Fee-for-service payment involves the provider billing the payer for each 'service' – an operation or other procedure, a laboratory test, or a visit for advice, counselling, or other treatment. Fee-for-service systems typically involve a fee schedule of thousands of items, including a mix of procedural and time-based items. Typically fee-for-service schedules over-reward procedural items relative to consultations (Hsiao et al. 1988; Ginsburg and Berenson 2007).

Fee-for-service is the quintessential 'professional' payment model: the professional establishes a one-to-one relationship with the client/patient, and there is a veneer of accountability of the professional to the patient. Assuming a functioning healthcare market – a questionable assumption as I have shown above – the consumer can change providers if unsatisfied with the care they receive or the responsiveness of the professional. In fact the professional model harks back to a yesteryear long past. Increasingly, the professional is part of a wider corporation – structured as a group practice or a commercial provider – and payment is not from the patient's pocket but from a third-party payer, either government or private insurer. The patient usually has little objective information on which to judge the relative merit of professionals and so choice is often illusory.

Fee-for-service payment assumes that each visit to the doctor or other professional is independent, and so the payment should logically be independent. With increasing prevalence of chronic disease, what is needed is continuity of care, with payment reflecting that. There is no financial incentive under fee-for-service for the professional/funded organisation to manage the number of visits or to emphasise prevention in each visit. Because professionals are paid for each separate interaction, they have an incentive to unbundle care – only deal with one problem at each visit and encourage the consumer to return to have second and subsequent problems dealt with. It suffers the same activity-increasing risks as episode payment, but with limited options to cap expenditure (see discussion on capping below).

To the extent the provider feels accountable and responsive to the patient, this is a consumer-oriented system, subject to the issues of continuity and unbundling referred to above, and the imperfections of the market, such as information asymmetry and weak effective choice.

Global Budgets

Some jurisdictions have maintained global budgets for hospitals and for some other providers. Under this model, a budget is set for each provider – based on history, politics, or some combination of those and other factors – and the provider is expected to manage within that budget.

Typically providers have a high degree of flexibility to facilitate budget management. Increases in demand for services typically result in pressure to increase the global budget and so the payer bears at least part of the utilisation risk. Efficiency risk is also borne by the payer, as the budgets are not set using DRGs or other activity measures and so hospitals funded under a global budget are probably less efficient than activity-based funded hospitals. As a result either the overall system will be more expensive – to the detriment of payers or taxpayers – or costs will be constrained by reducing access, to the detriment of consumers.

Value-Based Care and Paying for Outcomes

The ideal payment system would reward improvement in the patient's condition – payment for outcomes. The elements can be easily described: measure what patients want, and reward providers for meeting patients' concerns.

Originally termed value-based competition, reflecting the United States origins of the concept, the idea is that having organisations compete to meet patient needs would be in the patient's interest (Porter and Teisberg 2004, 2006). Overdiagnosis would also be a thing of the past: a focus on value would mean that low-value care would be eliminated, as patients would not want to pay for these medications or procedures. Although simple to describe, and despite innumerable conferences and consultancies, the idea has foundered in practice, and even more than a decade after the ideas first circulated, value-based care is still at the 'lessons learned' stage (Crook et al. 2021a, 2021b), with the very definition of 'value in healthcare' subject to multiple interpretations and definitions (Landon, Padikkala, and Horwitz 2021).

Good work has been done on how to measure what patients want with the development of so-called patient-reported outcome measures or PROMs (Maynard and Bloor 2010; Black 2013). Designing and implementing systems to measure improvement in outcomes is a non-trivial task, and, analogous to the observer effect in quantum mechanics, measurement has the potential to change what is measured (Mitchell, Cribb, and Entwistle 2021).

In England, PROMs were initially implemented as before and after measures for a handful of procedures. Between the design and execution, however, there was a large gap and the initial enthusiasm has waned, partly because of problems of patient heterogeneity, and partly because of technical problems of design (Boyce and Browne 2013; Tanenbaum 2016; Prodinger and Taylor 2018; Field, Holmes, and Newell 2019). Alternative, goal-based measures, may overcome some of these weaknesses (Giovannetti et al. 2021).

However, value-based healthcare does have a significant upside for consumers: it reorients the system to focus on what is important to them, and ask what their goals of treatment are. It focuses on measuring progress against those goals (Duckett 2019). This consumer focus may be able to be achieved, however, whether or not an attempt is made to use 'value-based payment' as the motivator of value-based healthcare.

Risk Mitigation and 'Adjunct Incentives'

No payment method is perfect, and indeed it should not be expected to be so. Even if perfectly designed – and there is no guarantee of that – policy implementation is critical and can be thwarted by local action (Pressman and Wildavsky 1973), poorly specified goals about what is to be achieved, and poor support to ensure that the implementation achieves the goal rather than is a 'quick fix', which unwinds shortly thereafter (Palmer et al. 2018a, 2018b, 2018c; Li et al. 2020).

Further, even well-designed implementations with clear goals may face hurdles. Policymakers generally pursue objectives about efficiency, quality, and access simultaneously, but policy instruments can generally only optimise one policy objective at a time and multiple policy objectives require multiple policy instruments (Tinbergen 1952).

Policymakers land on one payment strategy – capitation, episode payment, or fee-for-service – and obviously achieve the benefits of that strategy. But they should be aware of the risks of that strategy and take steps to minimise those risks and, if possible, achieve the benefit of the forgone payment strategy (Johnson 1996). Policymakers have multiple policy levers at their disposal, and funding and pricing policies are usually implemented with regulatory interventions and the provision of comparative information alongside the new funding policy.

Sometimes policymakers will use two different approaches to paying providers: capitation and fee-for-service, for example – so called blended payment (Robinson 2001) – as a way to harness the benefits of both approaches.

Pay-for-Performance

Increasingly the primary pricing incentive, capitation for example, is also accompanied by secondary pricing incentives, 'pay-for-performance', either to address additional 'adjunct' goals – most commonly quality or timeliness of care – or to mitigate design risks inherent in the payment system (Duckett 2008b).

Activity-based funding carries an inherent risk that providers might skimp on quality to improve recorded 'efficiency', even though the efficiency improvement is notional, redefining the product. In addition to evidence-based governance strategies to encourage quality improvement (Donabedian 2002; Langley et al. 2009; Tello, Barbazza, and Waddell 2020), payers mitigate this risk by supplementing the activity payment with additional payments against additional metrics. Importantly, pay-for-performance is described here as a *supplement*: the base payment needs to be adequate for everyone and the supplement is an add-on, to reward superior performance on the relevant dimension (Cattel and Eijkenaar 2020; Cattel, Eijkenaar, and Schut 2020), but many pay-for-performance implementations involve, at least in part, a reduction of base funding rather than a supplement. Pay-for-performance comes in many different forms with different objectives, including paying for additional information provision, paying for adherence to standards, or paying for meeting a particular quality threshold or quality improvement (Siciliani et al. 2021).

There is now an extensive literature about pay-for-performance and an array of potential pay-for-performance designs (Pope 2011; Conrad 2015), with the net impact of a specific implementation the result of the interplay of several factors, including gaming, target and reward setting, and health-increasing and health-decreasing substitutions (Friedman and Scheffler 2016). Perverse responses – including gaming (Carter, Newhouse, and Relles 1990; Rosenberg, Fryback, and Katz 2000; Bevan and Hood 2006; Steinbusch et al. 2007; Berta et al. 2010; Mannion and Braithwaite 2012;

Georgescu and Hartmann 2013) – may be mitigated with regulatory strategies including monitoring, and penalties.

Although intuitively and theoretically sound, in practice pay-for-performance implementations – especially those that focus on changing a single provider type (hospital or primary care) or specialty – have generally not lived up to the expectations and rhetoric (Tanenbaum 2009; Cromwell et al. 2011; Gillam, Siriwardena, and Steel 2012; Papanicolas 2012; Eijkenaar et al. 2013; Milstein and Schreyoegg 2016; Ogundeji, Bland, and Sheldon 2016; Markovitz and Ryan 2017; Mendelson et al. 2017; Yuan et al. 2017; Scott, Liu, and Yong 2018; Cattel and Eijkenaar 2020; Singh, Kovacs et al. 2021; Zaresani and Scott 2021). Song's summary of the state of evidence about 'accountable care' in the United States can equally apply to pay-for-performance

> Today, a verdict on payment reform resembles less the fork in the road between success or failure and more a work-in progress that has improved the value of care in some situations but needs refinement. (Song 2021, 574)

Unfortunately pay-for-performance, especially when poorly designed, can weaken intrinsic motivation of health professionals (Rosenbaum 2022a, 2022b, 2022c), and create perverse incentives as evidenced in both the mid-Staffordshire scandal in England (Francis 2013b) and the Bundaberg Hospital scandal in Queensland, Australia (Thomas 2007), and crowd out intrinsic professional motivation. However, well-designed performance monitoring and pay-for-performance can help to ensure that organisations pay appropriate attention to their processes and outcomes (Young and Conrad 2007; Conrad 2009; Smith et al. 2009), particularly as they impact on the most disadvantaged. Broader implementations – focusing on multidisciplinary provider groups – appear to have had more success, although this conclusion is based solely on implementations in the United States (Vlaanderen et al. 2019).

This is not to say that pay-for-performance is not worthwhile, but it is and should always be considered as part of payment design, mostly to ensure responsible stewardship. The cost of including a pay-for-performance component is often modest, especially where the cost of the ostensible reward is taken from the base payment. In these circumstances, pay-for-performance simply leads to a slightly different distribution of a capped budget. Pay-for-performance incentives serve a political and rhetorical purpose signalling that the payer values the metric rewarded and directing providers – who could be expected to respond to incentives at the margin – to pay attention to this metric too.

Applying the Three Principles to Payment Policy

A well-designed healthcare payment system will hold in tension all three of the underlying principles I have shown are fundamental to a Christian ethic of healthcare funding. The primary goal should always be about why care is being provided, derived from the compassion principle; the stewardship-related element should be a constraint on how care is provided, with the payment policy perhaps phrased as being about 'providing equitable care efficiently', rather than simply to drive efficiency.

A Christian ethic should always attempt to have all three principles at the forefront, not just one. It is too easy for funding policy to forget compassion, and de-emphasise equity, in pursuit of savings and efficiency targets. Stewardship should be considered as but one of a trinity of goals, alongside compassion and social justice.

As I argued above, payment policy will not simply involve a single pricing instrument but will require a combination of pricing and pay-for-performance. In this section, I will outline the key elements of how a Christian ethic of healthcare payment might inform funding design for three quite different types of care: primary care, dental care, and acute inpatient care.

Table 5.1 summarises the potential approaches to funding informed by a Christian ethic and incorporates consideration of compassion, social justice, and stewardship. Unlike common secular funding approaches, it does not start with efficiency or stewardship, but rather with compassion: compassion informs both the goal of the funding model and critical aspects of it.

A Christian ethic of healthcare funding is founded on assumptions about the dignity of all people: a compassionate society should aim to help all people in need. Funding models should promote and enhance the compassion of individual professionals and ensure their intrinsic motivation is not undermined (Friedman and Scheffler 2016).

Common to all three types of care is that care must be accessible and available to all. As discussed in Chapter 3, the evidence about out-of-pocket payments is clear: they inhibit use by the most disadvantaged and may be inefficient; they are not consistent with a principle of social justice and should be eschewed.

Primary Care

Both compassion and stewardship lead to blended payment to effect the twin goals for primary care identified in the table. There is an increasing prevalence of chronic disease in all countries and so the fee-for-service

Table 5.1 *Healthcare funding model as informed by a Christian ethic*

	Primary care	Dental care	Acute inpatient care
	Goals: • Manage acute presentations • Manage care of people with chronic illness, including ensuring care continuity	*Goals:* • Promote good oral health • Manage primary dental care needs	*Goals:* • Restore people to function
Compassion (access to high-quality services)	• Universal programme for access to holistic primary care • Pay-for-performance	• Universal programme for access to preventive dental care and oral health promotion • Universal programme for access to necessary dental care	• Universal programme for access to hospital care • Activity-based funding base rates need to be adequate for quality care • Pay-for-performance
Social justice (no financial barriers to access)	• No out-of-pocket payments • Social prescribing	No out-of-pocket payments	No out-of-pocket payments
Stewardship (responsible use of resources)	• Capitation and fee-for-service • Pay-for-performance	• Fee-for-service • Monitoring and pay-for-performance	Activity-based funding with caps

Source: Author's analysis.

funding model, based on its assumption of a sequence of independent visits, can no longer be the sole funding approach. Capitation, which rewards continuity, is the alternative starting point. However, managing chronic illness is not all that primary care does and so a blended approach, incorporating fee-for-service and capitation, with the former rewarding responsiveness for acute presentations and the latter continuity of care, is appropriate.

Responsible stewardship leads to incorporating pay-for-performance elements into primary care payment policy. Capitation involves patient enrolment with the practice and it then becomes possible to design incentives for personal prevention (e.g. screening and immunisation), monitoring patients' health, and reducing hospitalisations for conditions that could be prevented, so-called ambulatory-sensitive conditions or potentially preventable hospitalisations (Bindman et al. 1995; Ansari 2007; Rosano et al. 2013; Sundmacher et al. 2015; Busby, Purdy, and Hollingworth 2017; Sheryl Davies et al. 2017). There are a variety of approaches to patient enrolment funding, including whether enrolment is voluntary or not, and from enrolment payments being a small proportion of practice income to practices' main source of income being capitation payments (Marchildon et al. 2021).

Incentives can also be introduced to ensure high-quality practice – through practice accreditation and rewarding participation in quality improvement activities (Lester and Roland 2009) – and to ensure practices are geographically accessible (Wilson et al. 2009). Pay-for-performance incentives can also be used to reward desirable attributes of practice, and aspects of the patient experience (Marc N Elliott et al. 2016; Papanicolas et al. 2017). Capitation payment rates need to be set with an eye on social justice: to ensure that payment rates and risk adjustment do not discourage providers caring for people suffering social disadvantage.

As discussed earlier, a downside risk of capitation is under-provision. There are two risk mitigation strategies for this. Firstly, allow people to change their capitated provider: the time interval for this needs to be sufficiently frequent to ensure people are not locked in, but not too frequently so the benefits of capitation do not accrue. Most capitation policies involve annual re-enrolment. The second risk mitigation strategy involves monitoring: surveying patients regularly to assess their experience with providers and making this information public (Faber et al. 2009; Campanella et al. 2016).

Payment policy needs to ensure that addressing the social and economic determinants of health is part of clinical encounters. This includes encouraging – perhaps with financial incentives – documentation of social impacts in patient histories (Browne-Yung et al. 2019; Drake et al. 2021), and setting the scene for broadening the focus of the patient-professional encounter by incorporating the importance of upstream determinants in health professional education (Metzl and Hansen 2014; Castillo et al. 2020; Burson, Familusi, and Clapp 2021; Harvey et al. 2022). Social prescribing – linking patients to non-medical services – is an evolving strategy to help redress some social determinants, albeit with a weak evidence base (Alderwick et al. 2018; Chatterjee et al. 2018; Pescheny, Randhawa, and Pappas 2019) and requiring further policy development to determine the best funding approaches (Sandhu, Alderwick, and Gottlieb 2022 (in press)). Nevertheless has the potential to be incorporated in service design.

The critical contribution of a Christian ethic of healthcare funding is the emphasis on social justice – of no out-of-pocket payments – and compassion. Compassion should particularly inform the design of the pay-for-performance component of any blended payment so that continuity of care is rewarded and that there are no perverse incentives at play that impinge on the intrinsic motivation of healthcare professionals.

In addition, responsible stewardship would lead to a payment policy for healthcare that encourages the centrality of primary care, including strengthening the role of primary care in gatekeeping access to secondary care (Starfield 1992; Starfield, Shi, and Macinko 2005; Garrido, Zentner, and Busse 2011; Reibling and Wendt 2012; Sripa et al. 2019). Reducing unnecessary hospital admissions is both better for the patient and for the healthcare budget.

Dental Care

Dental care is an oft neglected part of healthcare, as if the mouth were disconnected from the rest of the body. Poor access to dental care can lead to poor physical health (Glurich and Acharya 2019), and also impacts on the social determinants of health, including employment (Halasa-Rappel et al. 2019).

Dental funding policy should incorporate two objectives: one about prevention, and one recognising that restorative treatment will sometimes be necessary (see Table 5.1).

Preventive care is an essential component of good dental care, and this may require specific attention in the design of dental care funding. But dental policy also needs to emphasise dental health education in the community (Fraihat et al. 2019), and strategies to prevent dental disease, such as fluoridation (Yeung 2008; Ran and Chattopadhyay 2016; Do et al. 2017; Spencer, Do, and Ha 2018), and pricing incentives to reduce consumption of sugary drinks (Allcott, Lockwood, and Taubinsky 2019; Teng et al. 2019; Dodd et al. 2020; Thow et al. 2022).

Funding design for dental *care* needs to balance compassion and social justice – ensuring all have access to care – and stewardship. The stewardship challenge relates to provider-side moral hazard – that uncapped fee-for-service creates perverse incentives which discourage prevention or conservative treatment – and that dental care and treatment includes both urgent restorative care and relief of pain and care for aesthetic reasons. Compassion and justice require the former to be accessible for all, stewardship would point to the latter not being publicly funded.

The need to distinguish care which is 'necessary' and that which is not has led to the quest to determine a list of 'essential' oral healthcare, paralleling lists for 'essential' drugs and healthcare generally. Morris, White, and Bradnock (2012, 96) have defined 'primary dental care as

> a service to the local community which provides the first point of access for advice and any necessary dental treatment and takes responsibility for assisting patients with oral health maintenance including recall for examination and co-ordination of dental treatment provided by other services.

Typically, national essential lists include care for the treatment of pain and preventive care.

Both major payments options – capitation and fee-for-service – have been proposed for dental care and both have strengths and weaknesses. Because the average number of dental visits per person per annum is low, and the distribution wide, capitation funding has a high selection risk, both for adverse selection for capitated organisations and deliberate strategies by providers to avoid high-need individuals ('cream skimming'), creating a funding risk for funders. Fee-for-service potentially creates an overservicing risk for funders.

The risk of fee-for-service can be mitigated by good monitoring and pay-for-performance strategies to minimise the risk of overservicing and encourage minimal intervention dentistry (Innes and Schwendicke 2017; Duckett, Cowgill, and Swerissen 2019; Laske et al. 2019).

Monitoring strategies should include obtaining feedback from patients on their experience of care and the outcomes of their care; monitoring adherence to evidence-based protocols, including risk and severity screening tools (Martin, Mills, and Foley 2018), for managing standard conditions in a cost-effective way (Warren et al. 2010; Warren et al. 2016); and requiring participation in quality improvement and utilisation review programmes (Byrne et al. 2019).

Acute Inpatient Care

Activity-based funding is now the most common approach to funding acute inpatient care, and appropriately so. The systems to describe hospital activity are now well developed and there is a rich literature on different implementations and their consequences (Kimberly and de Pouvourville 1993; Kimberly, de Pouvourville, and D'Aunno 2008; Busse et al. 2011; Palmer et al. 2014).

An issue in contemporary policy contention is the extent of bundling. Responsible stewardship would point to broader bundles – that physician and hospital payment should be bundled, and pre- and post-care bundled as well. The broader the bundles, the more that inefficient variations in physician services or post-acute care will be managed by the payee. There are technical complexities associated with funding bundles: episode design should lead to reasonably homogeneous bundles and, at least in the early stages of bundling implementation, this may not be the case. This increases the risk that payments may be unfair – that providers might not be paid appropriately for reasons outside their control, such as aberrant case-mix, potentially compromising quality of patient care.

Activity-based funding encourages additional activity, some of which may be of questionable value. Uncapped funding of hospital care is almost certain to crowd out expenditure on care of higher value outside the hospital or investments in other public sector services. In an era of flat of the curve medicine, the incremental benefit of additional hospital activity may be below the incremental cost and so adopting a principle of responsible stewardship would involve activity caps in activity-based funding. There are several ways to manage funding caps, but all involve negotiating volume caps or targets for each institution or group of institutions with above cap activity either not paid for or paid for at a lower rate. A common approach is to establish two thresholds, after the first additional activity is paid for at a discounted rate – potentially marginal cost – and after the second threshold, no payment at all. Funded services then must prioritise which patients are admitted. However, not all implementations of activity-based funding incorporate capping – the United States being the most obvious counter example.

Capped funding systems often have pay-for-performance elements to mitigate the key downside of capping, longer waiting times. Typically pay-for-performance includes incentives or penalties on services to ensure patients are admitted within specified times for elective procedures or managed within a specified time for emergencies (Street and Duckett 1996). Pay-for-performance needs to be structured carefully to avoid perverse, gaming responses, and an inappropriate focus only on that which is measured and rewarded, as Campbell's (Campbell 1979) and Goodhart's (Goodhart 1975, 5; Strathern 1997) laws warn. Capping is normally accompanied by standardised prioritisation systems to ensure equity in admission priority (Noseworthy et al. 2003; Curtis et al. 2010; Chan et al. 2016), and clinical agreement about what potential admissions are a low priority where the admission may not be justified (Elshaug et al. 2012).

Even in countries with capping of hospital activity, low or no value care is still provided (Badgery-Parker et al. 2019; Badgery-Parker, Pearson, and Elshaug 2020). In addition to nudges directed at clinicians, information and benchmarking strategies to discourage low value care (Cliff et al. 2021), and indicators of a hospital's propensity to admit care of low value, could be included in pay-for-performance metrics.

If capping is introduced fairly and waiting times are managed, capping principally results in reduction of low or lesser value care and will not conflict with either the compassion principle or social justice.

One special case where care should not be capped – either inpatient or in the community – is palliative care. Especially here compassion should come to the fore and people should have the services necessary to facilitate a good death (Duckett 2018a). Further, early access to palliative care, in addition to being life extending (Temel et al. 2010), also reduces non-beneficial health service utilisation in the last weeks of life (Khandelwal et al. 2015; May et al. 2017; Scheerens et al. 2020). Uncapping palliative care is consistent with a focus on stewardship as, in fact, palliative care will be only nominally uncapped as service access is effectively limited to those near death, which thus provides a natural cap.

Conclusion

A Christian ethic of healthcare funding adds a focus on compassion and social justice to the consideration of funding principles. As was argued in Chapter 2, a focus on efficiency and austerity can go too far – staff may not have the time to provide the interactions and care they are motivated to do. Adequate funding – needed to provide compassionate care – may in any event contribute to reduced readmissions or a quicker healing process and so be cost-effective.

Taken together, a Christian ethic of healthcare funding provides a different lens for the design of healthcare funding. In most countries, governments can be relied upon to focus on stewardship – although not necessarily with the consideration of distributional cost-effectiveness and the Rule of Rescue that the Christian conception of stewardship involves. The argument here is that authentic progress on funding reform is not simply about improving allocative efficiency or indeed social justice, all three goals need to be front and centre of policy and policy change, and policy reform should push the boundaries on all three dimensions simultaneously.

This chapter started with the person in the gutter by the wayside – reminding us that policy should focus on those in need. What is distinctive about a Christian ethic of healthcare funding is the contribution of compassion and social justice to inform all aspects of policy. Stewardship or economic efficiency without this focus on compassion and social justice is not consistent with treating *all* people with justice and dignity that we are called to do:

> And what does the Lord require of you?
> To act justly and to love mercy, and to walk humbly with your God (Micah 6:8).

CHAPTER 6

Envoi

> Then Jesus said to him, 'Go and constantly do the same.' (Luke 10:36–37; Amplified Bible translation)

Healthcare funding policy is a moral project – it is about trying to make things better, and better for everyone (Sanders 2021). Unfortunately, the moral basis, and moral direction for policy, is rarely made explicit, and, of course, there are competing moral foundations. I have argued that a Christian ethic of healthcare funding involves simultaneously facilitating and being founded on compassion, social justice, and stewardship. No one principle is pre-eminent.

In Chapter 1, I showed that these three principles are central to the parable of the 'Good' Samaritan, and this informed the explication of the three principles in Chapters 2, 3, and 4. In Chapter 5, I demonstrated application of the three principles. In this chapter, I returned briefly to another concern expressed in Chapter 1 – does a Christian perspective have a place in what is essentially a post-Christian society? My answer in Chapter 1 was twofold: Christians are called to participate in living and advocating the realm of God, and Christians working in modern healthcare systems may be struggling with the very issues I canvass.

Although there are many different approaches to public theology (Graham 2013), it is about

> addressing issues of public concern, urgency, and import to a religiously pluralistic and diverse audience of fellow members of a civic community in a way that is accessible to people of any or no faith tradition or commitment while rooted in and inspired by one's own faith perspective, commitments, and beliefs. (Massingale 2016, 352)

What I have advanced here is a work of public theology in that definition – Massingale specifically includes the parable of the 'Good' Samaritan as being 'accessible to people of any or no faith tradition or commitment' (page 354); Leget (2015) has a similar view describing the parable as the 'western role model of compassion par excellence' (Leget 2015, 677). Stone, writing about the parable, suggests that

> The story is so familiar, almost a universal folktale, that many people don't know its original context in the Christian Bible. (Stone 2008, 33)

The language of the three principles – compassion, social justice, and stewardship – is also shared between church and secular communities.

Carol Gilligan started her ground-breaking study of the way women's psychological development had been perceived, with this observation:

> Over the past 10 years, I have been listening to people talking about morality and about themselves. Halfway through that time, I began to hear a distinction in these voices, two ways of speaking about moral problems, two modes of describing the relationship between other and self. (Gilligan 1982, 1)

In a way, public theology should be doing the same: presenting a different voice in the public square, certainly a different way of thinking about moral problems and the relationship of I, Other-I, and the world, but with a language and a voice that resonates with all listeners.

Distinguished public policy theorist Aaron Wildavsky entitled one of his books *Speaking Truth to Power: The Art and Craft of Policy Analysis* (Wildavsky 1979), the first part of the title is a term first used by Quakers (American Friends Service Committee 1955). If public policy analysis is about speaking truth to power, so too is public theology, as it has been from earliest times (Graham 2013, Chapter 6). But public theology is also about speaking truth to everyone, and giving a voice to the voiceless, facilitating the voiceless to exercise their own voice in public policy debates.

Part of the work of the public theologian is to change the public discourse: to call out injustice, to emphasise where policies impinge on human dignity, or undermine social solidarity and fellowship. This may be done in 'big discourse' – in the public square – or in little discourse, in day-to-day encounters. Former Archbishop of Canterbury, William Temple, argued that 'Nine-tenths of the work of the church in the world is done by Christian people fulfilling responsibilities and performing tasks which in themselves are not part of the official system of the church at all' (Temple 1950/1976, 39).

The three principles I have advanced are particularly relevant to that 90 per cent, especially Christians working in healthcare and policy.

A New Language and New Priorities

A theology of healthcare funding needs to reclaim and reshape the contemporary policy terrain. The principal concern of the debate heretofore has been about efficiency and, indeed, that should always be a concern, but what I have argued here is that efficiency or stewardship should be only one concern, with compassion and social justice being the others. The efficiency discourse sometimes squeezes out the other concerns, and this skews the policy debate inappropriately.

One almost never hears or uses the word compassion in modern health policy discourse, even though it is a core motivator, and it is what patients are often looking for when they need to use healthcare. A focus on need or compassion has been derided by some as leading to priorities being distorted and subverting rational action (see the discussion of needology in Chapter 2). Christians should be unafraid to reclaim that discourse and to highlight the need for compassion, especially in terms of the need for a compassionate society. Compassion talk can be a bulwark against unbridled austerity and can also valorise those in the health sector who show compassion every day. In practical terms, compassion should shape performance measures and care should be taken not to pursue efficiency to such an extent that compassion is squeezed out of the healthcare system and staff. One of the founders of quality assessment in healthcare, Avedis Donabedian, was unafraid to talk about the importance of love in healthcare:

> Ultimately, the secret of quality is love. You have to love your patient, you have to love your profession, you have to love your God. If you have love, you can then work backward to monitor and improve the system. Commercialism should not be a principal force in the system. (Mullan 2001, 140)

Compassion and love – not commercial benefit – should be the context and motivator for improvement, guiding the quest todo better.

Social justice also needs to be highlighted constantly and consistently in the public discourse. The recent SARS-CoV-2 pandemic impacted people differently in different spheres: women and young people were more likely to lose their livelihoods; people in lower paid precarious employment often did not have an entitlement to stay at home and be paid while awaiting test results; lower status jobs were often those with higher rates of infection; and the pandemic affected poorer neighbourhoods more severely (Duckett 2020; Shadmi et al. 2020; Brandily et al. 2021; Stantcheva 2022), and the most vulnerable of all – older people in residential care – suffered a terrible death toll (Salcher-Konrad et al. 2020). And yet, it was not until months after the first infections in high-income countries that explicit attention began to be paid to the justice implications of what was occurring. Again, a Christian voice was sorely needed.

The Christian ethic is of a *social* justice, not simply about fairness for atomised individuals. Public theology needs to highlight person-in-community, reversing the process of what Sacks (2020) refers to as 'cultural climate change' – the shift in society from 'we' to 'I' – to refocus on what we have in common. The late Archbishop Desmond Tutu emphasises this in drawing on *ubuntu* theology:

> We say, 'a person is a person through other people'. It is not 'I think therefore I am'. It says rather: 'I am human because I belong.' I participate, I share. (Tutu 1999, 35)

Christian contributions to the public square need to challenge policy 'solutions' that rely on individuals pulling themselves up by their own bootstraps, victim-blaming approaches, and a narrow definition of 'neighbour'. Instead, the Christian voice should emphasise the role of community in both providing support through social justice and helping to define what humanity is, that a person is one who can participate, and that policy should be directed toward encouraging *social* engagement, creating a community of sharing, and belonging.

Public policy too often focuses narrowly, deemphasising needs of people who are not like us, pursuing a narrow definition of Other-I, and acting more like the priest and the Levite in passing by on the other side of the road. Policy de-emphasises our connectedness, and yet:

> We are linked with each other through trade, commerce, literature, language, music, arts, entertainment, religion, medicine, healthcare, politics, news reports, media communication and other ties … . We are increasingly linked not only by our mutual economic, social and political relations, but also by vaguely shared but far-reaching concerns about injustice and inhumanity that challenge our world, and the violence and terrorism that threaten it. Even our shared frustrations and shared thoughts on global helplessness can unite rather than divide. There are few non neighbours left in the world today. (Sen 2009, 172–173)

Finally, a Christian ethic can inform how stewardship is considered in health policy, perhaps using the more common language of 'responsible use of resources'. The Christian contribution here is to ensure that stewardship is held in tension with the other two principles – that austerity does not mean that compassion and social justice can be ignored, or distributional consequences erased from consideration.

As I have argued earlier, stewardship, and responsible use of resources, is not a 'set and forget' exercise – new technologies emerge, as does new evidence about old technologies. Stewardship is thus dynamic, recognising both the uncertainties inherent in our current knowledge and the gap between what might be shown to work in a controlled evaluation setting and what works in real life. In Chapter 2, I cited Walton's formulation that a need is recognised when state 'Y is incompatible with the values held in society Z' (Walton 1969, 14). Societal values change over time, which causes new needs to be recognised.

Responsible stewardship might also be a bulwark against those who seek to whittle away social provision as inevitably inefficient, creating excess because of purported moral hazard, and leading to unjust levels of taxation. Taxation itself is a moral project: 'Taxes are what we pay for civilized society' to use an aphorism coined by American jurist Oliver Wendell Holmes and popularised by United States President Franklin D, Roosevelt (Hellerstein 1945). The moral purpose of taxation is, *inter alia*, to raise revenues for the public good, and create a more equitable society (Frecknall-Hughes 2020). Demonstrating responsible stewardship – that spending is economically efficient and consistent with society's values – will increase public support for public spending.

All three principles developed here – of compassion, social justice, and stewardship – can and should inform policy. These three principles transcend the sterile debate about individualism versus collectivism: compassion requires us to recognise and valorise concern for the needs of, and response to, an individual; social justice raises our eyes and actions to focus on the needs of groups, particularly the 'quartet of the vulnerable', and the outcasts who Jesus welcomed; and stewardship draws our attention and policies to concerns for the whole of society, calling us to act to protect the whole of creation, now and into the future, with policies about how we exercise stewardship in healthcare.

In previous chapters, I have demonstrated a foundation from a Christian perspective for these three key principles to shape healthcare funding and payment decisions. The language used here, and the practical implications, have been crafted to be part of the discourse of a public theology and the secular policy debate.

The public theologian's role is a prophetic one, leading change through contribution to the public discourse. Stone highlights that

> the Good Samaritan parable in Luke's Gospel is as much a story about leadership as about morality. Jesus told the story of the Samaritan to illustrate

> a moral principle, but Luke told the story of Jesus's sermon to illustrate how Jesus led – by telling compelling stories that inspired people to behave rightly. (Stone 2008, 287)

Public theologians must therefore engage with and redefine the public narrative, but not to hector, rather to lead, 'carrying a summons as well as an involvement' (Heschel 2001). Public theologians must be close to the problems of 'the least of these', involved with 'the last', but able to speak out, telling stories and using quantitative data to call out how we ought to be.

A Theology of Healthcare Funding

A theology of healthcare funding is a theology of everyday life – it is about the policy decisions that are taken every day, decisions that prioritise social justice or not, decisions that hinder compassionate delivery or not, decisions that squander resources or not. These are big decisions, but the decisions also play out in little places – in hospitals, primary care, and ordinary workplaces, in schools and universities. A Christian ethic of healthcare funding as advanced here can contribute both to the big policy discourse – the public square – but can also contribute to how the realm of God is lived every day by all of us.

Temple argued that

> The method of the Church's impact upon society at large should be twofold. The Church must announce Christian principles and point out where the existing social order at any time is in conflict with them. It must then pass on to Christian citizens, acting in their civic capacity, the task of reshaping the existing order in closer conformity to principles. (Temple 1950/1976, 58)

In healthcare, there is particular role for Christian citizens who are healthcare workers to advance the three principles I have argued for in public debates and practice. I am not arguing here that a Christian position should have a special place in debates, especially in a post-Christian society, but rather what is offered is a coherent and balanced position, which recognises the multidimensional concerns of policy and people. The language – and policy prescriptions – of compassion, social justice, and stewardship can appeal to those who start with a Christian foundation and those who do not. They are in that sense 'bridging principles' (Gill 1997, 25), which can make a broader contribution to ethical debate.

Jesus' injunction to the lawyer in the parable of the 'Good' Samaritan is an active one: go and *do*. Jesus does not say go and cogitate, or go and talk, but go and act (Snodgrass 2008, 358–359). 'Do' here might also mean 'keep on doing' (Van Elderen 1978, 111; Bailey 1983, 38) or 'continue doing' (Bailey 2008, 285), a continuous, open ended injunction. In the light of the shift from object to subject in the parable, the injunction might also be phrased as to go and *be*.

The parable teaches us to be close to the afflicted. Unfortunately, however, many leaders

> Faced with the man left at the side of the road, some decide to walk on: distant from the situation, they prefer to ignore the facts and carry on as if nothing had happened. Imprisoned in various kinds of thinking and justifications, they pass on by. (Francis 2020b, 112–113)

Public theology challenges this, calling out this 'out-of-sight, out-of-mind' mindset, and emphasising that the 'least of these' are real people, with the same right to be treated with dignity as all other people. Christian third sector/not-for-profit organisations have a particular role in reducing the distance between decision-makers and the most disadvantaged, helping to give a voice to the voiceless.

Public theology is about attempting to change material conditions; it is about shaping how society functions. In the case of healthcare funding, it is about how, specifically, to make the health system more compassionate, more equitable, and more responsible in its use of resources. This is not just a task for the theologian, but rather, the theologian's task is to aid and work with others in mobilising to shift society in those directions. It means persuading Christians, those of other faiths, and those of none, and so must involve use of arguments that apply to people in all these categories. It involves 'strenuous, self-critical, intellectual and political engagement in the public sphere' (Sagovsky 2017, 268).

The Christian public theologian should seek to use a voice that affirms and calls to a person's SQ, their spiritual intelligence, which complements their IQ (intelligence as traditionally defined) and EQ, their 'emotional intelligence' with SQ defined as

> The intelligence with which we address and solve problems of meaning and value, the intelligence with which we can place our actions and our lives in a wider, richer, meaning-giving context, the intelligence with which we can assess that one course of action or life-path is more meaningful than another. (Zohar and Marshall 2000, 3–4)

Unfortunately, too many commentators in the public square do not build a community's capacity to 'solve problems of meaning and value', but instead emphasise individualism and encourage assessment of public policies in terms of me, the egoist's personal benefit.

In contrast, Christianity is a religion of selflessness (Gill 1997, Chapter 2), with an overwhelming concern for others, as Jesus demonstrated. It is not, and never has been, a religion of simple hidden private faith but is practised in community. It is about influencing and shaping today's world, as well as having an eye to the future. Public theology in a post-Christian world is about breaking out of the 'swarm of privateness' (Tracy 1981) that sometimes constrains Christian ethics and boxes Christian ethics into private morality, which makes concern about distributive justice and shaping policy debates illegitimate. SQ may be conceptualised as an attribute of an organisation (Zohar 2005) or possibly a whole society, with public theology then having an important role in addressing crucial problems of meaning and value, including on how to develop appropriate funding models for healthcare.

Public theology is a key manifestation of the prophetic role of the church, a role which has involved calling out leaders to be just over past millennia as documented in the Hebrew Scriptures. It is about challenging the view that a public decision-maker's motivation for 'health reform' is cost reduction balanced against their re-election prospects, with compassion and justice not in the equation (Zweifel 2019). But public theology is not only about the behaviour of (other) leaders but also about providing leadership in shaping the views of the public, to support the public both to influence leaders and in the day-to-day decisions made by everyone. I have argued that both public decisions of leaders and day-to-day decisions of Christians should be consistent with Jesus' 'do likewise' injunction to the questioning lawyer in the parable of the 'Good' Samaritan, which perhaps can be paraphrased as an injunction to be compassionate and just, and practise responsible stewardship.

I started this book with an ambitious goal of creating a new vision for health economics, informed by a theology of healthcare funding that goes beyond the old preoccupations of moral theology to address how the profession might function in an everyday world of its contributions to critical policy choices (Banner 2014, 202). The health economics profession is a heterogeneous one: some have always highlighted equity concerns; some have pioneered adding an equity lens to economic evaluation; and some are clearly motivated by social justice and attempting to ensure public money is used wisely so more needs can be met within the context of limited resources. As individuals, health economists will be as compassionate as the next person.

But unfortunately, the centre of gravity of the profession – particularly so in the United States – is skewed towards a position where compassion and social justice are not considered an intrinsic part of what we do; the economic evaluation engine ignores social justice, which is assumed to be dealt with separately, and compassion is not in the professional lexicon. In the parallel world of ethics and theology, the emphasis on compassion and social justice continues, but the concerns of stewardship and economic evaluation sit uneasily in the discourse.

Economics, healthcare, and theology can co-exist. For that to happen, the trinity of goals – compassion, social justice, and stewardship – must all be considered together. One goal cannot be pre-eminent.

The future path of health economics must change from the academic highway of *Homo economicus* to the Jericho Road where the health economist incorporates the same compassion, social justice, and stewardship shown by the outsider, the Samaritan. If the health economist stands with the wounded person by the wayside, health economics, and healthcare, will be all the stronger.

References

Aaron, Henry J., and William B. Schwartz. 1982. *The Painful Prescription: Rationing Hospital Care*. Washington, DC: Brookings Institution.

Achtemeier, Paul J. 1975. "The Lucan Perspective on the Miracles of Jesus: A Preliminary Sketch." *Journal of Biblical Literature* 94 (4): 547–562.

Advisory Council on the Implementation of National Pharmacare. 2019. *A Prescription for Canada: Achieving Pharmacare for All: Final Report of the Advisory Council on the Implementation of National Pharmacare*. Health Canada, Ottawa. http://publications.gc.ca/collections/collection_2019/sc-hc/H22-4-18-2019-eng.pdf.

Aghabarary, Maryam, and Nahid Dehghan Nayeri. 2016. "Medical Futility and Its Challenges: A Review Study." *Journal of Medical Ethics and History of Medicine* 9: 1–13.

Ailon, Galit. 2020. "The Phenomenology of Homo Economicus." *Sociological Theory* 38 (1): 36–50.

Airoldi, Mara. 2013. "Disinvestments in Practice: Overcoming Resistance to Change through a Sociotechnical Approach with Local Stakeholders." *Journal of Health Politics, Policy and Law* 38 (6): 1149–1171.

Akiyama, Kengo. 2018. *The Love of Neighbour in Ancient Judaism: The Reception of Leviticus 19: 18 in the Hebrew Bible, the Septuagint, the Book of Jubilees, the Dead Sea Scrolls, and the New Testament*. Leiden and Boston: Brill.

Aland, Barbara, Kurt Aland, Johannes Karavidopoulos, Carlo M. Martini, and Bruce M. Metzger, eds. 1994. *The Greek New Testament*. Stuttgart: Deutsche Bibelgesellschaft.

Aland, Kurt. 1982. *Synopsis of the Four Gospels*. New York: American Bible Society.

Albrecht, Gary L., and Patrick J. Devlieger. 1999. "The Disability Paradox: High Quality of Life against All Odds." *Social Science & Medicine* 48 (8): 977–988.

Alderwick, Hugh A. J., Laura M. Gottlieb, Caroline M. Fichtenberg, and Nancy E. Adler. 2018. "Social Prescribing in the U.S. and England: Emerging Interventions to Address Patients' Social Needs." *American Journal of Preventive Medicine* 54 (5): 715–718.

Allcott, Hunt, Benjamin Lockwood, and Dmitry Taubinsky. 2019. *Should We Tax Sugar-Sweetened Beverages? An Overview of Theory and Evidence*. Cambridge, MA: National Bureau of Economic Research.

Allin, Sara, Cristina Hernández-Quevedo, and Cristina Masseria. 2009. "Measuring Equity of Access to Health Care." In *Performance Measurement for Health System Improvement: Experiences, Challenges, and Prospects*, edited by Peter Smith, Elias Mossialos, Irene Papanicolas, and S. Leatherman, 187–221. Cambridge and New York: Cambridge University Press.

Allin, Sara, Julie Farmer, Carlos Quiñonez Allie Peckham, Gregory Marchildon, Dimitra Panteli, Cornelia Henschke, Giovanni Fattore, Demetrio Lamloum, Alexander C. L. Holden, and Thomas Rice. 2020. "Do Health Systems Cover the Mouth? Comparing Dental Care Coverage for Older Adults in Eight Jurisdictions." *Health Policy* 124 (9): 998–1007.

Allport, Gordon W., and J. Michael Ross. 1967. "Personal Religious Orientation and Prejudice." *Journal of Personality and Social Psychology* 5 (4): 432–443.

Alter, Robert. 2019a. *The Hebrew Bible: A Translation with Commentary. Volume 1: Torah*. New York: W. W. Norton & Company.

2019b. *The Hebrew Bible: A Translation with Commentary. Volume 3: Ketuvim*. New York: W. W. Norton & Company.

Alvey, James E. 1999. "A Short History of Economics as a Moral Science." *Journal of Markets & Morality* 2 (1): 53–73.

2000. "An Introduction to Economics as a Moral Science." *International Journal of Social Economics* 27 (12): 1231–1252.

American Friends Service Committee. 1955. *Speak Truth to Power. A Quaker Search for an Alternative to Violence*. Philadelphia, PA: American Friends Service Committee.

Amît, Ya'îra. 2012. *In Praise of Editing in the Hebrew Bible: Collected Essays in Retrospect*. Sheffield: Sheffield Phoenix Press.

Amundson, Ron. 2005. "Disability, Ideology, and Quality of Life: A Bias in Biomedical Ethics." In *Quality of Life and Human Difference: Genetic Testing, Health Care, and Disability*, edited by David Wasserman, Robert Wachbroit, and Jerome Bickenbach, 101–124. New York: Cambridge University Press.

Anand, Paul. 2001. "Social Choice as the Synthesis of Incommensurable Claims." In *The Social Economics of Health Care*, edited by John Bryan Davis, 61–93. London: Routledge.

Andersen, Ronald. 1968. *A Behavioral Model of Families' Use of Health Services*. Chicago: University of Chicago, Center for Health Administration Studies.

Andersen, Ronald, Joanna Kravits, and Odin W. Anderson. 1975. *Equity in Health Services: Empirical Analyses in Social Policy*. Cambridge, MA: Ballinger.

Andre, Judith. 1992. "Blocked Exchanges: A Taxonomy." *Ethics* 103 (1): 29–47.

Andreoni, James, Ann-Kathrin Koessler, and Marta Serr-Garcia. 2018. "Who Gives? The Role of Empathy and Impulsiveness." In *The Economics of Philanthropy: Donations and Fundraising*, edited by Kimberly A. Scharf and Mirco Tonin, 239–261. Cambridge: MIT Press.

Andrews, Christopher K. 2020. *The Overworked Consumer: Self-Checkouts, Supermarkets, and the Do-It-Yourself Economy*. Lanham, MD: Lexington Books.

Anesi, George L., Andrew J. Admon, Scott D. Halpern, and Meeta P. Kerlin. 2019. "Understanding Irresponsible Use of Intensive Care Unit Resources in the USA." *The Lancet Respiratory Medicine* 7 (7): 605–612.

Angell, Blake, Janani Muhunthan, Anne-Marie Eades, Joan Cunningham, Gail Garvey, Alan Cass, Kirsten Howard, Julie Ratcliffe, Sandra Eades, and Stephen Jan. 2016. "The Health-related Quality of Life of Indigenous Populations: A Global Systematic Review." *Quality of Life Research* 25 (9): 2161–2178.

Angner, Erik. 2016. *A Course in Behavioral Economics*. London, New York: Palgrave Macmillan.

Anik, Lalin, Lara B. Aknin, Michael I. Norton, and Elizabeth W. Dunn. 2009. "Feeling Good about Giving: The Benefits (and Costs) of Self-interested Charitable Behavior." *Harvard Business School Marketing Unit Working Paper* (10–012).

Anik, Lalin, Lara B. Aknin, Michael I. Norton, and Elizabeth W. Dunn. 2011. "Feeling Good about Giving: The Benefits (and Costs) of Self-interested Charitable Behavior." In *The Science of Giving: Experimental Approaches to the Study of Charity*, edited by Daniel M Oppenheimer and Christopher Y Olivola. New York, NY: Psychology Press.

Ansari, Zahid. 2007. "The Concept and Usefulness of Ambulatory Care Sensitive Conditions as Indicators of Quality and Access to Primary Health Care." *Australian Journal of Primary Health* 13 (3): 91–110.

Aristotle. 2014. "Complete Works of Aristotle, Volume 2: *The Revised Oxford Translation* (Translated by Jonathan Barnes)." http://kcl.eblib.com/patron/FullRecord.aspx?p=1632631.

Arrow, Kenneth J. 1963. "Uncertainty and the Welfare Economics of Medical Care." *American Economic Review* 53 (5): 941–973.

Asante, Augustine, Jennifer Price, Andrew Hayen, Stephen Jan, and Virginia Wiseman. 2016. "Equity in Health Care Financing in Low- and Middle-Income Countries: A Systematic Review of Evidence from Studies Using Benefit and Financing Incidence Analyses." *PLOS ONE* 11 (4): e0152866.

Asaria, Miqdad, Susan Griffin, and Richard Cookson. 2015. "Distributional Cost-Effectiveness Analysis: A Tutorial." *Medical Decision Making* 36 (1): 8–19.

Ashmore, Malcolm, Michael J. Mulkay, and Trevor J. Pinch. 1989. *Health and Efficiency: A Sociology of Health Economics*. Milton Keynes: Open University Press.

Asthana, Sheena, and Alex Gibson. 2020. "The National Health Service (NHS) in 'Crisis': The Role Played by a Shift from Horizontal to Vertical Principles of Equity." *Health Economics, Policy and Law* 15 (1): 1–17.

Ataguba, John E., Augustine D. Asante, Supon Limwattananon, and Virginia Wiseman. 2018. "How to Do (or Not to Do) … a Health Financing Incidence Analysis." *Health Policy and Planning* 33 (3): 436–444.

Atashzadeh-Shoorideh, Foroozan, Faraz Tayyar-Iravanlou, Zeynab Ahmadian Chashmi, Fatemeh Abdi, and Rosana Svetic Cisic. 2020. "Factors Affecting Moral Distress in Nurses Working in Intensive Care Units: A Systematic Review." *Clinical Ethics* 16 (1): 25–36.

Atkinson, A. B. 2009a. "Economics as a Moral Science." *Economica* 76 (s1): 791–804.

2009b. "Economics as a Moral Science." In *Lionel Robbins's Essay on the Nature and Significance of Economic Science: 75th Anniversary Conference Proceedings*, edited by Frank Cowell and Amos Witztum, 38–56. London: Suntory and Toyota International Centres for Economics and Related Disciplines.

Augustine. 2014. "On Christian Doctrine." In *The Complete Ante-Nicene & Nicene and Post-Nicene Church Fathers Collection: 3 Series, 37 Volumes, 65 Authors, 1,000 Books, 18,000 Chapters, 16 Million Words*, edited by Philip Schaff. London: Catholic Way Publishing.

Australian Bureau of Statistics. 2014. Australian Historical Population Statistics, 2014 (Cat no: 3105.0.65.001). ABS (Canberra).

Avanceña, Anton L. V., and Lisa A. Prosser. 2021. "Examining Equity Effects of Health Interventions in Cost-Effectiveness Analysis: A Systematic Review." *Value in Health* 24 (1): 136–143.

Averill, Richard F., Norbert I. Goldfield, James C. Vertrees, Elizabeth C. McCullough, Richard L. Fuller, and Jon Eisenhandler. 2010. "Achieving Cost Control, Care Coordination, and Quality Improvement through Incremental Payment System Reform." *Journal of Ambulatory Care Management* 33 (1): 2–23.

Ayres, Stephen M. 1992. "Rationality, Not Rationing, in Health Care." In *Rationing America's Medical Care, the Oregon Plan and Beyond*, edited by Martin A. Strosberg, Joshua M. Weiner, Robert Baker, and I. Alan Fein. Washington DC: Brookings Institution.

Bachrach, Peter, and Morton S. Baratz. 1963. "Decisions and Nondecisions: An Analytical Framework." *The American Political Science Review* 57 (3): 632–642.

Backhouse, Roger E., and Steve G. Medema. 2009. "Defining Economics: The Long Road to Acceptance of the Robbins Definition." *Economica* 76 (s1): 805–820.

Badgery-Parker, Tim, Sallie-Anne Pearson, and Adam G. Elshaug. 2020. "Hospital Characteristics Associated with Low-Value Care in Public Hospitals in New South Wales, Australia." *BMC Health Services Research* 20 (750): 1–7.

Badgery-Parker, Tim, Sallie-Anne Pearson, Kelsey Chalmers, Jonathan Brett, Ian A. Scott, Susan Dunn, Neville Onley, and Adam G. Elshaug. 2019. "Low-Value Care in Australian Public Hospitals: Prevalence and Trends over Time." *BMJ Quality & Safety* 28 (3): 205–214.

Badgery-Parker, Tim, Sallie-Anne Pearson, and Adam G. Elshaug. 2020. "Hospital Characteristics Associated with Low-Value Care in Public Hospitals in New South Wales, Australia." *BMC Health Services Research* 20 (750): 1–7.

Bahrampour, Mina, Joshua Byrnes, Richard Norman, Paul A. Scuffham, and Martin Downes. 2020. "Discrete Choice Experiments to Generate Utility Values for Multi-attribute Utility Instruments: A Systematic Review of Methods." *The European Journal of Health Economics* 21 (7): 983–992.

Baicker, Katherine, Sendhil Mullainathan, and Joshua Schwartzstein. 2015. "Behavioral Hazard in Health Insurance." *The Quarterly Journal of Economics* 130 (4): 1623–1667.

Bailey, Kenneth E. 1983. *Through Peasant Eyes [Bound as One Volume in Poet & Peasant and through Peasant Eyes: A Literary-Cultural Approach to the Parables in Luke]*. Grand Rapids, MI: Wm. B. Eeerdmans Publishing.

2008. *Jesus through Middle Eastern Eyes: Cultural Studies in the Gospels*. Downers Grove, IL: IVP Academic.

Baker, David L. 2005. "Last but Not Least: The Tenth Commandment." *Horizons in Biblical Theology* 27 (1): 3–24.

Baker, Dean. 2021. "The Future of the Pharmaceutical Industry: Beyond Government-Granted Monopolies." *Journal of Law, Medicine & Ethics* 49 (1): 25–29.

Baker, Hunter. 2012. "Reflections on Social Justice, Government, and Society." *Journal of Markets & Morality* 15 (1): 143–159.

Baker, Rachel, Helen Mason, Neil McHugh, and Cam Donaldson. 2021. "Public Values and Plurality in Health Priority Setting: What to Do When People Disagree and Why We Should Care about Reasons as Well as Choices." *Social Science & Medicine* 277 (113892): 1–9.

Balasooriya, Namal N., Jayatilleke S. Bandara, and Nicholas Rohde. 2021. "The Intergenerational Effects of Socioeconomic Inequality on Unhealthy Bodyweight." *Health Economics* 30 (4): 729–747.

Bann, David. 2021. "The Scope of Health Injustice." *European Journal of Public Health* 31 (3): 458–459.

Banner, Michael C. 2014. *The Ethics of Everyday Life: Moral Theology, Social Anthropology, and the Imagination of the Human*. Oxford: Oxford University Press.

Banting, Keith, and Will Kymlicka. 2017. "Introduction: The Political Sources of Solidarity in Diverse Societies." In *The Strains of Commitment: The Political Sources of Solidarity in Diverse Societies*, edited by Keith Banting and Will Kymlicka, 1–59. Oxford: Oxford University Press.

Banzhaf, H. Spencer. 2014. "The Cold-War Origins of the Value of Statistical Life." *The Journal of Economic Perspectives* 28 (4): 213–226.

Barbi, Elisabetta, Francesco Lagona, Marco Marsili, James W. Vaupel, and Kenneth W. Wachter. 2018. "The Plateau of Human Mortality: Demography of Longevity Pioneers." *Science* 360 (6396): 1459–1461.

Barnett, Arnold. 2020. "All The Same? On a Certain Pattern in Cross-National Death Risk." *Risk Analysis* 40 (9): 1831–1843.

Barr, Damian. 2020. "We Are Not All in the Same Boat. We Are All in the Same Storm. Some of Us Are on Super-Yachts. Some Have Just the One Oar." www.damianbarr.com/latest/https/we-are-not-all-in-the-same-boat.

Barr, James. 1968. "The Image of God in the Book of Genesis: A Study of Terminology." *Bulletin of the John Rylands Library, Manchester* 51 (1): 11–26.

Barr, Nicholas. 2001. *The Welfare State as Piggy Bank. Information, Risk, Uncertainty, and the Role of the State*. Oxford: Oxford University Press.

Barrera, Albino. 2005. *God and the Evil of Scarcity: Moral Foundations of Economic Agency*. Notre Dame: University of Notre Dame Press.

2007. *Economic Compulsion and Christian Ethics*. Cambridge: Cambridge University Press.

2011. *Market Complicity and Christian Ethics*. Cambridge: Cambridge University Press.

2013. *Biblical Economic Ethics: Sacred Scripture's Teachings on Economic Life*. Lanham, MD: Lexington.

Barth, Karl. 2004. *Church Dogmatics: The Doctrine of God, Volume 2, Part2: The Election of God; the Command of God*. London: Bloomsbury Publishing.

Bartholomew, Francis, and Justin of Canterbury. 2021. *A Joint Message for the Protection of Creation*. www.archbishopofcanterbury.org/sites/abc/files/2021-09/Joint%20Statement%20on%20the%20Environment.pdf.

Bartlett, Ben, and John Boffa. 2001. "Aboriginal Community Controlled Comprehensive Primary Health Care: The Central Australian Aboriginal Congress." *Australian Journal of Primary Health* 7 (3): 74–82.

2005. "The Impact of Aboriginal Community Controlled Health Service Advocacy on Aboriginal Health Policy." *Australian Journal of Primary Health* 11 (2): 53–62.

Barton, John. 1978. "Understanding Old Testament Ethics." *Journal for the Study of the Old Testament* 3 (9): 44–64.

1995. "The Basis of Ethics in the Hebrew Bible." In *Ethics and Politics in the Hebrew Bible*, edited by Douglas A. Knight, In Semeia, 11–22. Atlanta, GA: Scholars Press.

2003. *Understanding Old Testament Ethics: Approaches and Explorations*. Louisville, London: Westminster John Knox Press.

2014. *Ethics in Ancient Israel*. Oxford: Oxford University Press.

Barton, Stephen C. 2009. "Money Matters: Economic Relations and the Transformation of Value in Early Christianity." In *Engaging Economics: New Testament Scenarios and Early Christian Reception*, edited by Bruce W. Longenecker and Kelly D. Liebengood, 37–59. Grand Rapids, MI: Wm. B. Eerdmans Publishing.

Barton, Thomas D. 1998. "Troublesome Connections: The Law and Post-Enlightenment Culture." *Emory Law Journal* 47 (1): 163–236.

Bateman, Bradley W. 1998. "Clearing the Ground: The Demise of the Social Gospel Movement and the Rise of Neoclassicism in American Economics." *History of Political Economy* 30 (4): 29–52.

2001. "Make a Righteous Number: Social Surveys, the Men and Religion Forward Movement, and Quantification in American Economics." *History of Political Economy* 33, no. Winter Supplement: 57–85.

Bateman, Bradley W., and Ethan B. Kapstein. 1999. "Retrospectives: Between God and the Market: The Religious Roots of the American Economic Association." *Journal of Economic Perspectives* 13 (4): 249–258.

Batson, C. Daniel. 2017. "The Empathy-Altruism Hypothesis: What and So What?" In *The Oxford Handbook of Compassion Science*, edited by Emma M Seppälä, Emiliana Simon-Thomas, Stephanie L Brown, Monica C Worline, C Daryl Cameron, and James R Doty, 27–40. Oxford: Oxford University Press.

Batt, Sharon. 2017. *Health Advocacy, Inc.: How Pharmaceutical Funding Changed the Breast Cancer Movement*. Vancouver: UBC Press.

Battle, Michael. 2009. *Reconciliation: The Ubuntu Theology of Desmond Tutu*. Cleveland, OH: Pilgrim Press.

Bauckham, Richard. 1998. "The Scrupulous Priest and the Good Samaritan: Jesus' Parabolic Interpretation of the Law of Moses." *New Testament Studies* 44 (4): 475–489.

Baujard, Antoinette. 2009. "A Return to Bentham's Felicific Calculus: From Moral Welfarism to Technical Non-welfarism." *The European Journal of the History of Economic Thought* 16 (3): 431–453.

Baylis, Françoise, Nuala P. Kenny, and Susan Sherwin. 2008. "A Relational Account of Public Health Ethics." *Public Health Ethics* 1 (3): 196–209.

Beauchamp, Tom L., and James F. Childress. 1994. *Principles of Biomedical Ethics*. New York: Oxford University Press.

2013. *Principles of Biomedical Ethics*. New York: Oxford University Press.

Beck, Vanessa. 2018. "Capabilities and Choices of Vulnerable, Long-Term Unemployed Individuals." *Work, Employment and Society* 32 (1): 3–19.

Becker, Gary S. 1974. "A Theory of Marriage." In *Economics of the Family: Marriage, Children, and Human Capital*, edited by Theodore Schultz, 299–351. Chicago: University of Chicago Press.

1993. "Nobel Lecture: The Economic Way of Looking at Behavior." *Journal of Political Economy* 101 (3): 385–409.

Beckley, Harlan. 2011. "Christians and Economics." In *The Oxford Handbook of Theological Ethics*, edited by Gilbert Meilaender and William Werpehowski, 360–380. Oxford: Oxford University Press.

Bell, Eleanor, Margherita Neri, and Lotte Steuten. 2021. "Towards a Broader Assessment of Value in Vaccines: The BRAVE Way Forward." *Applied Health Economics and Health Policy*.

Benedict XVI. 2009. *Caritas in Veritate: Encyclical Letter on Integral Human Development in Charity and Truth*. Vatican City: The Holy See.

Benne, Robert. 2011. "Christians and Government." In *The Oxford Handbook of Theological Ethics*, edited by Gilbert Meilaender and William Werpehowski, 325–342. Oxford: Oxford University Press.

Bentley, Colene, Stuart Peacock, Julia Abelson, Michael M. Burgess, Olivier Demers-Payette, Holly Longstaff, Laura Tripp, John N. Lavis, and Michael G. Wilson. 2019. "Addressing the Affordability of Cancer Drugs: Using Deliberative Public Engagement to Inform Health Policy." *Health Research Policy and Systems* 17 (17).

Bentley, Tanya G. K., Rachel M. Effros, Kartika Palar, and Emmett B. Keeler. 2008. "Waste in the U.S. Health Care System: A Conceptual Framework." *Milbank Quarterly* 86 (4): 629–659.

Berdud, Mikel, Michael Drummond, and Adrian Towse. 2020. "Establishing a Reasonable Price for an Orphan Drug." *Cost Effectiveness and Resource Allocation* 18 (31): 1–18.

Bergant, Dianne. 2013. *Genesis: In the Beginning*. Collegeville, MN: Liturgical Press.

Bergthold, Linda A. 1995. "Medical Necessity: Do We Need It?" *Health Affairs* 14 (4): 180–190.

Berlant, Lauren, ed. 2004. *Compassion: The Culture and Politics of an Emotion*. New York: Routledge.

Bernstein, Peter L. 1996. *Against the Gods: The Remarkable Story of Risk*. New York: Wiley.

Berta, Paolo, Giuditta Callea, Gianmaria Martini, and Giorgio Vittadini. 2010. "The Effects of Upcoding, Cream Skimming and Readmissions on the Italian Hospitals Efficiency: A Population-Based Investigation." *Economic Modelling* 27 (4): 812–821.

Bertram, Melanie Y., Jeremy A. Lauer, Kees De Joncheere, Tessa Edejer, Raymond Hutubessy, Marie-Paule Kieny, and Suzanne R. Hill. 2016. "Cost–Effectiveness Thresholds: Pros and Cons." *Bulletin of the World Health Organization* 94 (12): 925–930.

Berwick, Donald M. 2020. "The Moral Determinants of Health." *JAMA* 324 (3): 225–226.

Berwick, Donald M., and Andrew D. Hackbarth. 2012. "Eliminating Waste in US Health Care." *JAMA – Journal of the American Medical Association* 307 (14): 1513–1516.

Bevan, Gwyn, and Christopher Hood. 2006. "What's Measured Is What Matters: Targets and Gaming in the English Public Health Care System." *Public Administration* 84 (3): 517–538.

Bhagwati, Jagdish. 2011. "Markets and Morality." *The American Economic Review* 101 (3): 162–165.

Bhattacharjya, Ashoke S., and Puneet K. Sapra. 2008. "Health Insurance in China and India: Segmented Roles for Public and Private Financing." *Health Affairs* 27 (4): 1005–1015.

Bhise, Viraj, Suja S. Rajan, Dean F. Sittig, Robert O. Morgan, Pooja Chaudhary, and Hardeep Singh. 2018. "Defining and Measuring Diagnostic Uncertainty in Medicine: A Systematic Review." *Journal of General Internal Medicine* 33 (1): 103–115.

Bibler, Trevor M., Devan Stahl, Sophia Fantus, Alex Lion, and Kyle B. Brothers. 2020. "A Process-Based Approach to Responding to Parents or Guardians Who Hope for a Miracle." *Pediatrics* 145 (3): e20192319.

Bichay, Nicolas. 2020. "Health Insurance as a State Institution: The Effect of Single-Payer Insurance on Expenditures in OECD Countries." *Social Science & Medicine* 265.

Bickerdyke, Ian, Robert Dolamore, Ian Monday, and Robb Preston. 2002. *Supplier-Induced Demand for Medical Services. Productivity Commission Staff Working Paper*. Canberra: Productivity Commission.

Bindman, Andrew B., Kevin Grumbach, Dennis Osmond, Miriam Komaromy, Karen Vranizan, Nicole Lurie, John Billings, and Anita Stewart. 1995. "Preventable Hospitalizations and Access to Health Care." *JAMA* 274 (4): 305–311.

Birch, Bruce C. 1991. *Let Justice Roll Down: The Old Testament, Ethics, and Christian Life*. Louisville: Westminster/John Knox Press.

Birch, Stephen, and Cam Donaldson. 2003. "Valuing the Benefits and Costs of Health Care Programmes: Where's the 'Extra' in Extra-Welfarism?" *Social Science & Medicine* 56 (5): 1121–1133.

Bird, Phyllis A. 2011. ""Male and Female He Created Them": Gen 1:27b in the Context of the Priestly Account of Creation." *Harvard Theological Review* 74 (2): 129–160.

Black, Nick. 2013. "Patient Reported Outcome Measures Could Help Transform Healthcare." *BMJ* 346: f167.

2017. "From Cutting Costs to Eliminating Waste: Reframing the Challenge." *Journal of Health Services Research & Policy* 22 (2): 73–74.

Blajer, Piotr. 2012. "The Parable of the Good Samaritan (Luke 10: 25–37): Its Function and Purpose within the Lukan Journey Section." *Doctor of Sacred Theology*, School of Theology and Religious Studies, Catholic University of America.

Bleichrodt, Han, and John Quiggin. 1999. "Life-Cycle Preferences over Consumption and Health: When Is Cost-Effectiveness Analysis Equivalent to Cost–Benefit Analysis?" *Journal of Health Economics* 18 (6): 681–708.

Blomberg, Karin, Peter Griffiths, Yvonne Wengström, Carl May, and Jackie Bridges. 2016. "Interventions for Compassionate Nursing Care: A Systematic Review." *International Journal of Nursing Studies* 62: 137–155.

Blum, Lawrence. 1980. "Compassion." In *Explaining Emotions*, edited by Amélie Oksenberg Rorty, 507–517. Berkeley, CA: University of California Press.

Boda, Mark J., and Shannon E. Baines. 2016. "Wisdom's Cry: Embracing the Vision of Justice in Bold Testament Wisdom Literature." In *The Bible and Social Justice: Old Testament and New Testament Foundations for the Church's Urgent Call*, edited by Cynthia Long Westfall and Bryan R. Dyer, 35–63. Eugene, OR: Pickwick publications.

Bohm, Natalie, Sarah Bermingham, Frank Grimsey Jones, Daniela C. Gonçalves-Bradley, Alex Diamantopoulos, Jessica R. Burton, and Hamish Laing. 2022. "The Challenges of Outcomes-Based Contract Implementation for Medicines in Europe." *PharmacoEconomics* 40 (1): 13–29.

Bohm, Peter. 1987. *Social Efficiency: A Concise Introduction to Welfare Economics*. London: Macmillan Education.

Boldrin, Michele, and David K. Levine. 2013. "The Case against Patents." *Journal of Economic Perspectives* 27 (1): 3–22.

Bolton, Sharon C. 2009. "The Lady Vanishes: Women's Work and Affective Labour." *International Journal of Work Organisation and Emotion* 3 (1): 72–80.

Booth, Christopher M., Ajay Aggarwal, and Richard Sullivan. 2022. "Commercial Determinants of Cancer Medicines." *Eurohealth* 28 (2): 18–21.

Booth, Neill. 2019. "On Value Frameworks and Opportunity Costs in Health Technology Assessment." *International Journal of Technology Assessment in Health Care* 35 (5): 367–372.

Boothe, Katherine. 2021. "(Re)defining Legitimacy in Canadian Drug Assessment Policy? Comparing Ideas over Time." *Health Economics, Policy and Law* 16 (4): 424–439.

Borg, Marcus J. 1998. *Conflict, Holiness, and Politics in the Teachings of Jesus.* London: Continuum.

2014. *Convictions: A Manifesto for Progressive Christians.* London: SPCK.

Borg, Marcus J., and John Dominic Crossan. 2009. *The First Paul: Reclaiming the Radical Visionary behind the Church's Conservative Icon.* New York: HarperOne.

Boulding, Kenneth E. 1966. "The Concept of Need for Health Services." *Milbank Memorial Fund Quarterly* 44 (4): 202–223.

1969. "Economics as a Moral Science." *The American Economic Review* 59 (1): 1–12.

Bourke, Christopher John, Henrietta Marrie, and Adrian Marrie. 2019. "Transforming Institutional Racism at an Australian Hospital." *Australian Health Review* 43 (6): 611–618.

Bovenberg, Josien, Hannah Penton, and Nasuh Buyukkaramikli. 2021. "10 Years of End-of-Life Criteria in the United Kingdom." *Value in Health* 24 (5): 691–698.

Bovens, Luc, and Adrien Lutz. 2019. "'From Each according to Ability; to Each according to Needs': Origin, Meaning, and Development of Socialist Slogans." *History of Political Economy* 51 (2): 237–257.

Bowe, Barbara E. 2017. *Biblical Foundations of Spirituality: Touching a Finger to the Flame* (2nd ed., with contributions by Laurie Brink and John R. Barker). Lanham MD: Rowman & Littlefield.

Boxall, Anne-Marie, and James A. Gillespie. 2013. *Making Medicare: The Politics of Universal Health Care in Australia.* Sydney: NewSouth Publishing.

Boyce, Maria B., and John P. Browne. 2013. "Does Providing Feedback on Patient-Reported Outcomes to Healthcare Professionals Result in Better Outcomes for Patients? A Systematic Review." *Quality of Life Research* 22 (9): 2266–2278.

Boyd, Richard. 2020. "The Early Modern Origins of Behavioral Economics." *Social Philosophy and Policy* 37 (1): 30–54.

Bradley, Elizabeth H., Maureen Canavan, Erika Rogan, Kristina Talbert-Slagle, Chima Ndumele, Lauren Taylor, and Leslie A. Curry. 2016. "Variation in Health Outcomes: The Role of Spending on Social Services, Public Health, and Health Care, 2000–09." *Health Affairs* 35 (5): 760–768.

Bradshaw, Jonathan. 1972. "Taxonomy of Social Need." In *Problems and Progress in Medical Care: Essays on Current Research,* edited by Gordon McLachlan, 71–82. London: Oxford University Press.

Braithwaite, Jeffrey, Paul Glasziou, and Johanna Westbrook. 2020. "The Three Numbers You Need to Know about Healthcare: The 60-30-10 Challenge." *BMC Medicine* 18 (102): 1–8.

Brandeis, Louis Dembitz. 1914. *Other People's Money: And How the Bankers Use It.* New York: Frederick A. Stokes Co.

Brandily, Paul, Clément Brébion, Simon Briole, and Laura Khoury. 2021. *A Poorly Understood Disease? The Impact of COVID-19 on the Income Gradient in Mortality over the Course of the Pandemic.* Paris: Paris School of Economics. halshs-02895908v2f.

Braveman, Paula, and Laura Gottlieb. 2014. "The Social Determinants of Health: It's Time to Consider the Causes of the Causes." *Public Health Reports* 129 (Supplement 2): 19–31. Braveman, Paula, Susan Egerter, and David R. Williams. 2011. "The Social Determinants of Health: Coming of Age." *Annual Review of Public Health* 32 (1): 381–398.

Braybrooke, David. 1987. *Meeting Needs.* Princeton: Princeton University Press.

Brenner, M. Harvey. 2017. "Years of Life Lost, Age Discrimination, and the Myth of Productivity." *American Journal of Public Health* 107 (10): 1535–1537.

Breton, Mylaine, Mélanie Ann Smithman, Martin Sasseville, Sara A. Kreindler, Jason M. Sutherland, Marie Beauséjour, Michael Green, Emily Gard Marshall, Jalila Jbilou, Jay Shaw, Astrid Brousselle, Damien Contandriopoulos, Valorie A. Crooks, and Sabrina T. Wong. 2020. "How the Design and Implementation of Centralized Waiting Lists Influence Their Use and Effect on Access to Healthcare – A Realist Review." *Health Policy* 124 (8): 787–795.

Brett, Jonathan, Adam G. Elshaug, R. Sacha Bhatia, Kelsey Chalmers, Tim Badgery-Parker, and Sallie-Anne Pearson. 2017. "A Methodological Protocol for Selecting and Quantifying Low-Value Prescribing Practices in Routinely Collected Data: An Australian Case Study." *Implementation Science* 12 (58).

Brook, Robert H., and Kathleen N. Lohr. 1986. "Will We Need to Ration Effective Health Care?" *Issues in Science and Technology* 3 (1): 68–77.

1991. *Will We Need to Ration Effective Health Care? Rand Note N-3375-HHS.* Santa Monica, CA: RAND.

Brooks, David B., Julie Trottier, and Giulia Giordano, eds. 2020. *Transboundary Water Issues in Israel, Palestine, and the Jordan River Basin: An Overview.* Singapore: Springer.

Broom, Dorothy H. 1991. *Damned If We Do: Contradictions of Women's Health.* Sydney: Allen and Unwin Pty Ltd.

1997. "The Best Medicine: Women Using Community Health Centres." *Australian and New Zealand Journal of Public Health* 21 (3): 275–280.

Broome, John. 1999. *Ethics Out of Economics.* Cambridge: University of Cambridge.

Broome, John. 2000. "Cost-Benefit Analysis and Population." *The Journal of Legal Studies* 29 (S2): 953–970.

Brot-Goldberg, Zarek C., Amitabh Chandra, Benjamin R. Handel, and Jonathan T. Kolstad. 2017. "What Does a Deductible Do? The Impact of Cost-Sharing on Health Care Prices, Quantities, and Spending Dynamics." *The Quarterly Journal of Economics* 132 (3): 1261–1318.

Brousselle, Astrid, and Chantale Lessard. 2011. "Economic Evaluation to Inform Health Care Decision-Making: Promise, Pitfalls and a Proposal for an Alternative Path." *Social Science & Medicine* 72 (6): 832–839.

Brown, Rebecca C. H., Hannah Maslen, and Julian Savulescu. 2019. "Against Moral Responsibilisation of Health: Prudential Responsibility and Health Promotion." *Public Health Ethics* 12 (2): 114–129.

Browne-Yung, Kathryn, Toby Freeman, Malcolm Battersby, Doug R. McEvoy, and Fran Baum. 2019. "Developing a Screening Tool to Recognise Social Determinants of Health in Australian Clinical Settings." *Public Health Research and Practice* 29 (4): 28341813.

Brownlee, Shannon M., and Deborah Korenstein. 2021. "Better Understanding the Downsides of Low Value Healthcare Could Reduce Harm." *British Medical Journal* 372: n117.

Brownlee, Shannon, Kalipso Chalkidou, Jenny Doust, Adam G. Elshaug, Paul Glasziou, Iona Heath, Somil Nagpal, Vikas Saini, Divya Srivastava, Kelsey Chalmers, and Deborah Korenstein. 2017. "Evidence for Overuse of Medical Services around the World." *The Lancet* 390 (10090): 156–168.

Brueggemann, Walter. 1997. *Theology of the Old Testament: Testimony, Dispute, Advocacy*. Minneapolis, MN: Fortress Press.

2016. *Money and Possessions*. Louisville, KY: Westminster John Knox Press.

Brunius, Teddy. 1958. "Jeremy Bentham's Moral Calculus." *Acta Sociologica* 3 (1): 73–85.

Buchanan, Allen. 1981. "Justice: A Philosophical Review." In *Justice and Health Care*, edited by Earl E. Shelp, 3–22. Dordrecht, Holland: D. Reidel.

Buchanan, David R. 2008. "Autonomy, Paternalism, and Justice: Ethical Priorities in Public Health." *American Journal of Public Health* 98 (1): 15–21.

Bulmer, Sandy, Jonathan Elms, and Simon Moore. 2018. "Exploring the Adoption of Self-service Checkouts and the Associated Social Obligations of Shopping Practices." *Journal of Retailing and Consumer Services* 42: 107–116.

Burger Araujo Santos, Diego, and Sangay Dorji. 2021. "Bhutan & Gross National Happiness." In *New Paths of Development: Perspectives from the Global South*, edited by Rahma Bourqia and Marcelo Sili, 161–168. Cham: Springer International Publishing.

Burridge, Richard A. 2007. *Imitating Jesus: An Inclusive Approach to New Testament Ethics*. Grand Rapids, MI: William B. Eerdmans Pub.

2021. "Is 'Biblical Ethics' a 'Genre Mistake'? Methodological Reflections on New Testament Ethics in Debate with Gustafson and Hays." In *Key Approaches to Biblical Ethics: An Interdisciplinary Dialogue*, edited by Volker Rabens, Jacqueline Grey, and Mariam Kamell Kovalishyn, 237–268. Leiden Boston: Brill.

Burson, Randall C., Olivia O. Familusi, and Justin T. Clapp. 2021. "Imagining the 'Structural' in Medical Education and Practice in the United States: A Curricular Investigation." *Social Science & Medicine: 114453*.

Burtch, Gordon, and Jason Chan. 2019. "Investigating the Relationship between Medical Crowdfunding and Personal Bankruptcy in the United States: Evidence of a Digital Divide." *MIS Quarterly* 43 (1): 237–262.

Busby, John, Sarah Purdy, and William Hollingworth. 2017. "Using Geographic Variation in Unplanned Ambulatory Care Sensitive Condition Admission Rates to Identify Commissioning Priorities: An Analysis of Routine Data from England." *Journal of Health Services Research & Policy* 22 (1): 20–27.

Busse, Reinhard, Alexander Geissler, Wilm Quentin, and Miriam Wiley, eds. 2011. *Diagnosis-Related Groups in Europe: Moving towards Transparency, Efficiency and Quality in Hospitals*. Maidenhead: Open University Press.

Busse, Reinhard, Jonas Schreyogg, and Christian Gericke. 2007. *Analyzing Changes in Health Financing Arrangements in High-Income Countries: A Comprehensive Framework Approach*. Washington: The World Bank.

Butler, John. 1999. *The Ethics of Health Care Rationing: Principles and Practices*. London: Cassell.

Butler, Tamara L., Kate Anderson, Gail Garvey, Joan Cunningham, Julie Ratcliffe, Allison Tong, Lisa J. Whop, Alan Cass, Michelle Dickson, and Kirsten Howard. 2019. "Aboriginal and Torres Strait Islander People's Domains of Wellbeing: A Comprehensive Literature Review." *Social Science & Medicine* 233: 138–157.

Buxbaum, Jason D., Michael E. Chernew, A. Mark Fendrick, and David M. Cutler. 2020. "Contributions of Public Health, Pharmaceuticals, and Other Medical Care to US Life Expectancy Changes, 1990–2015: Study Examines the Conditions Most Responsible for Changing US Life Expectancy and How Public Health, Pharmaceuticals, Other Medical Care, and Other Factors May Have Contributed to the Changes." *Health Affairs* 39 (9): 1546–1556.

Byrne, Matthew J., Martin Tickle, Anne-Marie Glenny, Stephen Campbell, Tom Goodwin, and Lucy O'Malley. 2019. "A Systematic Review of Quality Measures Used in Primary Care Dentistry." *International Dental Journal* 69 (4): 252–264.

Byrne, Patrick H. 1993. "Ressentiment and the Preferential Option for the Poor." *Theological Studies* 54 (2): 213–241.

Cafferky, Michael E. 2013. "Toward a Biblical Theology of Efficiency." *Journal of Biblical Integration in Business* 16 (2): 41–60.

Calabresi, Guido, and Philip Bobbitt. 1978. *Tragic Choices: The Conflicts Society Confronts in the Allocation of Tragically Scarce Resources*. New York: Norton.

Callison, Kevin, Robert Kaestner, and Jason Ward. 2021. "Do Supply-Side Forces Explain Geographic Variation in Health Care Use?" *Economic Inquiry* 59 (1): 119–139.

Calman, Kenneth. 2009. "Beyond the 'Nanny State': Stewardship and Public Health." *Public Health* 123 (1): e6–e10.

Cameron, C. Daryl. 2017a. "Compassion Collapse: Why We Are Numb to Numbers." In *The Oxford Handbook of Compassion Science*, edited by Emma M Seppälä, Emiliana Simon-Thomas, Stephanie L Brown, Monica C Worline, C Daryl Cameron and James R Doty, 261–271. Oxford: Oxford University Press.

Cameron, David, Jasper Ubels, and Fredrik Norström. 2018. "On What Basis Are Medical Cost-Effectiveness Thresholds Set? Clashing Opinions and an Absence of Data: A Systematic Review." *Global Health Action* 11 (1): 1447828.

Cameron, Kim S. 2017b. "Organizational Compassion: Manifestations through Organizations." In *The Oxford Handbook of Compassion Science*, edited by Emma M Seppälä, Emiliana Simon-Thomas, Stephanie L Brown, Monica C Worline, C Daryl Cameron, and James R Doty, 421–434. Oxford: Oxford University Press.

Camosy, Charles Christopher. 2012. *Peter Singer and Christian Ethic: Beyond Polarization*. Cambridge: Cambridge University Press.

Campanella, Paolo, Vladimir Vukovic, Paolo Parente, Adela Sulejmani, Walter Ricciardi, and Maria Lucia Specchia. 2016. "The Impact of Public Reporting on Clinical Outcomes: A Systematic Review and Meta-Analysis." *BMC Health Services Research* 16 (296).

Campbell, Donald T. 1979. "Assessing the Impact of Planned Social Change." *Evaluation and Program Planning* 2 (1): 67–90.

Campbell, Stephen M., Sven Nyholm, and Jennifer K. Walter. 2021. "Disability and the Goods of Life." *The Journal of Medicine and Philosophy: A Forum for Bioethics and Philosophy of Medicine* 46 (6): 704–728.

Caponi, Francis J. 2018. "Thomas Aquinas on the Parable of the Late-Come Workers (Matthew 20:1–16)." *Journal of Theological Interpretation* 12 (1): 90–109.

Cardona, Beatriz. 2021. "The Pitfalls of Personalization Rhetoric in Time of Health Crisis: COVID-19 Pandemic and Cracks on Neoliberal Ideologies." *Health Promotion International* 36 (3): 714–721.

Cardona-Morrell, Magnolia, James C. H. Kim, Mikkel Brabrand, Blanca Gallego-Luxan, and Ken Hillman. 2017. "What Is Inappropriate Hospital Use for Elderly People Near the End of Life? A Systematic Review." *European Journal of Internal Medicine* 42: 39–50.

Cardona-Morrell, Magnolia, James C. H. Kim, R. M. Turner, M. Anstey, I. A. Mitchell, and Ken Hillman. 2016. "Non-Beneficial Treatments in Hospital at the End of Life: A Systematic Review on Extent of the Problem." *International Journal for Quality in Health Care* 28 (4): 456–469.

Carlson, Colin J., Gregory F. Albery, Cory Merow, Christopher H. Trisos, Casey M. Zipfel, Evan A. Eskew, Kevin J. Olival, Noam Ross, and Shweta Bansal. 2022 (in press). "Climate Change Increases Cross-Species Viral Transmission Risk." *Nature*.

Carlson, Josh J., Elizabeth D. Brouwer, Eunice Kim, Phoebe Wright, and R. Brett McQueen. 2020. "Alternative Approaches to Quality-Adjusted Life-Year Estimation within Standard Cost-Effectiveness Models: Literature Review, Feasibility Assessment, and Impact Evaluation." *Value in Health* 23 (12): 1523–1533.

Carney, Frederick S. 1981. "Justice and Health Care: A Theological Review." In *Justice and Health Care*, edited by Earl E. Shelp, 37–50. Dordrecht, Holland: D. Reidel.

Carr, Brian. 2001. "Pity and Compassion as Social Virtues." *Philosophy* 74 (3): 411–429.

Carroll, John T. 1995. "Sickness and Healing in the New Testament Gospels." *Interpretation* 49 (2): 130–142.

Carroll, R., M. Daniel. 2016. "Seek Yahweh, Establish Justice: Probing Prophetic Ethics – An Orientation from Amos 5: 1–17." In *The Bible and Social Justice: Old Testament and New Testament Foundations for the Church's Urgent Call*, edited by Cynthia Long Westfall and Bryan R. Dyer, 1–34. Eugene, OR: Pickwick Publications.

Carter, Grace M., Joseph P. Newhouse, and Daniel A. Relles. 1990. "How Much Change in the Case Mix Index Is DRG Creep?" *Journal of Health Economics* 9 (4): 411–428.

Carter, Hannah Elizabeth, Xing Ju Lee, Cindy Gallois, Sarah Winch, Leonie Callaway, Lindy Willmott, Ben White, Malcolm Parker, Eliana Close, and Nicholas Graves. 2019. "Factors Associated with Non-beneficial Treatments in End of Life Hospital Admissions: A Multicentre Retrospective Cohort Study in Australia." *BMJ Open* 9 (11): e030955.

Carter, Hannah Elizabeth, Sarah Winch, Adrian G. Barnett, Malcolm Parker, Cindy Gallois, Lindy Willmott, Ben P. White, Mary Anne Patton, Letitia Burridge, Gayle Salkield, Eliana Close, Leonie Callaway, and Nicholas Graves. 2017. "Incidence, Duration and Cost of Futile Treatment in End-of-Life Hospital Admissions to Three Australian Public-Sector Tertiary Hospitals: A Retrospective Multicentre Cohort Study." *BMJ Open* 7 (10): e017661.

Case, Anne, and Angus Deaton. 2020. *Deaths of Despair and the Future of Capitalism*. Princeton: Princeton University Press.

Case, Donald O., and Lisa M. Given. 2016. *Looking for Information: A Survey of Research on Information Seeking, Needs, and Behavior*. Bingley, UK: Emerald.

Castaldo, Sandro, Katia Premazzi, and Fabrizio Zerbini. 2010. "The Meaning (s) of Trust. A Content Analysis on the Diverse Conceptualizations of Trust in Scholarly Research on Business Relationships." *Journal of Business Ethics* 96 (4): 657–668.

Castillo, Enrico G., Jessica Isom, Katrina L. DeBonis, Ayana Jordan, Joel T. Braslow, and Robert Rohrbaugh. 2020. "Reconsidering Systems-Based Practice: Advancing Structural Competency, Health Equity, and Social Responsibility in Graduate Medical Education." *Academic Medicine* 95 (12): 1817–1822.

Catillon, Maryaline, David Cutler, and Thomas Getzen. 2018. *Two Hundred Years of Health and Medical Care: The Importance of Medical Care for Life Expectancy Gains*. National Bureau of Economic Research. www.nber.org/papers/w25330.

Cattel, Daniëlle, and Frank Eijkenaar. 2020. "Value-Based Provider Payment Initiatives Combining Global Payments with Explicit Quality Incentives: A Systematic Review." *Medical Care Research and Review* 77 (6): 511–537.

Cattel, Daniëlle, Frank Eijkenaar, and Frederik T. Schut. 2020. "Value-Based Provider Payment: Towards a Theoretically Preferred Design." *Health Economics, Policy and Law* 15 (1): 94–112.

Caviola, Lucius, Stefan Schubert, and Joshua D. Greene. 2021. "The Psychology of (In)Effective Altruism." *Trends in Cognitive Sciences* 25 (7): 596–607.

Chadwick, Ruth F. 1989. "Playing God." *Cogito* 3 (3): 186–193.

Chalmers, Kelsey, Sallie-Anne Pearson, Tim Badgery-Parker, Jonathan Brett, Ian A. Scott, and Adam G. Elshaug. 2019. "Measuring 21 Low-Value Hospital Procedures: Claims Analysis of Australian Private Health Insurance Data (2010–2014)." *BMJ Open* 9 (3): e024142.

Chalmers, Kelsey, Tim Badgery-Parker, Sallie-Anne Pearson, Jonathan Brett, Ian A. Scott, and Adam G. Elshaug. 2018. "Developing Indicators for Measuring Low-Value Care: Mapping Choosing Wisely Recommendations to Hospital Data." *BMC Research Notes* 11 (163): 1–8.

Chalmers, Matthew. 2020. "Rethinking Luke 10: The Parable of the Good Samaritan Israelite." *Journal of Biblical Literature* 139 (3): 543–566.

Chamberlain, Charlotte, Amanda Owen-Smith, Fiona MacKichan, Jenny L. Donovan, and William Hollingworth. 2019. "'What's Fair to an Individual Is Not Always Fair to a Population': A Qualitative Study of Patients and Their Health Professionals Using the Cancer Drugs Fund." *Health Policy* 123 (8): 706–712.

Chamberlin, Peter, Jason Lambden, Elissa Kozlov, Renee Maciejewski, Lindsay Lief, David A. Berlin, Latrice Pelissier, Elina Yushuvayev, Cynthia X. Pan, and Holly G. Prigerson. 2019. "Clinicians' Perceptions of Futile or Potentially Inappropriate Care and Associations with Avoidant Behaviors and Burnout." *Journal of Palliative Medicine* 22 (9): 1039–1045.

Chan, Adrienne Y. L., Vivien K. Y. Chan, Sten Olsson, Min Fan, Mark Jit, Mengchun Gong, Shuyang Zhang, Mengqin Ge, Swathi Pathadka, Claudia C. Y. Chung, Brian H. Y. Chung, Celine S. L. Chui, Esther W. Chan, Gloria H. Y. Wong, Terry Y. Lum, Ian C. K. Wong, Patrick Ip, and Xue Li. 2020. "Access and Unmet Needs of Orphan Drugs in 194 Countries and 6 Areas: A Global Policy Review with Content Analysis." *Value in Health* 23 (12): 1580–1591.

Chan, Georgina, Louret Bezuidenhout, Logan Walker, and Robert Rowan. 2016. "The Impact on Life Questionnaire: Validation for Elective Surgery Prioritisation in New Zealand Prioritisation Criteria in Orthopaedic Surgery." *The New Zealand Medical Journal* 129 (1432): 26–32.

Chandra, Amitabh, and Douglas O. Staiger. 2020. "Identifying Sources of Inefficiency in Healthcare." *The Quarterly Journal of Economics* 135 (2): 785–843.

Chandra, Amitabh, Evan Flack, and Ziad Obermeyer. 2021. "The Health Costs of Cost-Sharing." *National Bureau of Economic Research Working Paper Series* 28439: 1–56.

Charlesworth, Anita, and Karen Bloor. 2018. "70 Years of NHS Funding: How Do We Know How Much Is Enough?" *BMJ* 361: k2373.

Charlton, Victoria. 2022 (in press). "The Normative Grounds for NICE Decision-Making: A Narrative Cross-Disciplinary Review of Empirical Studies." *Health Economics, Policy and Law*: 1–27.

Charlton, Victoria, and Albert Weale. 2021. "Exorcising the Positivist Ghost in the Priority-Setting Machine: NICE and the Demise of the 'Social Value Judgement'." *Health Economics, Policy and Law* 16 (4): 505–511.

Chatterjee, Helen J., Paul M. Camic, Bridget Lockyer, and Linda J. M. Thomson. 2018. "Non-Clinical Community Interventions: A Systematised Review of Social Prescribing Schemes." *Arts & Health* 10 (2): 97–123.

Chen, Jeng-Guo S. 2017. "'The Man Within': Adam Smith on Moral Autonomy and Religious Sentiments." *Journal of Scottish Philosophy* 15 (1): 47–64.

Chen, Simiao, Michael Kuhn, Klaus Prettner, David E. Bloom, and Chen Wang. 2021. "Macro-Level Efficiency of Health Expenditure: Estimates for 15 Major Economies." *Social Science & Medicine*: 114270.

Cheng, Terence Chai, Catherine M. Joyce, and Anthony Scott. 2013. "An Empirical Analysis of Public and Private Medical Practice in Australia." *Health Policy* 111 (1): 43–51.

Cheng, Terence Chai, Guyonne Kalb, and Anthony Scott. 2013. *Public Private or Both?: Analysing Factors Influencing the Labour Supply of Medical Specialists.* Melbourne: Melbourne Institute.

Chereches, Răzvan M., Marius I. Ungureanu, Petru Sandu, and Ioana A. Rus. 2013. "Defining Informal Payments in Healthcare: A Systematic Review." *Health Policy* 110 (2): 105–114.

Chernew, Michael E., Jessica Carichner, Jeron Impreso, J. Michael McWilliams, Thomas G. McGuire, Sartaj Alam, Bruce E. Landon, and Mary Beth Landrum. 2021. "Coding-Driven Changes in Measured Risk in Accountable Care Organizations." *Health Affairs* 40 (12): 1909–1917.

Childress, James F. 1986. "Compassion." In *A New Dictionary of Christian Ethics*, edited by John Macquarrie and James F Childress, 109. London: SCM Press.

Childress, James F., and Tom L. Beauchamp. 2021. "Common Morality Principles in Biomedical Ethics: Responses to Critics." *Cambridge Quarterly of Healthcare Ethics* 13 (2): 164–176.

Chim, Lesley, Glenn Salkeld, Patrick J. Kelly, Wendy Lipworth, Dyfrig A. Hughes, and Martin R. Stockler. 2019. "Community Views on Factors Affecting Medicines Resource Allocation: Cross-Sectional Survey of 3080 Adults in Australia." *Australian Health Review* 43 (3): 254–260.

Christen, Markus, Christian Ineichen, and Carmen Tanner. 2014. "How 'Moral' Are the Principles of Biomedical Ethics? – a Cross-Domain Evaluation of the Common Morality Hypothesis." *BMC Medical Ethics* 15 (47): 1–12.

Churruca, Kate, Chiara Pomare, Louise A. Ellis, Janet C. Long, Suzanna B. Henderson, Lisa E. D. Murphy, Christopher J. Leahy, and Jeffrey Braithwaite. 2021. "Patient-Reported Outcome Measures (PROMs): A Review of Generic and Condition-Specific Measures and a Discussion of Trends and Issues." *Health Expectations* 24 (4): 1015–1024.

Cipriani, Andrea, John P. A. Ioannidis, Peter M. Rothwell, Paul Glasziou, Tianjing Li, Adrian F. Hernandez, Anneka Tomlinson, John Simes, and Huseyin Naci. 2020. "Generating Comparative Evidence on New Drugs and Devices after Approval." *The Lancet* 395 (10228): 998–1010.

Clark, David J. 1996. "The Sermon on the Plain: Structure and Theme in Luke 6.20–49." *The Bible Translator* 47 (4): 428–434.

Clark, Patrick M. 2014. "Reversing the Ethical Perspective: What the Allegorical Interpretation of the Good Samaritan Parable Can Still Teach Us." *Theology Today* 71 (3): 300–309.

Claxton, Karl, Steve Martin, Marta Soares, Nigel Rice, Eldon Spackman, Sebastian Hinde, Nancy Devlin, Peter C. Smith, and Mark Sculpher. 2015. "Methods for the Estimation of the National Institute for Health and Care Excellence Cost-Effectiveness Threshold." *Health Technology Assessment* 19 (14): 1–503.

Clayton, Susan. 1983. "Social Need Revisited." *Journal of Social Policy* 12 (2): 215–234.

Cliff, Betsy Q., Anton L. V. Avanceña, Richard A. Hirth, and Shoou-Yih Daniel Lee. 2021. "The Impact of Choosing Wisely Interventions on Low-Value Medical Services: A Systematic Review." *The Milbank Quarterly* 99 (4):1024–1058.

Coady, C. A. J. 2009. "Playing God." In *Human Enhancement*, edited by Julian Savulescu and Nick Bostrom, 155–180. Oxford: Oxford University Press.

Coast, Joanna. 1997. "Rationing within the NHS Should Be Explicit: The Case Against." In *Rationing: Talk and Action in Health Care*, edited by B. New, 149–156. London: BMJ Publishing.

2000. "Explicit Rationing, Deprivation Disutility and Denial Disutility: Evidence from a Qualitative Study." In *The Global Challenge of Health Care Rationing*, edited by Angela Coulter and Chris Ham, 192–200. Buckingham: Open University Press.

2001. "Who Wants to Know If Their Care Is Rationed? Views of Citizens and Service Informants." *Health Expectations* 4 (4): 243–252.

Coast, Joanna, Cara Bailey, Alastair Canaway, and Philip Kinghorn. 2016. "Measuring and Valuing Outcomes for Care at the End of Life: The Capability Approach." In *Care at the End of Life: An Economic Perspective*, edited by Jeff Round. Cham: Adis.

2021. "'It Is Not a Scientific Number It Is Just a feeling': Populating a Multi-Dimensional End-of-Life Decision Framework Using Deliberative Methods." *Health Economics* 30 (5): 1033–1049.

Coast, Joanna, Jenny Donovan, Andrea Litva, John Eyles, Kieran Morgan, Michael Shepherd, and Jo Tacchi. 2002. "'If There Were a War Tomorrow, We'd Find the Money': Contrasting Perspectives on the Rationing of Health Care." *Social Science & Medicine* 54 (12): 1839–1851.

Cocker, Fiona, and Nerida Joss. 2016. "Compassion Fatigue among Healthcare, Emergency and Community Service Workers: A Systematic Review." *International Journal of Environmental Research and Public Health* 13 (6): 618.

Coetzee, Siedine K., and Heather K.S. Laschinger. 2018. "Toward a Comprehensive, Theoretical Model of Compassion Fatigue: An Integrative Literature Review." *Nursing & Health Sciences* 20 (1): 4–15.

Cohen, Joshua, and Peter Ubel. 2001. "Accounting for Fairness and Efficiency in Health Economics." In *The Social Economics of Health Care*, edited by John Bryan Davis, 94–109. London: Routledge.

Cohen, Nissim. 2012. "Informal Payments for Health Care – the Phenomenon and Its Context." *Health Economics, Policy and Law* 7 (3): 285–308.

2018. "How Culture Affects Street-Level Bureaucrats' Bending the Rules in the Context of Informal Payments for Health Care: The Israeli Case." *The American Review of Public Administration* 48 (2): 175–187.

Collins, John J. 2019. *What Are Biblical Values? What the Bible Says on Key Ethical Issues*. New Haven: Yale University Press.

Collins, Mary Elizabeth, Kate Cooney, and Sarah Garlington. 2011. "Compassion in Contemporary Social Policy: Applications of Virtue Theory." *Journal of Social Policy* 41 (2): 251–269.

Colvin, Jeffrey D., Troy Richardson, Donna K. Ginther, Matt Hall, and Paul J. Chung. 2020. "Economy-Sensitive Conditions: Are Some Pediatric Hospitalizations Triggered by Economic Recessions? Study Examines Whether Some Pediatric Hospitalizations Are Triggered by Economic Recessions." *Health Affairs* 39 (10): 1783–1791.

Commission on Social Determinants of Health. 2008. *Closing the Gap in a Generation: Health Equity through Action on the Social Determinants of Health*. Geneva: World Health Organization.

Congregation for the Doctrine of the Faith. 2008. *Instruction Dignitas Personae: On Certain Bioethical Questions*. Vatican City: Congregation for the Doctrine of the Faith.

Conrad, Douglas A. 2009. "Incentives for Health-Care Performance Improvement." In *Performance Measurement for Health System Improvement: Experiences, Challenges, and Prospects*, edited by Peter Smith, Elias Mossialos, Irene Papanicolas and S. Leatherman, 582–912. Cambridge, New York: Cambridge University Press.

2015. "The Theory of Value-Based Payment Incentives and Their Application to Health Care." *Health Services Research* 50 (S2): 2057–2089.

Conrad, Peter, and Joseph W. Schneider. 2010. *Deviance and Medicalization: From Badness to Sickness*. Philadelphia, PA: Temple University Press.

Cookson, Richard. 2013. "Can the NICE "End-of-Life Premium" Be Given a Coherent Ethical Justification?" *Journal of Health Politics, Policy and Law* 38 (6): 1129–1148.

Cookson, Richard, Anthony J. Culyer, and Ole F. Norheim. 2020. "Principles of Health Equity." In *Distributional Cost-Effectiveness Analysis Quantifying Health Equity Impacts and Trade-Offs*, edited by Richard Cookson, Susan Griffin, Ole Frithjof Norheim and Anthony J. Culyer. Oxford: Oxford University Press.

Cookson, Richard, Mike Drummond, and Helen Weatherly. 2009. "Explicit Incorporation of Equity Considerations into Economic Evaluation of Public Health Interventions." *Health Economics, Policy and Law* 4 (2): 231–245.

Cookson, Richard, Susan Griffin, Ole Frithjof Norheim, and Anthony J. Culyer, eds. 2020. *Distributional Cost-Effectiveness Analysis Quantifying Health Equity Impacts and Trade-Offs*. Oxford: Oxford University Press.

Cookson, Richard, Andrew J. Mirelman, Susan Griffin, Miqdad Asaria, Bryony Dawkins, Ole Frithjof Norheim, Stéphane Verguet, and Anthony J. Culyer. 2017. "Using Cost-Effectiveness Analysis to Address Health Equity Concerns." *Value in Health* 20 (2): 206–212.

Cooper-White, Michael L. 2009. "Christian Stewardship in Light of a Theology of the Cross." *Dialog* 48 (2): 202–206.

Copeland, M. Shawn. 2018. *Knowing Christ Crucified: The Witness of African American Religious Experience*. Maryknoll, NY: Orbis.
Costa-Font, Joan, and Frank Cowell. 2019. "Incorporating Inequality Aversion in Health-Care Priority Setting." *Social Justice Research* 32 (2): 172–185.
Costa-Font, Joan, and Sara Machado. 2021. "How Can Policy Interventions Encourage Pro-social Behaviours in the Health System?" *LSE Public Policy Review* 1 (3): 6.
Costello, Tim. 2020. *The Cost of Compassion*. Sydney: Acorn Press.
Cottingham, John. 1983. "Ethics and Impartiality." *Philosophical Studies* 43 (1): 83–99.
Coyle, Diane. 2014. *GDP: A Brief but Affectionate History*. Princeton: Princeton University Press.
Craig, Benjamin M., Kim Rand, Henry Bailey, and Peep F. M. Stalmeier. 2018. "Quality-Adjusted Life-Years without Constant Proportionality." *Value in Health* 21 (9): 1124–1131.
Crawford, Robert. 1977. "You Are Dangerous to Your Health: The Ideology and Politics of Victim Blaming." *International Journal of Health Services* 7 (4): 663–680.
Crespy, Georges. 1973. "La parabole dite: 'Le bon Samaritain.' Recherches structurales" *Études théologiques et religieuses* 48 (1): 61–79.
Cromwell, Jerry, Michael G. Trisolini, Gregory C. Pope, Janet B. Mitchell, and Leslie M. Greenwald, eds. 2011. *Pay for Performance in Health Care: Methods and Approaches*. Research Triangle Park, NC: RTI Press.
Crook, Hannah L., Robert S. Saunders, Rachel Roiland, Aparna Higgins, and Mark B. McClellan. 2021a. "A Decade of Value-Based Payment: Lessons Learned and Implications for the Center for Medicare and Medicaid Innovation, Part 1." *Health Affairs Blog (blog)*. www.healthaffairs.org/do/10.1377/hblog20210607.230763/full/.
2021b. "A Decade of Value-Based Payment: Lessons Learned and Implications for the Center for Medicare and Medicaid Innovation, Part 2." *Health Affairs Blog (blog)*. www.healthaffairs.org/do/10.1377/hblog20210607.656313/full/.
Crossan, John Dominic. 1992. *In Parables: The Challenge of the Historical Jesus*. Sonoma, CA: Polebridge Press.
2012. *The Power of Parable: How Fiction by Jesus Became Fiction about Jesus*. New York: HarperOne.
Cryder, Cynthia, and George Loewenstein. 2011. "The Critical Link between Tangibility and Generosity." In *The Science of Giving: Experimental Approaches to the Study of Charity*, edited by Daniel M Oppenheimer and Christopher Y Olivola. New York, NY: Psychology Press.
Cuadrado, Cristóbal, Francisca Crispi, Matías Libuy, Gregory Marchildon, and Camilo Cid. 2019. "National Health Insurance: A Conceptual Framework from Conflicting Typologies." *Health Policy* 123 (7): 621–629.
Cubi-Molla, Patricia, David Mott, Nadine Henderson, Bernarda Zamora, Mendel Grobler, and Martina Garau. 2021. *Resource Allocation in Public Sector Programmes: Does the Value of a Life Differ between Governmental Departments?*

London: Office of Health Economics. www.ohe.org/publications/resource-allocation-public-sector-programmes-does-value-life-differ-between.

Cubi-Molla, Patricia, Maria Errea, Kyann Zhang, and Martina Garau. 2020. *Are Cost-Effectiveness Thresholds Fit for Purpose for Real-World Decision Making*. London: Office of Health Economics. www.ohe.org/publications/are-cost-effectiveness-thresholds-fit-for-purpose.

Cubi-Molla, Patricia, Martin Buxton, and Nancy Devlin. 2021. "Allocating Public Spending Efficiently: Is There a Need for a Better Mechanism to Inform Decisions in the UK and Elsewhere?" *Applied Health Economics and Health Policy* 19 (5): 635–644.

Cullis, John G., and Peter A. West. 1979. *The Economics of Health: An Introduction*. Oxford: Martin Robertson.

Culyer, Anthony J. 1989. "The Normative Economics of Health Care Finance and Provision." *Oxford Review of Economic Policy* 5 (1): 34–58.

1991. "Conflicts between Equity Concepts and Efficiency in Health--A Diagrammatic Approach." *Osaka Economic Papers* 40 (3–4): 141–154.

1992. "The Morality of Efficiency in Health Care – Some Uncomfortable Implications." *Health Economics* 1 (1): 7–18.

2005. *The Dictionary of Health Economics*. Cheltenham: Edward Elgar.

Culyer, Anthony J., and Alan Maynard, eds. 1997. *Being Reasonable about the Economics of Health: Selected Essays by Alan Williams*. London: Edward Elgar.

Culyer, Anthony J., and Joseph P. Newhouse. 2000. "Introduction: The State and Scope of Health Economics." In *Handbook of Health Economics*, edited by A. J. Culyer and J. P. Newhouse. Amsterdam: Elsevier Science BV.

Culyer, Anthony J., R. J. Lavers, and Alan Williams. 1972. "Health Indicators." In *Social Indicators and Social Policy*, edited by Andrew Shonfield and Stella Shaw, 94–118. London: Heinemann.

Curran, Charles E. 1985. "Just Taxation in the Roman Catholic Tradition." *The Journal of Religious Ethics* 13 (1): 113–133. www.jstor.org/stable/40015003.

Curtis, Andrea J., Colin O. H. Russell, Johannes U. Stoelwinder, and John J. McNeil. 2010. "Waiting Lists and Elective Surgery: Ordering the Queue." *Medical Journal of Australia* 192 (4): 217–220.

Cyr, Pascale Renée, Vageesh Jain, Kalipso Chalkidou, Trygve Ottersen, and Unni Gopinathan. 2021. "Evaluations of Public Health Interventions Produced by Health Technology Assessment Agencies: A Mapping Review and Analysis by Type and Evidence Content." *Health Policy* 125 (8): 1054–1064.

D'Andreamatteo, Antonio, Luca Ianni, Federico Lega, and Massimo Sargiacomo. 2015. "Lean in Healthcare: A Comprehensive Review." *Health Policy* 119 (9): 1197–1209.

Dabbous, Monique, Mondher Toumi, Steven Simoens, Juergen Wasem, Gauri Saal, Yitong Wang, José Luis Huerta Osuna, Clément François, Lieven Annemans, Johann-Matthias Graf von der Schulenburg, Oriol Sola-Morales, Daniel Malone, and Louis P. Garrison. 2022. "Amortization of Gene Replacement Therapies: A Health Policy Analysis Exploring a Mechanism for Mitigating Budget Impact of High-Cost Treatments." *Health Policy* 126 (1): 49–59.

Dakin, Helen, Nancy Devlin, Yan Feng, Nigel Rice, Phill O'Neill, and David Parkin. 2015. "The Influence of Cost-Effectiveness and Other Factors on Nice Decisions." *Health Economics* 24 (10): 1256–1271.

Daniels, Norman, Donald W. Light, and Ronald L. Caplan. 1996. *Benchmarks of Fairness for Health Care Reform.* New York: Oxford University Press.

Daniels, Norman, and James Sabin. 1997. "Limits to Health Care: Fair Procedures, Democratic Deliberation, and the Legitimacy Problem for Insurers." *Philosophy and Public Affairs* 26 (4): 303–350.

2002. *Setting Limits Fairly: Can We Learn to Share Medical Resources?* New York: Oxford University Press.

Danis, Marion, and Donald L. Patrick. 2002. "Health Policy, Vulnerability and Vulnerable Populations." In *Ethical Dimensions of Health Policy*, edited by Marion Danis, Carolyn M Clancy and Larry R Churchill. New York: Oxford University Press.

Danzon, Patricia M., Michael F. Drummond, Adrian Towse, and Mark V. Pauly. 2018. "Objectives, Budgets, Thresholds, and Opportunity Costs – A Health Economics Approach: An ISPOR Special Task Force Report." *Value in Health* 21 (2): 140–145.

Daraz, Lubna, Allison S. Morrow, Oscar J. Ponce, Bradley Beuschel, Magdoleen H. Farah, Abdulrahman Katabi, Mouaz Alsawas, Abdul M. Majzoub, Raed Benkhadra, Mohamed O. Seisa, Jingyi Ding, Larry Prokop, and M. Hassan Murad. 2019. "Can Patients Trust Online Health Information? A Meta-narrative Systematic Review Addressing the Quality of Health Information on the Internet." *Journal of General Internal Medicine* 34 (9): 1884–1891.

Darley, John M., and C. Daniel Batson. 1973. ""From Jerusalem to Jericho": A Study of Situational and Dispositional Variables in Helping Behavior." *Journal of Personality and Social Psychology* 27 (1): 100–108.

Daroudi, Rajabali, Ali Akbari Sari, Azin Nahvijou, and Ahmad Faramarzi. 2021. "Cost per DALY Averted in Low, Middle- and High-Income Countries: Evidence from the Global Burden of Disease Study to Estimate the Cost-Effectiveness Thresholds." *Cost Effectiveness and Resource Allocation* 19 (7): 1–9. https://doi.org/10.1186/s12962-021-00260-0.

das Neves, João César. 2017. "The Economics of Pope Francis." *Catholic Social Science Review* 22: 157–170. https://search.ebscohost.com/login.aspx?direct=true&db=a9h&AN=124789122&site=ehost-live.

Davids, Peter H. 2005. "The Test of Wealth in James and Paul." In *The Missions of James, Peter, and Paul: Tensions in Early Christianity*, edited by Bruce D. Chilton and Craig A. Evans, 355–384. Leiden: Brill.

Davidson, Bob. 2018. "The Marketisation of Aged Care in Australia." In *Wrong Way: How Privatisation and Economic Reform Backfired*, edited by Damien Cahill and Phillip Toner, 101–116. Melbourne: La Trobe University Press in Conjunction with Black Inc.

Davies, Ben, and Julian Savulescu. 2019. "Solidarity and Responsibility in Health Care." *Public Health Ethics* 12 (2): 133–144.

Davies, Oliver. 2016. *A Theology of Compassion: Metaphysics of Difference and the Renewal of Tradition*. Eugene, OR: Wipf and Stock Publishers.

Davies, Sally, and Jonathan Pearson-Stuttard. 2021. *Whose Health Is It, Anyway?* Oxford: Oxford University Press.

Davies, Sheryl, Ellen Schultz, Maria Raven, Nancy Ewen Wang, Carol L. Stocks, Mucio Kit Delgado, and Kathryn M. McDonald. 2017. "Development and Validation of the Agency for Healthcare Research and Quality Measures of Potentially Preventable Emergency Department (ED) Visits: The ED Prevention Quality Indicators for General Health Conditions." *Health Services Research* 52 (5): 1667–1684.

Davis, Courtney, Huseyin Naci, Evrim Gurpinar, Elita Poplavska, Ashlyn Pinto, and Ajay Aggarwal. 2017. "Availability of Evidence of Benefits on Overall Survival and Quality of Life of Cancer Drugs Approved by European Medicines Agency: Retrospective Cohort Study of Drug Approvals 2009–13." *BMJ* 359: j4530.

Davis, John B. 1991. "Keynes's View of Economics as a Moral Science." In *Keynes and Philosophy: Essays on the Origins of Keynes's Thought*, edited by Bradley W. Bateman and John B. Davis, 89–103. Aldershot: Edward Elgar.

Day, Rebecca Trowman, Richard Norman, and Suzanne Robinson. 2016. "Challenges and Opportunities for Disinvestment in Australia: A Need to Evaluate the Implementation and Impact of Choosing Wisely in Australia." *Journal of Health Organization and Management*." *Journal of Health Organization and Management* 30 (8): 1301–1307.

de Beer, Joop, Anastasios Bardoutsos, and Fanny Janssen. 2017. "Maximum Human Lifespan May Increase to 125 Years." *Nature* 546: E16.

de Bekker-Grob, Esther W., Mandy Ryan, and Karen Gerard. 2012. "Discrete Choice Experiments in Health Economics: A Review of the Literature." *Health Economics* 21 (2): 145–172.

de Vries, Linda M., Pieter H. M. van Baal, and Werner B. F. Brouwer. 2019. "Future Costs in Cost-Effectiveness Analyses: Past, Present, Future." *PharmacoEconomics* 37 (2): 119–130.

de Zulueta, Paquita. 2013. "Compassion in 21st Century Medicine: Is It Sustainable?" *Clinical Ethics* 8 (4): 119–128.

2016. "Developing Compassionate Leadership in Health Care: An Integrative Review." *Journal of Healthcare Leadership* 8: 1–10.

2021. "How Do We Sustain Compassionate Healthcare? Compassionate Leadership in the Time of the COVID-19 Pandemic." *Clinics in Integrated Care* 8: 100071.

Dean, James M., and Andrew Michael Charles Waterman. 1999. "Summary If Not Conclusions." In *Religion and Economics: Normative Social Theory*, edited by James M. Dean and Andrew Michael Charles Waterman, 175–183. Dordrecht: Kluwer Academic.

Deane-Drummond, Celia. 2017. *A Primer in Ecotheology Theology for a Fragile Earth*. Eugene, OR: Wipf and Stock.

Deane-Drummond, Celia, and Barbara Rossing. 2013. "The Eco-Theological Significance of John 10:10." *Ecumenical Review* 65 (1): 83–97.

Deeble, John Stewart, and Richard Bailey Scotton. 1968. *Health Care under Voluntary Insurance: Report of a Survey*. Melbourne: Institute of Applied Economic Research.

Dees, Marianne, Myrra Vernooij-Dassen, Wim Dekkers, and Chris van Weel. 2010. "Unbearable Suffering of Patients with a Request for Euthanasia or Physician-Assisted Suicide: An Integrative Review." *Psycho-Oncology* 19 (4): 339–352.

Deming, W. Edwards. 1993. *The New Economics for Industry, Government, Education*. Cambridge, MA: Massachusetts Institute of Technology, Center for Advanced Engineering Study.

Denburg, Avram E., Wendy J. Ungar, Shiyi Chen, Jeremiah Hurley, and Julia Abelson. 2020. "Does Moral Reasoning Influence Public Values for Health Care Priority Setting?: A Population-Based Randomized Stated Preference Survey." *Health Policy* 124 (6): 647–658.

DeNicola, Nathaniel G., Curtis L. Lowery, Kathryn I. Marko, and Daniel Aaron Grossman. 2019. "A Systematic Review of Telehealth on Clinical Outcomes in Obstetrics & Gynecology." *Obstetrics & Gynecology* 133: 58S.

Dennison, William David. 1976. "Miracles As "Signs" Their Significance for Apologetics." *Biblical Theology Bulletin* 6 (2–3): 190–202.

Department of Health and Human Services. Centers for Medicare & Medicaid Services. 2020. "Medicaid Program; Establishing Minimum Standards in Medicaid State Drug Utilization Review (DUR) and Supporting Value-Based Purchasing (VBP) for Drugs Covered in Medicaid, Revising Medicaid Drug Rebate and Third Party Liability (TPL) Requirements." *Federal Register* 85 (251): 87000–87104.

Department of Health. Pharmaceutical Benefits Advisory Committee. 2016. Guidelines for Preparing Submissions to the Pharmaceutical Benefits Advisory Committee (PBAC) – version 5.0. PBAC (Canberra).

Derickson, Gary W. 1998. "The Cessation of Healing Miracles in Paul's Ministry." *Bibliotheca Sacra* 155 (Jul–Sep): 299–315.

DeRock, Daniel. 2021. "Hidden in Plain Sight: Unpaid Household Services and the Politics of GDP Measurement." *New Political Economy* 26 (1): 20–35.

Derrett, J. Duncan M. 1964. "Law in the New Testament: Fresh Light on the Parable of the Good Samaritan." *New Testament Studies* 11 (1): 22–37.

Dewar, Belinda, and Mike Nolan. 2013. "Caring about Caring: Developing a Model to Implement Compassionate Relationship Centred Care in an Older People Care Setting." *International Journal of Nursing Studies* 50 (9): 1247–1258.

Dewar, Belinda, Simon Pullin, and Ria Tocheris. 2011. "Valuing Compassion through Definition and Measurement." *Nursing Management (Harrow)* 17 (9): 32–37.

Dewitt, Barry, and George W. Torrance. 2020. "Incorporating Mortality in Health Utility Measures." *Medical Decision Making* 40 (7): 862–872.

Dhami, Sanjit. 2016. *The Foundations of Behavioral Economic Analysis*. Oxford: Oxford University Press.

Dickman, Samuel L., David U. Himmelstein, and Steffie Woolhandler. 2017. "Inequality and the Health-Care System in the USA." *The Lancet* 389 (10077): 1431–1441.

Dijkstra, Ilse, and Klasien Horstman. 2021. "'Known to Be Unhealthy': Exploring How Social Epidemiological Research Constructs the Category of Low Socioeconomic Status." *Social Science & Medicine* 285: 114263.

Do, Loc, Diep Ha, Marco A. Peres, John Skinner, Roy Byun, and A. John Spencer. 2017. "Effectiveness of Water Fluoridation in the Prevention of Dental Caries across Adult Age Groups." *Community Dentistry and Oral Epidemiology* 45 (3): 225–232.

Dobkin, Carlos, Amy Finkelstein, Raymond Kluender, and Matthew J. Notowidigdo. 2018. "Myth and Measurement – The Case of Medical Bankruptcies." *The New England Journal of Medicine* 378 (12): 1076–1078.

Dobrow, Mark J., Victoria Hagens, Roger Chafe, Terrence Sullivan, and Linda Rabeneck. 2018. "Consolidated Principles for Screening Based on a Systematic Review and Consensus Process." *Canadian Medical Association Journal* 190 (14): E422–E429.

Dodd, Charles H. 1961. *The Parables of the Kingdom.* New York, NY: Charles Scribner.

Dodd, Rebecca, Joseph Alvin Santos, Monique Tan, Norm R. C. Campbell, Cliona Ni Mhurchu, Laura Cobb, Michael F. Jacobson, Feng J. He, Kathy Trieu, Sutayut Osornprasop, and Jacqui Webster. 2020. "Effectiveness and Feasibility of Taxing Salt and Foods High in Sodium: A Systematic Review of the Evidence." *Advances in Nutrition.*

Dodd, Sarah Drakopoulou, and George N. Gotsis. 2000. "Some Economic Implications of Synoptic Gospel Theology: A Short Overview." *History of Economic Ideas* 8 (2): 7–34.

Dolan, Paul. 2000. "The Measurement of Health-Related Quality of Life." In *Handbook of Health Economics. Volume 1B*, edited by A. J. Culyer and J. P. Newhouse, 1723–1760. Amsterdam: Elsevier Science B.V.

Dolan, Paul, Robert Metcalfe, Vicki Munro, and Michael C. Christensen. 2008. "Valuing Lives and Life Years: Anomalies, Implications, and an Alternative." *Health Economics, Policy and Law* 3 (3): 277–300.

Dolan, Paul, and Jan Abel Olsen. 2002. *Distributing Health Care: Economic and Ethical Issues.* Oxford: Oxford University Press.

Donabedian, Avedis. 1973. *Aspects of Medical Care Administration: Specifying Requirements for Health Care.* Cambridge, MA: Harvard University Press.

2002. *An Introduction to Quality Assurance in Health Care.* New York: Oxford University Press.

Donahue, John R. 1988. *The Gospel in Parable: Metaphor, Narrative, and Theology in the Synoptic Gospels.* Philadelphia, PA: Fortress Press.

Donaldson, Cam, Angela Bate, Peter Bramblegy, and Howard Waldner. 2008. "Moving Forward on Rationing: An Economic View." *BMJ* 337: a1872.

Dong, Xiao, Brandon Milholland, and Jan Vijg. 2016. "Evidence for a Limit to Human Lifespan." *Nature* 538 (7624): 257–259.

Donne, John. 1624. *Devotions upon Emergent Occasions, and Severall Steps in My Sicknesse. Digested into 1. Meditations, upon Our Humane Condition. 2. Expostulations, and Debatements with God. 3. Prayers, upon the Severall Occasions to Him*. London: Printed by A[ugustine] M[athewes] for Thomas Jones.

Dormandy, Richard. 2002. "Unjust Steward or Converted Master?" *Revue Biblique* 109 (4): 512–527.

Doucouliagos, Chris. 1994. "A Note on the Evolution of Homo Economicus." *Journal of Economic Issues* 28 (3): 877–883.

Dougherty, Charles J., and Ruth Purtilo. 1995. "Physicians' Duty of Compassion." *Cambridge Quarterly of Healthcare Ethics* 4 (4): 426–433.

Dowd, Sharyn. 2000. "Faith That Works: James 2:14–26." *Review & Expositor* 97 (2): 195–205.

Downar, James, John J. You, Sean M. Bagshaw, Eyal Golan, Francois Lamontagne, Karen Burns, S. Kavita Sridhar, Andrew Seely, Maureen O. Meade, Alison Fox-Robichaud, Deborah Cook, Alexis F. Turgeon, Peter Dodek, Wei Xiong, Rob Fowler, and on Behalf of the Canadian Critical Care Trials Group. 2015. "Nonbeneficial Treatment Canada: Definitions, Causes, and Potential Solutions from the Perspective of Healthcare Practitioners." *Critical Care Medicine* 43 (2): 270–281.

Downie, Jocelyn, Lindy Willmott, and Ben White. 2014. "Cutting the Gordian Knot of Futility: A Case for Law Reform on Unilateral Withholding and Withdrawal of Potentially Life-Sustaining Treatment." *New Zealand Universities Law Review* 26 (1): 24–59.

Downie, Jocelyn, Lindy Willmott, and Ben P. White. 2017. "Next Up: A Proposal for Values-Based Law Reform on Unilateral Withholding and Withdrawal of Potentially Life-Sustaining Treatment." *Alberta Law Review* 54 (3): 803–830.

Downs, David J. 2016. *Alms: Charity, Reward, and Atonement in Early Christianity*. Waco, TX: Baylor University Press.

Dowse, Leanne. 2009. "'Some People Are Never Going to Be Able to Do That'. Challenges for People with Intellectual Disability in the 21st Century." *Disability & Society* 24 (5): 571–584.

Drake, Connor, Heather Batchelder, Tyler Lian, Meagan Cannady, Morris Weinberger, Howard Eisenson, Emily Esmaili, Allison Lewinski, Leah L. Zullig, Amber Haley, David Edelman, and Christopher M. Shea. 2021. "Implementation of Social Needs Screening in Primary Care: A Qualitative Study Using the Health Equity Implementation Framework." *BMC Health Services Research* 21 (975): 1–16.

Dreifus, Claudia, ed. 1977. *Seizing Our Bodies: The Politics of Women's Health*. New York: Vintage Books.

Drummond, Michael F., David A. Wilson, Panos Kanavos, Peter Ubel, and Joan Rovira. 2007. "Assessing the Economic Challenges Posed by Orphan Drugs." *International Journal of Technology Assessment in Health Care* 23 (1): 36–42.

Drummond, Michael, Mark Sculpher, Karl Claxton, Greg Stoddart, and George Torrance. 2015. *Methods for the Economic Evaluation of Health Care Programmes* (4th ed). Oxford: Oxford University Press.

Drummond, Michael, and Adrian Towse. 2019. "Is Rate of Return Pricing a Useful Approach When Value-Based Pricing Is Not Appropriate?" *The European Journal of Health Economics* 20 (7): 945–948.

Duckett, Stephen. 2005. "Private Care and Public aiting." *Australian Health Review* 29 (1): 87–93.

2008a. "The Continuing Contest of Values in the Australian Health Care System." In *International Health Law: Solidarity and Justice in Health Care*, edited by A. den Exter, 177–199. Antwerpen: Maklu.

2008b. "Design of Price Incentives for Adjunct Policy Goals in Formula Funding for Hospitals and Health Services." *BMC Health Services Research* 8 (72): 1–9.

2018a. "Aligning Policy Objectives and Payment Design in Palliative Care." *BMC Palliative Care* 17 (42): 1–10.

2018b. "Coercing, Subsidising and Encouraging: Two Decades of Support for Private Health Insurance." In *Wrong Way: How Privatisation and Economic Reform Backfired*, edited by Damien Cahill and Phillip Toner, 40–58. Melbourne, Victoria: La Trobe University Press in conjunction with Black Inc.

2019. "Value-Based Health Care – Fad or Fabulous?" *Healthcare Papers* 18 (3): 15–21.

2020. "Waves of Inequity in the Coronavirus Pandemic." *Gesher* 6 (2): 10–13.

Duckett, Stephen, and Cheri Nijssen-Jordan. 2012. "Using Quality Improvement Methods at the System Level to Improve Hospital Emergency Department Treatment Times." *Quality Management in Healthcare* 21 (1): 29–33.

Duckett, Stephen, and Kristina Nemet. 2019. *The History and Purposes of Private Health Insurance*. Melbourne, Victoria: Grattan Institute.

Duckett, Stephen, and Michael Ward. 2008. "Developing 'Robust Performance Benchmarks' for the Next Australian Health Care Agreement: The Need for a New Framework. " *Australian and New Zealand Health Policy* 5 (1): 1–8.

Duckett, Stephen, Hal Swerissen, and Trent Wiltshire. 2016. *A Sugary Drinks Tax: Recovering the Community Costs of Obesity*. Melbourne: Grattan Institute.

Duckett, Stephen, Matt Cowgill, and Hal Swerissen. 2019. *Filling the Gap: A Universal Dental Scheme for Australia*. Melbourne: Grattan Institute.

Duckett, Stephen, Will Mackey, and Anika Stobart. 2020. *Climate Change and Health: Preparing for the Next Disaster*. Melbourne, Victoria.: Grattan Institute.

Dukhanin, Vadim, Alexandra Searle, Alice Zwerling, David W. Dowdy, Holly A. Taylor, and Maria W. Merritt. 2018. "Integrating Social Justice Concerns into Economic Evaluation for Healthcare and Public Health: A Systematic Review." *Social Science & Medicine* 198: 27–35.

Duncan, Bruce. 2014. "Pope Francis's Call for Social Justice in the Global Economy." *Australasian Catholic Record* 91 (2): 178–193.

2017. "The Economics behind the Social Thought of Pope Francis." *Australasian Catholic Record* 94 (2): 148–166.

Dutton, Jane E., Monica C. Worline, Peter J. Frost, and Jacoba Lilius. 2006. "Explaining Compassion Organizing." *Administrative Science Quarterly* 51 (1): 59–96.

Dwyer, Judith, K. O'Donnell, E. Willis, and J. Kelly. 2016. "Equitable Care for Indigenous People: Every Health Service Can Do It." *Asia Pacific Journal of Health Management* 11 (3): 11–17.

Dyer, Bryan R. 2016. "Good News to the Poor: Social Upheaval, Strong Warnings, and Sincere Giving in Luke-Acts." In *The Bible and Social Justice: Old Testament and New Testament Foundations for the Church's Urgent Call*, edited by Cynthia Long Westfall and Bryan R. Dyer, 102–124. Eugene, OR: Pickwick Publications.

Eberl, Jason T. 2012. "Religious and Secular Perspectives on the Value of Suffering." *National Catholic Bioethics Quarterly* 12 (2): 251–261.

Eckelman, Matthew J., and Jodi D. Sherman. 2018. "Estimated Global Disease Burden from US Health Care Sector Greenhouse Gas Emissions." *American Journal of Public Health* 108 (S2): S120–S122.

Edelman, Murray. 1988. *Constructing the Political Spectacle*. Chicago: University of Chicago Press.

Edney, Laura, Hossein Haji Ali Afzali, Terence Chai Cheng, and Jonathan Karnon. 2018. "Estimating the Reference Incremental Cost-Effectiveness Ratio for the Australian Health System." *PharmacoEconomics* 36 (2): 239–252.

Edney, Laura, Hossein Haji Ali Afzali, and Jonathan Karnon. 2019. "Are the Benefits of New Health Services Greater Than Their Opportunity Costs?" *Australian Health Review* 43 (5): 508–510.

Edney, Laura C., James Lomas, Jonathan Karnon, Laura Vallejo-Torres, Niek Stadhouders, Jonathan Siverskog, Mike Paulden, Ijeoma P. Edoka, and Jessica Ochalek. 2022.

"Empirical Estimates of the Marginal Cost of Health Produced by a Healthcare System: Methodological Considerations from Country-Level Estimates." *PharmacoEconomics* 40 (1): 31–43.

Ehrenreich, Barbara, and Deirdre English. 2011. *Complaints and Disorders: The Sexual Politics of Sickness*. New York: Feminist Press.

Eijkenaar, Frank, Martin Emmert, Manfred Scheppach, and Oliver Schöffski. 2013. "Effects of Pay for Performance in Health Care: A Systematic Review of Systematic Reviews." *Health Policy* 110 (2–3): 115–130.

Einav, Liran, and Amy Finkelstein. 2018. "Moral Hazard in Health Insurance: What We Know and How We Know It." *Journal of the European Economic Association* 16 (4): 957–982.

Einav, Liran, Amy Finkelstein, Sendhil Mullainathan, and Ziad Obermeyer. 2018. "Predictive Modeling of U.S. Health Care Spending in Late Life." *Science* 360 (6396): 1462–1465.

Einmahl, Jesson J., John H. J. Einmahl, and Laurens de Haan. 2019. "Limits to Human Life Span through Extreme Value Theory." *Journal of the American Statistical Association* 114 (527): 1075–1080.

Ekeh, Peter P. 1974. *Social Exchange Theory: The Two Traditions*. London: Heinemann.

Ekman, Björn. 2004. "Community-Based Health Insurance in Low-Income Countries: A Systematic Review of the Evidence." *Health Policy and Planning* 19 (5): 249–270.

Elliott, Marc N., David E. Kanouse, Q. Burkhart, Gary A. Abel, Georgios Lyratzopoulos, Megan K. Beckett, Mark A. Schuster, and Martin Roland. 2015. "Sexual Minorities in England Have Poorer Health and Worse Health Care Experiences: A National Survey." *Journal of General Internal Medicine* 30 (1): 9–16.

Elliott, Marc N., Megan K. Beckett, William G. Lehrman, Paul Cleary, Christopher W. Cohea, Laura A. Giordano, Elizabeth H. Goldstein, and Cheryl L. Damberg. 2016. "Understanding the Role Played by Medicare's Patient Experience Points System in Hospital Reimbursement." *Health Affairs* 35 (9): 1673–1680.

Ellis, Randall P., Bruno Martins, and Sherri Rose. 2018. "Risk Adjustment for Plan Payment." In *Risk Adjustment, Risk Sharing and Premium Regulation in Health Insurance Markets*, edited by Thomas G. McGuire and Richard C. van Kleef, 55–104. London: Academic Press.

Ellis, Randall P., Gregory C. Pope, Lisa I. Iezzoni, John Z. Ayanian, David W. Bates, H. Burstin, and Arlene S. Ash. 1996. "Diagnosis-Based Risk Adjustment for Medicare Capitation Payments." *Health Care Financing Review* 17 (3): 101–128.

Elovainio, Riku, and David B. Evans. 2017. "Raising More Domestic Money for Health: Prospects for Low- and Middle-Income Countries." *Health Economics, Policy and Law* 12 (2): 139–157.

Elshaug, Adam G., A. M. Watt, L. Mundy, and C. D. Willis. 2012. "Over 150 Potentially Low-Value Health Care Practices: An Australian Study." *The Medical Journal of Australia* 197 (10): 556–560.

Elverum, Kris, and Maria Whitman. 2020. "Delivering Cellular and Gene Therapies to Patients: Solutions for Realizing the Potential of the Next Generation of Medicine." *Gene Therapy* 27 (12): 537–544.

Emanuel, Ezekiel. 2002. "Patient v. Population: Resolving the Ethical Dilemmas Posed by Treating Patients as Members of Populations." In *Ethical Dimensions of Health Policy*, edited by Marion Danis, Carolyn M Clancy and Larry R Churchill. New York: Oxford University Press.

2019. "When Is the Price of a Drug Unjust? The Average Lifetime Earnings Standard." *Health Affairs* 38 (4): 604–612.

Embuldeniya, Gayathri, Jennifer Gutberg, and Walter P. Wodchis. 2021. "The Reimagination of Sustainable Integrated Care in Ontario, Canada." *Health Policy* 125 (1): 83–89.

Engelhardt Jr, H Tristram. 2002. "Infinite Expectations and Finite Resources: A Roman Catholic Perspective on Setting Limits to Critical Care, or, Can Roman Catholic Moral Theology Offer More than Secular Morality Provides?" In *Allocating Scarce Medical Resources: Roman Catholic Perspectives*, edited by H Tristram Engelhardt Jr and Mark J Cherry, 3–18. Washington, DC: Georgetown University Press.

Enthoven, Alain. 2019. "How Systems Analysis, Cost-Effectiveness Analysis, or Benefit-Cost Analysis First Became Influential in Federal Government Program Decision-Making." *Journal of Benefit-Cost Analysis* 10 (2): 146–155.

Erickson, Rebecca J., and Clare L. Stacey. 2012. "Attending to Mind and Body: Engaging the Complexity of Emotion Practice among Caring Professionals." In *Emotional Labor in the 21st Century: Diverse Perspectives on Emotion Regulation at Work*, edited by Alicia Grandey, James Diefendorff, and Deborah E. Rupp, 175–196. London: Taylor & Francis Group.

Esler, Philip Francis. 1998a. "Introduction: Christianity for the Twenty-First Century." In *Christianity for the Twenty-First Century*, edited by Philip Francis Esler, 1–21. Edinburgh: T & T Clark.

1998b. "Poverty and Riches in the Bible and the Third World." In *Christianity for the Twenty-First Century*, edited by Philip Francis Esler, 145–179. Edinburgh: T & T Clark.

2000. "Jesus and the Reduction of Intergroup Conflict: The Parable of the Good Samaritan in the Light of Social Identity Theory." *Biblical Interpretation* 8 (4): 325–357.

Esserman, Laura, Jeffrey Belkora, and Leslie Lenert. 1995. "Potentially Ineffective Care: A New Outcome to Assess the Limits of Critical Care." *JAMA* 274 (19): 1544–1551.

Etzioni, Amitai. 1988. *The Moral Dimension: Towards a New Economics*. New York: Free Press.

1999. *Essays in Socio-Economics*. Berlin: Springer.

Evans, Craig A. 2006. "Paul the Exorcist and Healer." In *Paul and His Theology*, edited by Stanley E. Porter, 363–379. Leiden: Brill.

Evans, Paul S. 2016a. "Imagining Justice for the Marginalized: A Suspicious Reading of the Covenant Code (Exodus 21:1–23:33) in Its Ancient near Eastern Context." In *The Bible and Social Justice: Old Testament and New Testament Foundations for the Church's Urgent Call*, edited by Cynthia Long Westfall and Bryan R. Dyer, 1–34. Eugene, OR: Pickwick Publications.

Evans, Robert G. 1974. "Supplier-Induced Demand: Some Empirical Evidence and Implications." In *The Economics of Health and Medical Care: Proceedings of a Conference Held by the International Economic Association at Tokyo*, edited by Mark Perlman. London: Palgrave Macmillan.

1997. "Going for the Gold: The Redistributive Agenda behind Market-Based Health Care Reform." *Journal of Health Politics Policy and Law* 22 (2): 427–465.

2016b. "Supplier-Induced Demand: Some Empirical Evidence and Implications." In *An Undisciplined Economist: Robert G. Evans on Health Economics, Health Care Policy, and Population Health*, edited by Morris L Barer, Greg L Stoddart, Kimberlyn M McGrail and Chris B McLeod. Montreal and Kingston: McGill-Queen's Press.

Evans, Robert G., Morris L. Barer, and Ted R. Marmor, eds. 1994. *Why Are Some People Healthy and Others Not? The Determinants of Health Populations*. New York: de Gruyter.

Evans, Robert G., Morris L. Barer, and Greg L. Stoddart. 1995. "User Fees for Health Care: Why a Bad Idea Keeps Coming Back (or, What's Health Got to Do With It?)." *Canadian Journal on Aging* 14 (2): 360–390.

2016a. "Modelling the Benefits of Insurance: Here Comes the Insurance Salesman." In *An Undisciplined Economist*, edited by Morris L. Barer, Greg L. Stoddart, Kimberlyn M. McGrail and Chris B. McLeod, In Robert G. Evans on Health Economics, Health Care Policy, and Population Health, 235–263. Montreal and Kingston: McGill-Queen's University Press.

2016b. "User Fees for Health Care: Why a Bad Idea Keeps Coming Back (or, What's Health Got to Do with It?)." In *An Undisciplined Economist*, edited by Morris L. Barer, Greg L. Stoddart, Kimberlyn M. McGrail and Chris B. McLeod, In Robert G. Evans on Health Economics, Health Care Policy, and Population Health, 154–191. Montreal and Kingston: McGill-Queen's University Press.

Evans, Tim, and Hilary Brown. 2003. "Road Traffic Crashes: Operationalizing Equity in the Context of Health Sector Reform." *Injury Control and Safety Promotion* 10 (1–2): 11–12.

Eykelenboom, Michelle, Maartje M. van Stralen, Margreet R. Olthof, Linda J. Schoonmade, Ingrid H. M. Steenhuis, Carry M. Renders, Joerg Meerpohl, and P. E. N. Consortium on behalf of the. 2019. "Political and Public Acceptability of a Sugar-Sweetened Beverages Tax: A Mixed-Method Systematic Review and Meta-Analysis." *International Journal of Behavioral Nutrition and Physical Activity* 16 (78): 1–19.

Faber, Marjan, Marije Bosch, Hub Wollersheim, Sheila Leatherman, and Richard Grol. 2009. "Public Reporting in Health Care: How Do Consumers Use Quality-of-Care Information? A Systematic Review." *Medical care* 47 (1): 1–8.

Faden, Ruth, Justin Bernstein, and Sirine Shebaya. 2020. "Public Health Ethics." In *Stanford Encyclopedia of Philosophy (Spring edition)*, edited by Edward N. Zalta. Stanford, CA: Metaphysics Research Lab, Center for the Study of Language and Information, Stanford University. https://stanford.library.sydney.edu.au/entries/publichealth-ethics/.

Falgueras-Sorauren, Ignacio. 2009. "Is Robbins's Definition Necessarily Imperialistic? The Demarcation of Economics in Robbins's Essay and the Concepts of Real and Formal Scarcity." In *Lionel Robbins's Essay on the Nature and Significance of Economic Science: 75th Anniversary Conference Proceedings*, edited by Frank Cowell and Amos Witztum, 16–37. London: Suntory and Toyota International Centres for Economics and Related Disciplines.

Fan, Victoria Y., and William D. Savedoff. 2014. "The Health Financing Tansition: A Conceptual Framework and Empirical Evidence." *Social Science & Medicine* 105: 112–121.

Färdow, Joakim, Linus Broström, and Mats Johansson. 2019. "Co-payment for Unfunded Additional Care in Publicly Funded Healthcare Systems: Ethical Issues." *Journal of Bioethical Inquiry* 16 (4): 515–524.

Farley, Margaret A. 2002. *Compassionate Respect: A Feminist Approach to Medical Ethics and Other Questions. Madeleva Lectures in Spirituality*. New York: Paulist Press.

Farnood, Annabel, Bridget Johnston, and Frances S. Mair. 2020. "A Mixed Methods Systematic Review of the Effects of Patient Online Self-Diagnosing in the 'Smart-Phone Society' on the Healthcare Professional-Patient Relationship and Medical Authority." *BMC Medical Informatics and Decision Making* 20 (253): 1–14.

Fein, Rashi. 2010. *Learning Lessons: Medicine, Economics, and Public Policy*. New Brunswick, NJ: Transaction.

Feiring, Eli, and Hege Wang. 2018. "Rationing Cancer Treatment: A Qualitative Study of Perceptions of Legitimate Limit-Setting." *BMC Health Services Research* 18 (342): 1–10.

Feng, Xue, David D. Kim, Joshua T. Cohen, Peter J. Neumann, and Daniel A. Ollendorf. 2020. "Using QALYs versus DALYs to Measure Cost-Effectiveness: How Much Does It Matter?" *International Journal of Technology Assessment in Health Care* 36 (2): 96–103.

Ferguson, Jenny, Emma A. Craig, and Katerina Dounavi. 2019. "Telehealth as a Model for Providing Behaviour Analytic Interventions to Individuals with Autism Spectrum Disorder: A Systematic Review." *Journal of Autism and Developmental Disorders* 49 (2): 582–616.

Ferngren, Gary B. 1992. "Early Christianity as a Religion of Healing." *Bulletin of the History of Medicine* 66 (1): 1–15.

Fetter, Robert B., Donald A. Brand, and Dianne Gamache, eds. 1991. *DRGs: Their Design and Development* (1st ed). Ann Arbor, MI: Health Administration Press.

Fetter, Robert B., Youngsoo Shin, Jean L. Freeman, Ricahard F. Averill, and James. D. Thompson. 1980. "Case Mix Definition by Diagnosis Related Groups." *Medical Care* 18 (2 (supplement)): 1–53.

Field, Jonathan, Michelle M. Holmes, and Dave Newell. 2019. "PROMs Data: Can It Be Used to Make Decisions for Individual Patients? A Narrative Review." *Patient Related Outcome Measures* 10: 233–241.

Figueroa, Jose F., Irene Papanicolas, Kristen Riley, Olukorede Abiona, Mina Arvin, Femke Atsma, Enrique Bernal-Delgado, Nicholas Bowden, Carl Rudolf Blankart, Sarah Deeny, Francisco Estupiñán-Romero, Robin Gauld, Philip Haywood, Nils Janlov, Hannah Knight, Luca Lorenzoni, Alberto Marino, Zeynep Or, Anne Penneau, Kosta Shatrov, Onno van de Galien, Kees van Gool, Walter Wodchis, and Ashish K. Jha. 2021 (in press). "International Comparison of Health Spending and Utilization among People with Complex Multimorbidity." *Health Services Research* 56, no. Suppl 3: 1317–1334.

Finn, Daniel K. 2013. *Christian Economic Ethics: History and Implications*. Minneapolis, MN: Fortress Press.

Fioretti, Michele, and Hongming Wang. 2019. *Subsidizing Inequality: Performance Pay and Risk Selection in Medicare*. Paris: Sciences Po Departement of Economics.

Firth, Isabel, Hannah Schirrmacher, Kyann Zhang, Grace Hampson, and Adrian Towse. 2021. *Exploring the Financial Sustainability of Gene Therapies*. London: Office of Health Economics. www.ohe.org/publications/exploring-financial-sustainability-gene-therapies#.

Fitzpatrick, Ray. 2009. "Patient Reported Outcome Measures and Performance Measurement." In *Performance Measurement for Health System Improvement: Experiences, Challenges, and Prospects*, edited by Peter Smith, Elias Mossialos, Irene Papanicolas, and S. Leatherman, 63–86. Cambridge; New York: Cambridge University Press.

Flood, Colleen M. 2021. "Two-Tier Healthcare after Cambie." *Healthcare Management Forum* 34 (4): 221–224.

Flood, Colleen M., Bryan Thomas, and Kelli White. 2020. "The Courts and Two-Tier Medicare." *Healthcare Policy* 5 (4): 13–20.

Flynn, Maria, and Dave Mercer. 2013. "Is Compassion Possible in a Market-Led NHS?" *Nursing Times* 109 (7): 12–14.

Forrester, Duncan B. 1997. *Christian Justice and Public Policy*. Cambridge: Cambridge University Press.

2012. "Social Justice and Welfare." In *The Cambridge Companion to Christian Ethics*, edited by Robin Gill, 205–218. Cambridge: Cambridge University Press.

Foster, Ruth Ann. 1995. "Stewardship: Sign and Substance of the Christian Life as Taught in the New Testament." *South Western Journal of Theology* 37 (2): 15–22.

Fotaki, Marianna. 2015. "Why and How Is Compassion Necessary to Provide Good Quality Healthcare?" *International Journal of Health Policy and Management* 4 (4): 199–201.

Fraihat, Nadine, Saba Madae'en, Zsuzsa Bencze, Adrienn Herczeg, and Orsolya Varga. 2019. "Clinical Effectiveness and Cost-Effectiveness of Oral-Health Promotion in Dental Caries Prevention among Children: Systematic Review and Meta-Analysis." *International Journal of Environmental Research and Public Health* 16 (15).

Frakt, Austin B., and Rick Mayes. 2012. "Beyond Capitation: How New Payment Experiments Seek to Find the 'Sweet Spot' in Amount of Risk Providers and Payers Bear." *Health Affairs* 31 (9): 1951–1958.

Francis. 2013a. *Evangelii Gaudium, Apostolic Exhortation on the Proclamation of the Gospel in Today's World*. Vatican City: The Holy See.

2015. *Laudato si': Encyclical Letter of the Holy Father Francis on Care for Our Common Home*. Vatican City: Vatican Press.

2020a. *Fratelli Tutti: Encyclical Letter of the Holy Father Francis on the Fraternity and Social Friendship*. Vatican City: Vatican Press.

2020b. *Let Us Dream: The Path to a Better Future*. London: Simon and Schuster.

Francis, James. 1993. "Some Reflections from the Perspective of Ministry in Secular Employment." In *God and the Marketplace: Essays on the Morality of Wealth Creation*, edited by Jon Davies, 125–140. London: IEA Health and Welfare Unit.

Francis, Robert. 2013b. *Report of the Mid Staffordshire NHS Foundation Trust public Inquiry*. London: The Stationery Office.

Frankel, Stephen. 1991. "Health Needs, Health-Care Requirements, and the Myth of Infinite Demand." *The Lancet* 337 (8757): 1588–1590.

Fraser, Nancy, and Linda Gordon. 1994a. ""Dependency" Demystified: Inscriptions of Power in a Keyword of the Welfare State." *Social Politics: International Studies in Gender, State & Society* 1 (1): 4–31.

1994b. "A Genealogy of Dependency: Tracing a Keyword of the U.S. Welfare State." *Signs: Journal of Women in Culture and Society* 19 (2): 309–336.

Frean, Molly, Jonathan Gruber, and Benjamin D. Sommers. 2017. "Premium Subsidies, the Mandate, and Medicaid Expansion: Coverage Effects of the Affordable Care Act." *Journal of Health Economics* 53: 72–86.

Frecknall-Hughes, Jane. 2020. "The Moral Basis for Taxation." In *Ethics and Taxation*, edited by Robert F. van Brederode, 23–45. Singapore: Springer Singapore.

Freedland, Mark, and Lucy Vickers. 2016. "Age Discrimination and EU Labour Rights Law." In *Research Handbook on EU Labour Law*, edited by Alan Bogg, Cathryn Costello and Anne CL Davies, 527–546. Cheltenham: Edward Elgar Publishing.

Freidson, Eliot. 2007. *Professional Dominance: The Social Structure of Medical Care*. New Brunswick, NJ: Aldine Transaction.

Friedberg, Mark, Bernard Saffran, Tammy J. Stinson, Wendy Nelson, and Charles L. Bennett. 1999. "Evaluation of Conflict of Interest in Economic Analyses of New Drugs Used in Oncology." *JAMA* 282 (15 (20.10.99)): 1453–57.

Friedman, Jed, and Richard M. Scheffler. 2016. "Pay for Performance in Health Systems: Theory, Evidence and Case Studies." In *World Scientific Handbook of Global Health Economics and Public Policy*, edited by Richard M. Scheffler, 295–332. Singapore: World Scientific Publishing.

Frost, Jeana H., and Michael P. Massagli. 2008. "Social Uses of Personal Health Information within PatientsLikeMe, an Online Patient Community: What Can Happen When Patients Have Access to One Another's Data." *Journal of Medical Internet Research* 10 (3): e15.

Fuchs, Victor R. 1998. *Who Shall Live? Health, Economics and Social Choice*. Singapore: World Scientific Publishing.

2004. "More Variation in Use of Care, More Flat-of-the-Curve Medicine." *Health Affairs* 23: VAR104–VAR107.

Fuller, Reginald H. 1978. "The Double Commandment of Love: A Test Case for the Criteria of Authenticity." In *Essays on the Love Commandment*, edited by Luise Schottroff, Christoph Burchard, Reginald H. Fuller, and Ilse Fuller, 41–56. Philadelphia: Fortress Press.

Funk, Robert W. 1974. "The Good Samaritan as Metaphor." *Semeia* 2 (2): 74–81.

Furnish, Victor Paul. 1973. *The Love Command in the New Testament*. London: SCM Press.

Gaál, Péter 2006. "Gift, Fee or Bribe? Informal Payments in Hungary." In *Global Corruption Report 2006*, edited by Jana Kotalik and Diana Rodriguez, 71–73. London: Pluto Press in association with Transparency International.

Gaal, Peter, Paolo Carlo Belli, Martin McKee, and Miklós Szócska. 2006. "Informal Payments for Health Care: Definitions, Distinctions, and Dilemmas." *Journal of Health Politics, Policy and Law* 31 (2): 251–293.

Gaal, Peter, and Martin McKee. 2004. "Informal Payment for Health Care and the Theory of 'INXIT'." *The International Journal of Health Planning and Management* 19 (2): 163–178.

Gabbay, Ezra, Jose Calvo-Broce, Klemens B. Meyer, Thomas A. Trikalinos, Joshua Cohen, and David M. Kent. 2010. "The Empirical Basis for Determinations of Medical Futility." *Journal of General Internal Medicine* 25 (10): 1083–1089.

Gabe, Jonathan, Kirsten Harley, and Michael Calnan. 2015. "Healthcare Choice: Discourses, Perceptions, Experiences and Practices." *Current Sociology* 63 (5): 623–635.

Gagnon, Robert A. J. 1998. "A Second Look at Two Lukan Parables: Reflections on the Unjust Steward and the Good Samaritan." *Horizons in Biblical Theology* 20 (1): 1–11.

Gallie, Walter Bryce. 1955. "Essentially Contested Concepts." *Proceedings of the Aristotelian Society* 56 (1): 167–198.

Gandjour, Afschin, and Nadja Chernyak. 2011. "A New Prize System for Drug Innovation." *Health Policy* 102 (2–3): 170–177.

García, Leidy Y., and Arcadio A. Cerda. 2020. "Contingent Assessment of the COVID-19 Vaccine." *Vaccine* 38 (34): 5424–5429.

Garner, Sarah, and Peter Littlejohns. 2011. "Disinvestment from Low Value Clinical Interventions: NICEly Done?" *BMJ* 343.

Garrett, Laurie, A. Mushtaque R. Chowdhury, and Ariel Pablos-Méndez. 2009. "All for Universal Health Coverage." *The Lancet* 374 (9697): 1294–1299.

Garrido, Marcial Velasco, Annette Zentner, and Reinhard Busse. 2011. "The Effects of Gatekeeping: A Systematic Review of the Literature." *Scandinavian Journal of Primary Health Care* 29 (1): 28–38.

Garrison, Louis P., Sachin Kamal-Bahl, and Adrian Towse. 2017. "Toward a Broader Concept of Value: Identifying and Defining Elements for an Expanded Cost-Effectiveness Analysis." *Value in Health* 20 (2): 213–216.

Garrison, Louis P., Adrian Towse, Andrew Briggs, Gerard de Pouvourville, Jens Grueger, Penny E. Mohr, J. L. Severens, Paolo Siviero, and Miguel Sleeper. 2013. "Performance-Based Risk-Sharing Arrangements – Good Practices for Design, Implementation, and Evaluation: Report of the ISPOR Good Practices for Performance-Based Risk-Sharing Arrangements Task Force." *Value in Health* 16 (5): 703–719.

Gawande, Atul. 2009a. "The Cost Conundrum – What a Texas Town Can Teach Us about Health Care." *The New Yorker*, 36–40.

2009b. "The Cost Conundrum: What a Texas Town Can Teach Us about Health Care " *The New Yorker* 1 (June): 36–44.

2014. *Being Mortal: Medicine and What Matters in the end.* New York, NY: Hamish Hamilton.

GBD 2016 Causes of Death Collaborators. 2017. "Global, Regional, and National Age-Sex Specific Mortality for 264 Causes of Death, 1980–2016: A Systematic Analysis for the Global Burden of Disease Study 2016." *The Lancet* 390 (10100): 1151–1210.

Gee, Laura K., and Jonathan Meer. 2020. "The Altruism Budget: Measuring and Encouraging Charitable Giving." In *The Nonprofit Sector: A Research Handbook* (3rd ed), edited by Walter W. Powell and Patricia Bromley, 558–565. Stanford, CA: Stanford University Press.

George, Bethan, Anthony Harris, and Andrew Mitchell. 2001. "Cost-Effectiveness Analysis and the Consistency of Decision Making: Evidence from Pharmaceutical Reimbursement in Australia (1991 to 1996)." *PharmacoEconomics* 19 (11): 1103–1109.

George, Timothy. 1986. "'A Right Strawy Epistle': Reformation Perspectives on James." *Review & Expositor* 83 (3): 369–382.

Georgescu, Irène, and Frank G. H. Hartmann. 2013. "Sources of Financial Pressure and up Coding Behavior in French Public Hospitals." *Health Policy* 110 (2–3): 156–163.

Gérard-Varet, Louis-André, Serge-Christophe Kolm, and Jean Mercier Ythier, eds. 2000. *The Economics of Reciprocity, Giving, and Altruism*. Basingstoke, Hampshire: Macmillan.

Geruso, Michael, and Timothy Layton. 2020. "Upcoding: Evidence from Medicare on Squishy Risk Adjustment." *Journal of Political Economy* 128 (3): 984–1026.

Ghijben, Peter, Yuanyuan Gu, Emily Lancsar, and Silva Zavarsek. 2018. "Revealed and Stated Preferences of Decision Makers for Priority Setting in Health Technology Assessment: A Systematic Review." *PharmacoEconomics* 36 (3): 323–340.

Ghinea, Narcyz, Wendy Lipworth, and Ian Kerridge. 2016. "Propaganda or the Cost of Innovation? Challenging the High Price of New Drugs." *BMJ* 352.

2020. "Does Consumer Engagement in Health Technology Assessment Enhance or Undermine Equity?" *Journal of Bioethical Inquiry* 17 (1): 87–94.

Ghinea, Narcyz, Miles Little, and Wendy Lipworth. 2017. "Access to High Cost Cancer Medicines through the Lens of an Australian Senate Inquiry – Defining the "Goods" at Stake." *Journal of Bioethical Inquiry* 14 (3): 401–410.

Gilbert, Paul. 2019. "Explorations into the Nature and Function of Compassion." *Current Opinion in Psychology* 28: 108–114.

Gill, Robin. 1997. *Moral Leadership in a Postmodern Age*. Edinburgh: T & T Clark.

2004. *Christian Ethics in Secular Worlds*. London: T & T Clark International.

2006. *Health Care and Christian Ethics*. Cambridge: Cambridge University Press.

ed. 2012. *The Cambridge Companion to Christian Ethics*. Cambridge: Cambridge University Press.

2020. "Was Jesus an Ethical Revolutionary?" In *Revolutionary. Who Was Jesus? Why Does He Still Matter?*, edited by Tom Holland, 34–51. London: SPCK Publishing.

Gillam, Stephen J., A. Niroshan Siriwardena, and Nicholas Steel. 2012. "Pay-for-Performance in the United Kingdom: Impact of the Quality and Outcomes Framework: A Systematic Review." *Annals of Family Medicine* 10 (5): 461–468.

Gilligan, Carol. 1982. *In a Different Voice: Psychological Theory and Women's Development*. Cambridge, MA: Harvard University Press.

Ginsburg, Paul B., and Robert A. Berenson. 2007. "Revising Medicare's Physician Fee Schedule – Much Activity, Little Change." *New England Journal of Medicine* 356 (12): 1201–1203.

Giovannetti, Erin R., Catherine A. Clair, Lee A. Jennings, Shana F. Sandberg, Angelia Bowman, David B. Reuben, and Sarah H. Scholle. 2021. "Standardised Approach to Measuring Goal-Based Outcomes among Older Disabled Adults: Results from a Multisite Pilot." *BMJ Quality & Safety* 30 (2): 157–166.

Giroux, Henry A. 2021. "The Covid-19 Pandemic Is Exposing the Plague of Neoliberalism." In *Collaborative Futures in Qualitative Inquiry: Research in a Pandemic*, edited by Norman K. Denzin, Michael D. Giardina, 16–27. New York: Routledge.

Givel, Michael S. 2015. "Gross National Happiness in Bhutan: Political Institutions and Implementation." *Asian Affairs* 46 (1): 102–117.

Glanville, Mark. 2018. "The Gēr (Stranger) in Deuteronomy: Family for the Displaced." *Journal of Biblical Literature* 137 (3): 599–623.

Global Burden of Disease Health Financing Collaborator Network. 2019. "Past, Present, and Future of Global Health Financing: A Review of Development Assistance, Government, Out-of-Pocket, and Other Private Spending on Health for 195 countries, 1995–2050." *The Lancet* 393 (10187): 2233–2260.

Glurich, Ingrid, and Amit Acharya. 2019. "Updates from the Evidence Base Examining Association between Periodontal Disease and Type 2 Diabetes Mellitus: Current Status and Clinical Relevance." *Current Diabetes Reports* 19 (11): 121.

Goetz, Jennifer L, Dacher Keltner, and Emiliana Simon-Thomas. 2010. "Compassion: An Evolutionary Analysis and Empirical Review." *Psychological Bulletin* 136 (3): 351–374.

Goetz, Jennifer L, and Emiliana Simon-Thomas. 2017. "The Landscape of Compassion: Definitions and Scientific Approaches." In *The Oxford Handbook of Compassion Science*, edited by Emma M Seppälä, Emiliana Simon-Thomas, Stephanie L Brown, Monica C Worline, C Daryl Cameron and James R Doty, 3–15. Oxford: Oxford University Press.

Gold, Marthe R., David Stevenson, and Dennis G. Fryback. 2002. "HALYs and QALYs and DALYs, Oh My: Similarities and Differences in Summary Measures of Population Health." *Annual Review of Public Health* 23 (1): 115–134.

Golding, Martin P. 1981. "Justice and Rights: A Study in Relationship." In *Justice and Health Care*, edited by Earl E. Shelp. Dordrecht, Holland: D. Reidel.

González, Paula. 2020. "On the Design of Equity-Oriented Pharmaceutical Copayments." *SERIEs – Journal of the Spanish Economic Association* 11 (2): 179–202.

Goodacre, Mark. 2001. *The Synoptic Problem: A Way through the Maze.* London: Continuum.

Goodchild, Philip. 2009. *Theology of Money.* Durham, NC: Duke University Press.

Goodhart, Charles. 1975. "Problems of Monetary Management: The U.K. Experience." In *Papers in Monetary Economics vol 1.* Sydney: Reserve Bank of Australia.

Goodrich, John K. 2012. "Voluntary Debt Remission and the Parable of the Unjust Steward (Luke 16: 1–13)." *Journal of Biblical Literature* 131 (3): 547–566.

Gordon, Barry J. 1982. "Lending at Interest: Some Jewish, Greek, and Christian Approaches, 800 BC–AD 100." *History of Political Economy* 14 (3): 406–426.

1989. *The Economic Problem in Biblical and Patristic Thought.* Leiden: E. J. Brill.

Goswami, Reena, Gayatri Subramanian, Liliya Silayeva, Isabelle Newkirk, Deborah Doctor, Karan Chawla, Saurabh Chattopadhyay, Dhyan Chandra, Nageswararao Chilukuri, and Venkaiah Betapudi. 2019. "Gene Therapy Leaves a Vicious Cycle." *Frontiers in Oncology* 9: 297–297.

Gotsis, George N., and Sarah Drakopoulou Dodd. 2002. "Economic Ideas in the Pauline Epistles of the New Testament." *History of Economics Review* 35 (1): 13–34.

2004. "Economic Ideas in the Epistle of James." *History of Economic Ideas* 12 (1): 7–35.

Gotsis, George N., and Gerasimos Merianos. 2012. "Early Christian Representations of the Economy: Evidence from New Testament Texts." *History and Anthropology* 23 (4): 467–505.

Gøtzsche, Peter C. 2018. "Patients Not Patents: Drug Research and Development as a Public Enterprise." *European Journal of Clinical Investigation* 48 (2): e12875.

Gourgues, Michel. 1998. "The Priest, the Levite, and the Samaritan Revisited: A Critical Note on Luke 10:31–35." *Journal of Biblical Literature* 117 (4): 709–713.

Graham, Elaine. 2013. *Between a Rock and a Hard Place: Public Theology in a Post-Secular Age.* London: SCM press.

Grassi, Joseph A. 2003. *Informing the Future: Social Justice in the New Testament.* New York: Paulist Press.

Graystone, Andrew. 2022. *Falling among Thieves: Understanding and Responding to Church-related Abuse.* Chester: William Temple Foundation.

Gray, Alastair M., and Thomas Wilkinson. 2016. "Economic Evaluation of Healthcare Interventions: Old and New Directions." *Oxford Review of Economic Policy* 32 (1): 102–121.

Greek Orthodox Archdiocese of America. 2020. *For the Life of the World: Toward a Social Ethos of the Orthodox Church.* New York, NY: Greek Orthodox Archdiocese of America. www.goarch.org/social-ethos.

Green, Joel B. 2014. "Good News to the Poor: A Lukan Leitmotif." *Review & Expositor* 111 (2): 173–179.

Green, Ronald M. 2020. "Head, Proportional, or Progressive Taxation: An Evaluation Based on Jewish and Christian Ethics." In *Ethics and Taxation*, edited by Robert F. van Brederode, 115-144. Singapore: Springer Singapore.

Greenhalgh, Trisha. 2021. "Moral Uncertainty: A Case Study of Covid-19." *Patient Education and Counseling* 104 (11): 2643–2647.

Greenwald, Bruce C., and Joseph E. Stiglitz. 1986. "Externalities in Economies with Imperfect Information and Incomplete Markets." *The Quarterly Journal of Economics* 101 (2): 229–264.

Gribble, Jennifer. 2004. "Why the Good Samaritan Was a Bad Economist: Dickens' Parable for Hard Times." *Literature and Theology* 18 (4): 427–441.

Griffin, Susan. 2020. "Uncertainty about Facts and Heterogeneity in Values." In *Distributional Cost-Effectiveness Analysis Quantifying Health Equity Impacts and Trade-offs*, edited by Richard Cookson, Susan Griffin, Ole Frithjof Norheim, and Anthony J. Culyer. Oxford: Oxford University Press.

Griffin, Susan, James Love-Koh, Becky Pennington, and Lesley Owen. 2019. "Evaluation of Intervention Impact on Health Inequality for Resource Allocation." *Medical Decision Making* 39 (3): 171–182.

Grignon, Michel, Jeremiah Hurley, David Feeny, Emmanuel Guindon, and Christina Hackett. 2018. "Moral Hazard in Health Insurance." *Œconomia. History, Methodology, Philosophy* 8 (3): 367–405.

Grimm, Sabine E., Xavier Pouwels, Bram L. T. Ramaekers, Ben Wijnen, Saskia Knies, Janneke Grutters, and Manuela A. Joore. 2020. "Development and Validation of the TRansparent Uncertainty ASsessmenT (TRUST) Tool for Assessing Uncertainties in Health Economic Decision Models." *PharmacoEconomics* 38 (2): 205–216.

Grimshaw, Jeremy M., Andrea M. Patey, Kyle R. Kirkham, Amanda Hall, Shawn K. Dowling, Nicolas Rodondi, Moriah Ellen, Tijn Kool, Simone A. van Dulmen, Eve A. Kerr, Stefanie Linklater, Wendy Levinson, and R. Sacha Bhatia. 2020. "De-implementing Wisely: Developing the Evidence Base to Reduce Low-Value Care." *BMJ Quality & Safety* 29 (5): 409–417.

Grinnell, Andrew. 2021. *Wisdom Cries Out: Public Theology from the Margins*. London: William Temple Foundation.

Groopman, Jerome. 2009. "Diagnosis: What Doctors Are Missing." *The New York Review of Books* 56 (17).

Gu, Yuanyuan, Emily Lancsar, Peter Ghijben, James R. G. Butler, and Cam Donaldson. 2015. "Attributes and Weights in Health Care Priority Setting: A Systematic Review of What Counts and to What Extent." *Social Science & Medicine* 146: 41–52.

Guindo, Lalla Aïda, Monika Wagner, Rob Baltussen, Donna Rindress, Janine van Til, Paul Kind, and Mireille M. Goetghebeur. 2012. "From Efficacy to Equity: Literature Review of Decision Criteria for Resource Allocation and Healthcare Decisionmaking." *Cost Effectiveness and Resource Allocation* 10 (9): 1–13.

Guo, Ping, Mendwas Dzingina, Alice M. Firth, Joanna M. Davies, Abdel Douiri, Suzanne M. O'Brien, Cathryn Pinto, Sophie Pask, Irene J. Higginson, Kathy Eagar, and Fliss E. M. Murtagh. 2018. "Development and Validation of a Casemix Classification to Predict Costs of Specialist Palliative Care Provision across Inpatient Hospice, Hospital and Community Settings in the UK: A Study Protocol." *BMJ Open* 8 (3): e020071.

Gurwitz, Jerry H., and Steven D. Pearson. 2019. "Novel Therapies for an Aging Population: Grappling with Price, Value, and Affordability." *JAMA* 321 (16): 1567–1568.

Gusmano, Michael K., Miriam Laugesen, Victor G. Rodwin, and Lawrence D. Brown. 2020. "Getting the Price Right: How Some Countries Control Spending in a Fee-For-Service System." *Health Affairs* 39 (11): 1867–1874.

Gustafson, James M. 1977. "Interdependence, Finitude, and Sin: Reflections on Scarcity." *The Journal of Religion* 57 (2): 156–168.

1986. "Christian Ethics." In *A New Dictionary of Christian Ethics*, edited by John Macquarrie and James F Childress, 87–90. London: SCM Press.

Gyrd-Hansen, Dorte. 2018. "Is There Additional Value Attached to Health Gains at the End of Life? A Revisit." *Health Economics* 27 (1): e71–e75.

Haas, Marion, Jane Hall, Rosalie Viney, and Gisselle Gallego. 2012. "Breaking Up Is Hard to Do: Why Disinvestment in Medical Technology Is Harder than Investment." *Australian Health Review* 36 (2): 148–152.

Habermas, Jürgen. 2006. "Religion in the Public Sphere." *European Journal of Philosophy* 14 (1): 1–25.

2008. *Between Naturalism and Religion: Philosophical Essays*. London: Routledge.

Habibov, Nazim, and Alex Cheung. 2017. "Revisiting Informal Payments in 29 Transitional Countries: The Scale and Socio-Economic Correlates." *Social Science & Medicine* 178: 28–37.

Hadorn, David C. 1991. "Setting Health Care Priorities in Oregon: Cost-Effectiveness Meets the Rule of Rescue." *JAMA* 265 (17): 2218–2225.

1996. "The Oregon Priority-Setting Exercise: Cost-Effectiveness and the Rule of Rescue, Revisited." *Medical Decision Making* 16 (2): 117–119.

Hagner, Donald A. 1998. "Law, Righteousness, and Discipleship in Matthew." *Word and World* 18 (4): 364–371.

Halasa-Rappel, Yara A., Cynthia A. Tschampl, Mary Foley, Martha Dellapenna, and Donald S. Shepard. 2019. "Broken Smiles: The Impact of Untreated Dental Caries and Missing Anterior Teeth on Employment." *Journal of Public Health Dentistry* 79 (3): 231–237.

Hall, Jane, Richard De Abreu Lourenco, and Rosalie Viney. 1999. "Carrots and Sticks – the Fall and Fall of Private Health Insurance in Australia." *Health Economics* 8 (8): 653–60.

Hallett, Garth L. 1998. *Priorities and Christian Ethics*. Cambridge: Cambridge University Press.

Hamad, Rita, Holly Elser, Duy C. Tran, David H. Rehkopf, and Steven N. Goodman. 2018. "How and Why Studies Disagree about the Effects of Education on Health: A Systematic Review and Meta-analysis of Studies of Compulsory Schooling Laws." *Social Science & Medicine* 212: 168–178.

Hammitt, James K., and Nicolas Treich. 2007. "Statistical vs. Identified Lives in Benefit-Cost Analysis." *Journal of Risk and Uncertainty* 35 (1): 45–66.

Hanna, Eve, Moundher Toumi, Claude Dussart, Borislav Borissov, Omar Dabbous, Karloina Badora, and Pascal Auquier. 2018. "Funding Breakthrough Therapies: A Systematic Review and Recommendation." *Health Policy* 122 (3): 217–229.

Hansen, Lise Desireé, and Trine Kjær. 2019. "Disentangling Public Preferences for Health Gains at End-of-Life: Further Evidence of No Support of an End-of-Life Premium." *Social Science & Medicine* 236: 112375.

Harcourt, Geoffrey Colin 1992. "Markets, Madness and a Middle Way." *The Australian Quarterly* 64 (1): 1–17.

1994. "Comment." In *Economics and Religion: Are They Distinct?*, edited by H. Geoffrey Brennan and Anthony Michael Charles Waterman. Dordrecht: Kluwer Academic.

Hardin, Garrett. 1968. "The Tragedy of the Commons." *Science* 162 (3859): 1243–1248.

Hardin, Leslie T. 2015. "Is a Pauline Spirituality Still Viable?" *Journal of Spiritual Formation and Soul Care* 8 (2): 132–146.

Harding, Nancy. 2015. "Why the Critics of Poor Health Service Delivery Are the Causes of Poor Service Delivery: A Need to Train the Policy-makers; Comment on 'Why and How Is Compassion Necessary to Provide Good Quality Healthcare?'." *International Journal of Health Policy and Management* 4 (9): 633–634.

Hardon, John A. 1954. "The Miracle Narratives in the Acts of the Apostles." *The Catholic Biblical Quarterly* 16 (3): 303–318.

Harink, Douglas Karel. 2020. *Resurrecting Justice: Reading Romans for the Life of the World.* Downers Grove, IL: IVP Academic.

Harrison, Peter. 1999. "Subduing the Earth: Genesis 1, Early Modern Science, and the Exploitation of Nature." *The Journal of Religion* 79 (1): 86–109.

2009. "Miracles, Early Modern Science, and Rational Religion." *Church History* 75 (3): 493–510.

Harsanyi, John C. 1955. "Cardinal Welfare, Individualistic Ethics, and Interpersonal Comparisons of Utility." *Journal of Political Economy* 63 (4): 309–321.

Hart, Oliver. 2003. "Incomplete Contracts and Public Ownership: Remarks, and an Application to Public-Private Partnerships." *The Economic Journal* 113 (486): C69–C76.

Hart, Oliver, and John Moore. 1999. "Foundations of Incomplete Contracts." *The Review of Economic Studies* 66 (1): 115–138.

2007. "Incomplete Contracts and Ownership: Some New thoughts." *American Economic Review* 97 (2): 182–186.

Harvard, Stephanie, Gregory R. Werker, and Diego S. Silva. 2020. "Social, Ethical, and Other Value Judgments in Health Economics Modelling." *Social Science & Medicine* 253: 112975.

Harvey, Anthony Ernest. 1990. *Strenuous Commands: The Ethic of Jesus.* London: SCM Press.

Harvey, Clare, Eileen Willis, Julie Henderson, Patti Hamilton, Luisa Toffoli, Claire Verrall, Ian Blackman, and Elizabeth Abery. 2016. "Priced to Care: Factors Underpinning Missed Care." *Journal of Industrial Relations* 58 (4): 510–526.

Harvey, Michael, Joshua Neff, Kelly R. Knight, Joia S. Mukherjee, Sriram Shamasunder, Phuoc V. Le, Robin Tittle, Yogesh Jain, Héctor Carrasco, Daniel Bernal-Serrano, Tinashe Goronga, and Seth M. Holmes. 2022. "Structural Competency and Global Health Education." *Global Public Health*— 17 (3): 341–362.

Hauck, Katharina, Ranjeeta Thomas, and Peter C. Smith. 2016. "Departures from Cost-Effectiveness Recommendations: The Impact of Health System Constraints on Priority Setting." *Health Systems & Reform* 2 (1): 61–70.

Hauerwas, Stanley. 1983. *The Peaceable Kingdom: A Primer in Christian Ethics*. Notre Dame, Indiana: University of Notre Dame Press.

2011. *Working with Words: On Learning to Speak Christian*. Eugene, OR: Cascade Books.

Havrilesky, Thomas. 1993. "Life Philosophy: Ethics and Economists." *The American Economist* 37 (2): 32–36.

Häyry, Matti. 2002. "Utilitarian Approaches to Justice in Health Care." In *Medicine and Social Justice. Essays on the Distribution of Health Care*, edited by R. Rhodes, M. P. Battin and A. Silvers, 53–64. New York: Oxford University Press.

2021. "Just Better Utilitarianism." *Cambridge Quarterly of Healthcare Ethics* 30 (2): 343–367.

Hays, Christopher M. 2010. *Luke's Wealth Ethics: A Study in Their Coherence and Character*. Tübingen: Mohr Siebeck.

Hays, Christopher M. 2012. "Slaughtering Stewards and Incarcerating Debtors: Coercing Charity in Luke 12:35–13:9." *Neotestamentica* 46 (1): 41–60.

Hays, Richard B. 1996. *The Moral Vision of the New Testament: Community, Cross, New Creation. A Contemporary Introduction to New Testament Ethics*. New York, NY: HarperOne.

Hazra, Nisha C., Martin C. Gulliford, and Caroline Rudisill. 2017. "'Fair Innings' in the Face of Ageing and Demographic Change." *Health Economics, Policy and Law* 13 (2): 209–217.

Heggie, Robert, Kathleen Boyd, and Olivia Wu. 2021. "How Has Implementation Been Incorporated in Health Technology Assessments in the United Kingdom? A Systematic Rapid Review." *Health Research Policy and Systems* 19 (118): 1–15.

Heider, Ann-Kathrin, and Harald Mang. 2020. "Effects of Monetary Incentives in Physician Groups: A Systematic Review of Reviews." *Applied Health Economics and Health Policy* 18 (5): 655–667.

Hellerstein, Jerome R. 1945. "Federal Tax Policy during the Roosevelt Era Roosevelt Issue." *Lawyers Guild Review* 5 (3): 160–171.

Hellowell, Mark, John Appleby, and Mark Taylor. 2018. "What Models of Funding Are Best for a Healthy and Just Society?" *BMJ* 361.

Henderson, Julie, and Eileen Willis. 2019. "The Marketisation of Aged Care: The Impact of Aged Care Reform in Australia." In *Navigating Private and Public Healthcare: Experiences of Patients, Doctors and Policy-Makers*, edited by Fran Collyer and Karen Willis, 249–267. Singapore: Springer Nature.

Henderson, Julie, Eileen Willis, Ian Blackman, Luisa Toffoli, and Claire Verrall. 2016. "Causes of Missed Nursing Care: Qualitative Responses to a Survey of Australian Nurses." *Labour & Industry* 26 (4): 281–297.

Henderson, Nadine, Isobel Firth, Maria Errea, Chris Skedgel, and Mireia Jofre-Bonet. 2021. *A Case Study Analysis: Challenges in the NICE Evaluation of Multi-Indication Medicines for Rare and Ultra-Rare Diseases*. London: Office of Health Economics.

Hendrickx, Herman. 1987. *The Parables of Jesus*. London: Geoffrey Chapman.

Hensher, Martin, Ben Canny, Craig Zimitat, Julie Campbell, and Andrew Palmer. 2020. "Health Care, Overconsumption and Uneconomic Growth: A Conceptual Framework." *Social Science & Medicine* 266: 113420.

Hensher, Martin, John Tisdell, Ben Canny, and Craig Zimitat. 2020. "Health Care and the Future of Economic Growth: Exploring Alternative Perspectives." *Health Economics, Policy and Law* 15 (4): 419–439.

Hernández-Quevedo, Cristina, and Helen Weatherly. 2015. "Health Promotion, Disease Prevention and Health Inequalities." In *Promoting Health, Preventing Disease: The Economic Case*, edited by David McDaid, Franco Sassi and Sherry Merkur, 259–278. Maidenhead: Open University Press.

Hernandez Alava, Monica, Allan Wailoo, Sabine Grimm, Stephen Pudney, Manuel Gomes, Zia Sadique, David Meads, John O'Dwyer, Garry Barton, and Lisa Irvine. 2018. "EQ-5D-5L versus EQ-5D-3L: The Impact on Cost Effectiveness in the United Kingdom." *Value in Health* 21 (1): 49–56.

Hero, Joachim O., Alan M. Zaslavsky, and Robert J. Blendon. 2017. "The United States Leads Other Nations in Differences by Income in Perceptions of Health and Health Care." *Health Affairs* 36 (6): 1032–1040.

Herzog, William R. 1994. *Parables as Subversive Speech: Jesus as Pedagogue of the Oppressed*. Louisville, Kentucky: Westminster/ John Knox Press.

Heschel, Abraham Joshua. 2001. *The Prophets*. New York: Perennial Classics.

Hicks, Douglas A. 2000. *Inequality and Christian Ethics*. Cambridge: Cambridge University Press.

Hiers, Richard H. 2009. *Justice and Compassion in Biblical Law*. New York: Continuum.

Higton, Mike. 2003. "Boldness and Reserve: A Lesson from St. Augustine." *Anglican Theological Review* 85 (3): 447–456.

Himmelstein, David U., Robert M. Lawless, Deborah Thorne, Pamela Foohey, and Steffie Woolhandler. 2019. "Medical Bankruptcy: Still Common Despite the Affordable Care Act." *American Journal of Public Health* 109 (3): 431–433.

Himmelstein, David U., Deborah Thorne, Elizabeth Warren, and Steffie Woolhandler. 2009. "Medical Bankruptcy in the United States, 2007: Results of a National Study." *The American Journal of Medicine* 122 (8): 741–746.

Hinde, Sebastian, Helen Weatherly, Gabriella Walker, and Lorna K. Fraser. 2021. "What Does Economic Evaluation Mean in the Context of Children at the End of Their Life?" *International Journal of Environmental Research and Public Health* 18 (11562): 1–11.

Hipgrave, David B., Katarzyna Bolsewicz Alderman, Ian Anderson, and Eliana Jimenez Soto. 2014. "Health Sector Priority Setting at Meso-level in Lower and Middle Income Countries: Lessons Learned, Available Options and Suggested Steps." *Social Science & Medicine* 102: 190–200.

Hirsch, Joshua A., H. Benjamin Harvey, Robert M. Barr, William D. Donovan, Richard Duszak, Gregory N. Nicola, Pamela W. Schaefer, and Laxmaiah Manchikanti. 2016. "Sustainable Growth Rate Repealed, MACRA Revealed: Historical Context and Analysis of Recent Changes in Medicare Physician Payment Methodologies." *American Journal of Neuroradiology* 37 (2): 210–214.

Hirschman, Albert O. 1970. *Exit, Voice and Loyalty: Responses to Decline in Firms, Organizations and States*. Cambridge: Harvard University Press.

Hochschild, Arlie Russell. 2009. "Invited Commentary: Can Emotional Labour Be Fun?" *International Journal of Work Organisation and Emotion* 3 (2): 112–119.

2012. *The Managed Heart: Commercialization of Human Feeling*. Berkerley, CA: University of California Press.

2013. *So How's the Family? And Other Essays*. 1 ed. Berkeley, CA: University of California Press.

Hofmann, Bjørn. 2020. "Biases Distorting Priority Setting." *Health Policy* 124 (1): 52–60.

2021. "Internal Barriers to Efficiency: Why Disinvestments Are So Difficult. Identifying and Addressing Internal Barriers to Disinvestment of Health Technologies." *Health Economics, Policy and Law* 16 (4): 473–488.

Hole, Barnaby, and Joseph Salem. 2016. "How Long Do Patients with Chronic Disease Expect to Live? A Systematic Review of the Literature." *BMJ Open* 6 (12).

Hollenbach, David. 2002. *The Common Good and Christian Ethics*. Cambridge: Cambridge University Press.

Hollis, Martin. 1998. *Trust within Reason*. Cambridge: Cambridge University Press.

Hong, Phebe, Aaron S. Kesselheim, and Ameet Sarpatwari. 2019. "Transformative Models to Promote Prescription Drug Innovation and Access: A Landscape Analysis." *Yale Journal of Health Policy Law & Ethics* 19 (2): 56–95.

Hope, Tony. 2001. "Rationing and Life-Saving Treatments: Should Identifiable Patients Have Higher Priority?" *Journal of Medical Ethics* 27 (3): 179–185.

Hordern, Joshua. 2013. "What's Wrong with 'Compassion'? Towards a Political, Philosophical and Theological Context." *Clinical Ethics* 8 (4): 91–97.

Hornsby-Smith, Michael P. 2006. *An Introduction to Catholic Social Thought*. Cambridge: Cambridge University Press.

Horodnic, Adrian V., and Colin C. Williams. 2018. "Informal Payments by Patients for Health Services: Prevalence and Determinants." *The Service Industries Journal* 38 (11–12): 841–855.

Horrell, David G. 2015. *The Bible and the Environment: Towards a Critical Ecological Biblical Theology*. Oxford: Routledge.

Horsell, Chris. 2017. "A Politics of Compassion: Informing a New Social Policy for Homelessness?" *International Social Work* 60 (4): 966–975.

Housset, Emmanuel. 2011. "The Paradoxes of Pity." In *Care, Compassion and Recognition: An Ethical Discussion*, edited by Carlo Leget, Chris Gastmans and Marian Verkerk, 70–87. Leuven: Peeters.

Houston, C. Stuart 2002. *Steps on the Road to Medicare: Why Saskatchewan Led the Way*. Montréal: McGill-Queen's University Press.

Howe, Peter E. 2013. "Adam Smith and the Missing Distribution Function." *Faith and Economics* 61/62: 72–77.

Hoyer, Stephen, and Patrice McDaniel. 1990. "From Jericho to Jerusalem: The Good Samaritan from a Different Direction." *Journal of Psychology and Theology* 18 (4): 326–333.

Hrynkow, Christopher William. 2017. "Greening God? Christian Ecotheology, Environmental Justice, and Socio-Ecological Flourishing." *Environmental Justice* 10 (3): 81–87.

Hsiao, William C., Peter Braun, Daniel Dunn, Edmund R. Becker, Margaret DeNicola, and Thomas R. Ketcham. 1988. "Results and Policy Implications of the Resource-Based Relative-Value Study." *New England Journal of Medicine* 319 (13): 881–888.

Hughes, David, and Donald Light, eds. 2002. *Rationing: Constructed Realities and Professional Practices*. Surrey, UK: Blackwell.

Hui, David, John P. Maxwell, and Carlos Eduardo Paiva. 2019. "Dealing with Prognostic Uncertainty: The Role of Prognostic Models and Websites for Patients with Advanced Cancer." *Current Opinion in Supportive and Palliative Care* 13 (4): 360–368.

Hultgren, Arland J. 2017. "Enlarging the Neighborhood: The Parable of the Good Samaritan (Luke 10:25–37)." *Word & World* 37 (1): 71–78.

Humphries, Brittany, and Feng Xie. 2019. "Canada's Amendment to Patented Drug Price Regulation: A Prescription for Global Drug Cost Control?" *JAMA* 321 (16): 1565–1566

Hunter, Rachael Maree. 2016. "The Role of the Health Economist in the Evaluation and Development of Complex Interventions in End-of-Life Care." In *Care at the End of Life: An Economic Perspective*, edited by Jeff Round, 31–45. Cham: Springer International Publishing.

Hurley, Jeremiah. 2000. "An Overview of the Normative Economics of the Health Sector." In *Handbook of Health Economics*, edited by Anthony J. Culyer and Joseph P. Newhouse, 55–118. Amsterdam: Elsevier Science BV.

2001. "Ethics, Economics, and Public Financing of Health Care." *Journal of Medical Ethics* 27 (4): 234–239.

2020. "Borders, Fences, and Crossings: Regulating Parallel Private Finance in Health Care." In *Is Two-Tier Health Care the Future?*, edited by Colleen M. Flood and Bryan Thomas, 69–91. Ottawa: University of Ottawa Press.

Hurst, Martin. 2019. "The Green Book: Central Government Guidance on Appraisal and Evaluation." *Journal of Mega Infrastructure & Sustainable Development* 1 (1): 101–103.

Husereau, Don, Michael Drummond, Federico Augustovski, Esther de Bekker-Grob, Andrew H. Briggs, Chris Carswell, Lisa Caulley, Nathorn Chaiyakunapruk, Dan Greenberg, Elizabeth Loder, Josephine Mauskopf, C. Daniel Mullins, Stavros Petrou, Raoh-Fang Pwu, and Sophie Staniszewska. 2022. "Consolidated Health Economic Evaluation Reporting Standards 2022 (CHEERS 2022) Statement: Updated Reporting Guidance for Health Economic Evaluations." *BMJ* 376: e067975.

Iacobucci, Gareth. 2021. "Covid-19: How Will a Waiver on Vaccine Patents Affect Global Supply?" *BMJ: British Medical Journal* 373: n1182.

Iezzoni, Lisa I., ed. 2013. *Risk Adjustment for Measuring Health Care Outcomes.* Chicago, IL: Health Administration Press.

Immergut, Ellen M., and Simone M. Schneider. 2020. "Is It Unfair for the Affluent to Be Able to Purchase "Better" Healthcare? "Existential Standards" and "Institutional Norms" in Healthcare Attitudes across 28 Countries." *Social Science & Medicine* 267: 113146.

Incandela, Joseph M. 1996. "Playing God: Divine Activity, Human Activity, and Christian Ethics." *CrossCurrents* 46 (1): 59–76.

Innes, Nicola P. T., and Falk Schwendicke. 2017. "Restorative Thresholds for Carious Lesions: Systematic Review and Meta-analysis." *Journal of Dental Research* 96 (5): 501–508.

Institute of Medicine. Committee on Understanding and Eliminating Racial and Ethnic Disparities in Health Care. 2009. *Unequal Treatment: Confronting Racial and Ethnic Disparities in Health Care.* Washington, D.C.: National Academy Press.

Ireland, Dennis J. 1992. *Stewardship and the Kingdom of God: An Historical, Exegetical, and Contextual Study of the Parable of the Unjust Steward in Luke 16:1–13*. Leiden: E. J. Brill.

Isasi-Diaz, Ada Maria. 1998. "Love of Neighbor in the 21st Century." In *Lift Every Voice: Constructing Christian Theologies from the Underside*, edited by Susan Brooks Thistlethwaite and Mary Potter Engel, 30–52. Maryknoll: Orbis.

Jackson, Terri. 2001a. "The Politics of Crisis in the Funding of Hospital Intensive Care Services." In *Technologies and Health Critical Compromises*, edited by Jeanne Daly, Marilys Guillemin and Sophie Hill. Melbourne: Oxford University Press.

2001b. "Rationing versus Rationality: Observations from Outside the United States." *Medical Decision Making* 21 (4): 324–328.

Jackson, Terri J. 2001b. "The Politics of Crisis in the Funding of Hospital Intensive Care Services." In *Technologies and Health: Critical Compromises*, edited by Jeanne Daly, Marilys Guillemin and Sophie Hill, 202–218. South Melbourne: Oxford University Press.

Jackson, Terri, Sally Mitchell, and Maria Wright. 1989. "The Community Development Continuum." *Community Health Studies* XIII (1): 66–73.

Jacobs, Alan M. 2011. *Governing for the Long Term: Democracy and the Politics of Investment.* Cambridge; New York: Cambridge University Press.

Jacobs, Rowena, Martin Chalkley, Jan R. Böhnke, Michael Clark, Valerie Moran, and M. J. Aragón. 2019. "Measuring the Activity of Mental Health Services in England: Variation in Categorising Activity for Payment Purposes." *Administration and Policy in Mental Health and Mental Health Services Research* 46 (6): 847–857.

Jacobson, Rolf A., and Karl Jacobson. 2017. "The Old Testament and the Neighbor." *Word & World* 37 (1): 16–26.

Jalali, Faride Sadat, Parisa Bikineh, and Sajad Delavari. 2021. "Strategies for Reducing Out of Pocket Payments in the Health System: A Scoping Review." *Cost Effectiveness and Resource Allocation* 19 (47): 1–22.

James, Brent C., and Gregory P. Poulsen. 2016. "The Case for Capitation." *Harvard Business Review* 94 (7): 102–111.

James, Jack E. 2020. "Generational Lifespan Convergence and the Longevity Revolution: Are People Truly Living Longer?" *European Journal of Clinical Investigation* 50 (1): e13185.

Jecker, Nancy S. 1991. "Knowing When to Stop: The Limits of Medicine." *Hastings Center Report* 21 (3): 5–8.

Jegers, Marc, Katrien Kesteloot, Diana De Graeve, and Willem Gilles. 2002. "A Typology for Provider Payment Systems in Health Care." *Health Policy* 60 (3): 255–273.

Jiang, Wei, and Rainer Marggraf. 2021. "The Origin of Cost–Benefit Analysis: A Comparative View of France and the United States." *Cost Effectiveness and Resource Allocation* 19 (74): 1–11.

Jin, Kai, Sahar Khonsari, Robyn Gallagher, Patrick Gallagher, Alexander M. Clark, Ben Freedman, Tom Briffa, Adrian Bauman, Julie Redfern, and Lis Neubeck. 2019. "Telehealth Interventions for the Secondary Prevention of Coronary Heart Disease: A Systematic Review and Meta-Analysis." *European Journal of Cardiovascular Nursing* 18 (4): 260–271.

Johannesson, Magnus, Bengt Jonsson, Linus Jonsson, Gisela Kobelt, and Niklas Zethraeus. 2009. *Why Should Economic Evaluations of Medical Innovations Have a Societal Perspective?* London: Office of Health Economics.

Johar, Meliyanni, Glenn Jones, and Elizabeth Savage. 2014. "What Explains the Quality and Price of GP Services? An Investigation Using Linked Survey and Administrative Data." *Health Economics* 23 (9): 1115–1133.

John Paul, II. 1991. *Centesimus Annus* Vatican City: The Holy See.

Johnson, Barry. 1996. *Polarity Management: Identifying and Managing Unsolvable Problems.* Amherst: HRD Press.

Johnson, Elizabeth A. 1992. *She Who Is: The Mystery of God in Feminist Theological Discourse.* New York: Crossroad.

Johnson, Luke Timothy. 2016. "James." In *The Catholic Study Bible*, edited by Donald Senior, John Collins and Mary Ann Getty, RG550–RG554. New York: Oxford University Press.

Johnston, Bridget M. 2016. "The Application of Economic Evaluation Techniques to Studies of Palliative and End-of-Life Care." In *Care at the End of Life: An Economic Perspective*, edited by Jeff Round, 19–30. Cham: Springer International Publishing.

Johnston, Fabian M., and Michael Beckman. 2019. "Navigating Difficult Conversations." *Journal of Surgical Oncology* 120 (1): 23–29.

Jones, Holly Miller. 2020. "Life-Prolonging Medical Care and Religiosity at the End of Life." MA, University of Otago.

Jonsen, Albert R. 1986. "Bentham in a Box: Technology Assessment and Health Care Allocation." *Law, Medicine and Health Care* 14 (3–4): 172–174.

Jordan, Roberta I., Matthew J. Allsop, Yousuf ElMokhallalati, Catriona E. Jackson, Helen L. Edwards, Emma J. Chapman, Luc Deliens, and Michael I. Bennett. 2020. "Duration of Palliative Care before Death in International Routine Practice: A Systematic Review and Meta-Analysis." *BMC Medicine* 18 (368): 1–25.

Joumard, Isabelle, Peter Hoeller, Christophe André, and Chantal Nicq. 2010. *Health Care Systems: Efficiency and Policy Settings*. Paris: OECD.

Juhnke, Christin, Susanne Bethge, and Axel C. Mühlbacher. 2016. "A Review on Methods of Risk Adjustment and Their Use in Integrated Healthcare Systems." *International Journal of Integrated Care* 16 (4): 1–18.

Justman, Stewart. 2015. *The Nocebo Effect: Overdiagnosis and Its Costs*. New York, NY: Palgrave.

Kahn, Jeffrey, and Anna Mastroianni. 2009. "The Implications of Public Health for Bioethics." In *The Oxford Handbook of Bioethics*, edited by Bonnie Steinbock. New York, NY: Oxford University Press.

Kahneman, Daniel. 2011. *Thinking, Fast and Slow*. London: Penguin.

Kahneman, Daniel, Jack L. Knetsch, and Richard H. Thaler. 1986. "Fairness and the Assumptions of Economics." *Journal of Business* 59 (4): S285–S300.

Kaldjian, Lauris C., Ann E. Curtis, Laura A. Shinkunas, and Katrina T. Cannon. 2008. "Goals of Care Toward the End of Life: A Structured Literature Review." *American Journal of Hospice and Palliative Medicine* 25 (6): 501–511.

Kalson, Nicholas S., John A. Mathews, Andrew D. Toms, and James R. D. Murray. 2021. "Clinical Prioritisation of Revision Knee Surgical Procedures: BASK Working Group Consensus Document." *The Knee* 28: 57–63.

Kanagaraj, Jey J. 2001. "The Implied Ethics of the Fourth Gospel: A Reinterpretation of the Decalogue." *Tyndale Bulletin* 52 (1): 33–60.

Kankeu, Hyacinthe Tchewonpi, and Bruno Ventelou. 2016. "Socioeconomic Inequalities in Informal Payments for Health Care: An Assessment of the 'Robin Hood' Hypothesis in 33 African Countries." *Social Science & Medicine* 151: 173–186.

Kanov, Jason, Sally Maitlis, Monica C. Worline, Jane E. Dutton, Peter J. Frost, and Jacoba M. Lilius. 2004. "Compassion in Organizational Life." *American Behavioral Scientist* 47 (6): 808–827.

Kanov, Jason, Edward H. Powley, and Neil D. Walshe. 2017. "Is It OK to Care? How Compassion Falters and Is Courageously Accomplished in the Midst of Uncertainty." *Human Relations* 70 (6): 751–777.

Kapczynski, Amy, and Aaron S. Kesselheim. 2016. "'Government Patent Use': A Legal Approach to Reducing Drug Spending." *Health Affairs* 35 (5): 791–797.

Kapiriri, Lydia, and Donya Razavi. 2017. "How Have Systematic Priority Setting Approaches Influenced Policy Making? A Synthesis of the Current Literature." *Health Policy* 121 (9): 937–946.

Kaplan, Robert M., and Arnold Milstein. 2019. "Contributions of Health Care to Longevity: A Review of 4 Estimation Methods." *The Annals of Family Medicine* 17 (3): 267–272.

Karnon, Jonathan, Laura Edney, and Hossein Afzali. 2018. "The Political Economy of the Assessment of Value of New Health Technologies." *Journal of Health Services Research & Policy* 23 (2): 116–122.

Kaufman, Sharon R., Janet K. Shim, and Ann J. Russ. 2004. "Revisiting the Biomedicalization of Aging: Clinical Trends and Ethical Challenges." *The Gerontologist* 44 (6): 731–738.

Kaveny, M. Cathleen. 2002. "Developing the Doctrine of Distributive Justice: Methods, of Distribution, Redistribution, and the Role of Time in Allocating Intensive Care Resources." In *Allocating Scarce Medical Resources: Roman Catholic Perspectives*, edited by H Tristram Engelhardt Jr and Mark J Cherry, 177–199. Washington, DC: Georgetown University Press.

Kay, John Anderson, and Mervyn A. King. 2020. *Radical Uncertainty: Decision-Making for an Unknowable Future*. London: Bridge Street Press.

Kayal, Philip M. 2018. *Bearing Witness: Gay Men's Health Crisis and the Politics of AIDS*. New York: Routledge.

Keeling, Michael. 1998. "Christian Ethics in a Secular Context." In *Christianity for the Twenty-First Century*, edited by Philip Francis Esler, 123–143. Edinburgh: T & T Clark.

Keith, Katie. 2020. "Senate Passes COVID-19 Package# 3: The Coverage Provisions." *Health Affairs Blog (blog)*. 26 March 2020.

Kelly, Conor. 2019. "Grace at the End of Life: Rethinking Ordinary and Extraordinary Means in a Global Context." *Journal of Moral Theology* 8 (1): 89–113.

Kelly, Henry Ansgar. 2017. "Love of Neighbor as Great Commandment in the Time of Jesus: Grasping at Straws in the Hebrew Scriptures." *Journal of the Evangelical Theological Society* 60 (2): 265–281.

Kerasidou, Angeliki. 2019. "Empathy and Efficiency in Healthcare at Times of Austerity." *Health Care Analysis* 27 (3): 171–184.

Kerridge, Ian, Kenneth Mitchell, and John McPhee. 1996. "Defining Medical Futility in Ethics, Law and Clinical Practice: An Exercise in Futility? (1997)." *Journal of Law and Medicine* 4: 235–242.

Keynes, John Maynard. 1978. *The Collected Writings of John Maynard Keynes* (edited by Elizabeth Johnson, and Donald Moggridge). Volume 14: The

General Theory and After: Part II. Defence and Development. Vol. 14. The Collected Writings of John Maynard Keynes: Royal Economic Society.

Khandelwal, Nita, Erin K. Kross, Ruth A. Engelberg, Norma B. Coe, Ann C. Long, and J. Randall Curtis. 2015. "Estimating the Effect of Palliative Care Interventions and Advance Care Planning on ICU Utilization: A Systematic Review." *Critical Care Medicine* 43 (5): 1102–1111.

Kickbusch, Ilona, Luke Allen, and Christian Franz. 2016. "The Commercial Determinants of Health." *The Lancet Global Health* 4 (12): e895–e896.

Kiil, Astrid, and Kurt Houlberg. 2014. "How Does Copayment for Health Care Services Affect Demand, Health and Redistribution? A Systematic Review of the Empirical Evidence from 1990 to 2011." *The European Journal of Health Economics* 15 (8): 813–828.

Kilner, John Frederic. 2015. *Dignity and Destiny: Humanity in the Image of God.* Grand Rapids, MI: William B. Eerdmans Publishing Company.

Kim, Kyoung-Jin. 1993. "Stewardship and Almsgiving in Luke's Theology: A Study in Luke's Theology of Wealth." Department of Biblical Studies, University of Glasgow.

Kimberly, John R., and Gérard de Pouvourville, eds. 1993. *The Migration of Managerial Innovation: Diagnosis Related Groups and Health Care Administration in Western Europe.* San Francisco: Jossey-Bass.

Kimberly, John R., Gérard de Pouvourville, and Thomas D'Aunno, eds. 2008. *The Globalization of Managerial Innovation in Health Care.* Cambridge: Cambridge University Press.

Kind, Paul, Geoffrey Hardman, and Susan Macran. 1999. *UK Population Norms for EQ-5D.* York: Centre for Health Economics, University of York.

King Jr, Martin Luther. 1967. Beyond Vietnam – A Time to Break Silence (Sermon Delivered Riverside Church, New York City, 4 April 1967). www.americanrhetoric.com/speeches/mlkatimetobreaksilence.htm.

Kirby, Emma, Alex Broom, John MacArtney, Sophie Lewis, and Phillip Good. 2021. "Hopeful Dying? The Meanings and Practice of Hope in Palliative Care Family Meetings." *Social Science & Medicine* 291: 114471.

Kitchen, Merrill. 2014. "Luke's Gospel: Economics of Restorative Justice." In *The Bible, Justice and Public Theology*, edited by David Neville, 45–58. Sheffield: Sheffield Phoenix Press.

Kitson, Alison. 2018. "The Fundamentals of Care Framework as a Point-of-Care Nursing Theory." *Nursing Research* 67 (2): 99–107.

Kitson, Alison, Tiffany Conroy, Kerry Kuluski, Louise Locock, and Renee Lyons. 2013. *Reclaiming and Redefining the Fundamentals of Care: Nursing's Response to Meeting Patients' Basic Human Needs.* Adelaide: School of Nursing, University of Adelaide.

Kleinhout-Vliek, Tineke, Antoinette de Bont, and Bert Boer. 2021. "Necessity under Construction – Societal Weighing Rationality in the Appraisal of Health Care Technologies." *Health Economics, Policy and Law* 16 (4): 457–472.

Kluge, Eike-Henner W. 2007. "Resource Allocation in Healthcare: Implications of Models of Medicine as a Profession." *MedGenMed: Medscape General Medicine* 9 (1): 57.

Kniesner, Thomas J. 2019. "Behavioral Economics and the Value of a Statistical Life." *Journal of Risk and Uncertainty* 58 (2): 207–217.

Knoppers, Gary N. 2013. *Jews and Samaritans: The Origins and History of Their Early Relations*. New York: Oxford University Press.

Knowles, Michael P. 2004. "What Was the Victim Wearing? Literary, Economic, and Social Contexts for the Parable of the Good Samaritan." *Biblical Interpretation* 12 (2): 145–174.

Knutsson, Daniel, and Björn Tyrefors. 2022 (in press). "The Quality and Efficiency of Public and Private Firms: Evidence from Ambulance Services." *The Quarterly Journal of Economics*: qjac014. https://doi.org/10.1093/qje/qjac014. https://doi.org/10.1093/qje/qjac014.

Koch, Kira, and Dheepa Rajan. 2021. "Representation in Participation." In *Voice, agency, empowerment – handbook on social participation for universal health coverage*, edited by Dheepa Rajan, Katja Rohrer-Herold, Kira Koch and Agnès Soucat, 59–103. Geneva: World Health Organization.

Kogut, Tehila, and Ilana Ritov. 2005. "The 'Identified Victim' Effect: An Identified Group, or Just a Single Individual?" *Journal of Behavioral Decision Making* 18 (3): 157–167.

Kogut, Tehila, and Ilana Ritove. 2011. "The Identifiable Victim Effect: Causes and Boundary Conditions." In *The Science of Giving: Experimental Approaches to the Study of Charity*, edited by Daniel M Oppenheimer and Christopher Y Olivola. New York, NY: Psychology Press.

Kolers, Avery. 2016. *A Moral Theory of Solidarity*. Oxford: Oxford University Press.

Kolm, Serge-Christophe. 2000. "The Theory of Reciprocity." In *The Economics of Reciprocity, Giving, and Altruism*, edited by Louis-André Gérard-Varet, Serge-Christophe Kolm and Jean Mercier Ythier, 115–141. Basingstoke, Hampshire: Macmillan.

Korenstein, Deborah, Susan Chimonas, Brooke Barrow, Salomeh Keyhani, Aaron Troy, and Allison Lipitz-Snyderman. 2018. "Development of a Conceptual Map of Negative Consequences for Patients of Overuse of Medical Tests and Treatments." *JAMA Internal Medicine* 178 (10): 1401–1407.

Korenstein, Deborah, Russell Harris, Adam G. Elshaug, Joseph S. Ross, Daniel J. Morgan, Richelle J. Cooper, Hyung J. Cho, and Jodi B. Segal. 2021. "To Expand the Evidence Base about Harms from Tests and Treatments." *Journal of General Internal Medicine* 36 (7): 2105–2110.

Kosecoff, J., K. L. Kahn, W. H. Rogers, E. J. Reinisch, M. J. Sherwood, L. V. Rubenstein, D. Draper, C. P. Roth, C. Chew, and R. H. Brook. 1990. "Prospective Payment System and Impairment at Discharge. The 'Quicker-and-Sicker' Story Revisited." *JAMA* 264 (15): 1995–1996.

Kragten, Nigel, and Jesper Rözer. 2017. "The Income Inequality Hypothesis Revisited: Assessing the Hypothesis Using Four Methodological Approaches." *Social Indicators Research* 131 (3): 1015–1033.

Krahn, Murray, Fiona Miller, Ahmed Bayoumi, Ann-Sylvia Brooker, Frank Wagner, Shawn Winsor, Mita Giacomini, Ron Goeree, Holger Schünemann, Gabrielle van der Velde, Stephen Petersen, Nancy Sikich, and

Irfan Dhalla. 2018. "Development of the Ontario Decision Framework: A Values Based Framework for Health Technology Assessment." *International Journal of Technology Assessment in Health Care* 34 (3): 290–299.

Krames, Jeffrey. 2014. *Lead with Humility: 12 Leadership Lessons from Pope Francis.* New York: AMACOM.

Kristensen, Finn Børlum, Don Husereau, Mirjana Huić, Michael Drummond, Marc L. Berger, Kenneth Bond, Federico Augustovski, Andrew Booth, John F. P. Bridges, Jeremy Grimshaw, Maarten J. Ijzerman, Egon Jonsson, Daniel A. Ollendorf, Alric Rüther, Uwe Siebert, Jitendar Sharma, and Allan Wailoo. 2019. "Identifying the Need for Good Practices in Health Technology Assessment: Summary of the ISPOR HTA Council Working Group Report on Good Practices in HTA." *Value in Health* 22 (1): 13–20.

Kröger, Teppo, Jiby Mathew Puthenparambil, and Lina Van Aerschot. 2019. "Care Poverty: Unmet Care Needs in a Nordic Welfare State." *International Journal of Care and Caring* 3 (4): 485–500.

Krohmal, Benjamin J., and Ezekiel J. Emanuel. 2007. "Access and Ability to Pay: The Ethics of a Tiered Health Care System." *Archives of Internal Medicine* 167 (5): 433–437.

2009. "Tiers without Tears: The Ethics of a Two-Tiered Health Care System." In *The Oxford Handbook of Bioethics*, edited by Bonnie Steinbock. New York, NY: Oxford University Press.

Kugel, James L. 2008. *How to Read the Bible: A Guide to Scripture, Then and Now.* New York: Free Press.

Kuhse, Helga. 1987. *The Sanctity-of-Life Doctrine in Medicine: A Critique*. Oxford: Clarendon Press.

Kutzin, Joseph. 2013. "Health Financing for Universal Coverage and Health System Performance: Concepts and Implications for Policy." *Bulletin of the World Health Organization* 91 (8): 602–11.

Laffont, Jean-Jacques. 1989. "Externalities." In *Allocation, Information and Markets*, edited by John Eatwell, Murray Milgate and Peter Newman, 112–116. London: Palgrave Macmillan UK.

Laffont, Jean-Jacques, and Jean Tirole. 1993. *A Theory of Incentives in Procurement and Regulation*. Cambridge: MIT Press.

Lago, Santiago, David Cantarero, Berta Rivera, Marta Pascual, Carla Blázquez-Fernández, Bruno Casal, and Francisco Reyes. 2018. "Socioeconomic Status, Health Inequalities and Non-communicable Diseases: A Systematic Review." *Journal of Public Health* 26 (1): 1–14

Lal, Anita, Marjory Moodie, Anna Peeters, and Rob Carter. 2018. "Inclusion of Equity in Economic Analyses of Public Health Policies: Systematic Review and Future Directions." *Australian and New Zealand Journal of Public Health* 42 (2): 207–213.

Lal, Anita, Mohammad Siahpush, Marjory Moodie, Anna Peeters, and Robert Carter. 2018. "Weighting Health Outcomes by Socioeconomic Position Using Stated Preferences." *PharmacoEconomics – Open* 2 (1): 43–51.

Lambden, Jason P., Peter Chamberlin, Elissa Kozlov, Lindsay Lief, David A. Berlin, Latrice A. Pelissier, Elina Yushuvayev, Cynthia X. Pan, and Holly G. Prigerson. 2019. "Association of Perceived Futile or Potentially Inappropriate Care with Burnout and Thoughts of Quitting among Health-Care Providers." *American Journal of Hospice and Palliative Medicine* 36 (3): 200–206.

Lampert, Khen. 2014. *Traditions of Compassion: From Religious Duty to Social Activism*. Basingstoke: Palgrave Macmillan.

Lancsar, Emily, Yuanyuan Gu, Dorte Gyrd-Hansen, Jim Butler, Julie Ratcliffe, Liliana Bulfone, and Cam Donaldson. 2020. "The Relative Value of Different QALY Types." *Journal of Health Economics* 70 (102303): 1–13.

Landon, Susan n, Jane Padikkala, and Leora i Horwitz. 2021. "Defining Value in Health Care: A Scoping Review of the Literature." *International Journal for Quality in Health Care* 33 (4): mzab140.

Lang, Dany. 2008. "Why Economists Should Choose Their Inheritance: Physics and Path-Independence in Economic Systems." *Review of Political Economy* 20 (3): 405–420.

Langley, Gerald J., Ronald Moen, Kevin M. Nolan, Thomas W. Nolan, Clifford L. Norman, and Lloyd P. Provost. 2009. *The Improvement Guide: A Practical Approach to Enhancing Organizational Performance* (2nd ed). San Francisco: Jossey-Bass.

Lapidus, John. 2022 (in press). "Privatising, Liberalising and Dividing a Welfare State without Affecting Universality? Debunking the Myths Surrounding the Rapid Rise of Private Health Insurance in Sweden." *Health Economics, Policy and Law*. 1–13.

Laske, Mark, Niek J. M. Opdam, Ewald M. Bronkhorst, Jozé C. C. Braspenning, Wil J. M. van der Sanden, Marie Charlotte D. N. J. M. Huysmans, and Josef J. Bruers. 2019. "Minimally Invasive Intervention for Primary Caries Lesions: Are Dentists Implementing This Concept?" *Caries Research* 53 (2): 204–216.

Lasswell, Harold Dwight. 1936. *Politics: Who Gets What, When, How*. New York: Whittlesey House.

Latimer, Tara, Joseph Roscamp, and Andrew Papanikitas. 2017. "Patient-Centredness and Consumerism in Healthcare: An Ideological Mess." *Journal of the Royal Society of Medicine* 110 (11): 425–427.

Lauenroth, Victoria D., Aaron S. Kesselheim, Ameet Sarpatwari, and Ariel D. Stern. 2020. "Lessons from the Impact of Price Regulation on the Pricing of Anticancer Drugs in Germany." *Health Affairs* 39 (7): 1185–1193.

Lawford-Smith, Holly. 2015. "Unethical Consumption and Obligations to Signal." *Ethics & International Affairs* 29 (3): 315–330.

Le, Van Anh, and Leah Samson. 2021. "Are IPRs and Patents the Real Barriers to COVID-19 Vaccine Supplies?" *Manchester Journal of International Economic Law* 15 (2): 192–204.

Ledley, Fred D., Sarah Shonka McCoy, Gregory Vaughan, and Ekaterina Galkina Cleary. 2020. "Profitability of Large Pharmaceutical Companies Compared with Other Large Public Companies." *JAMA* 323 (9): 834–843.

Le Grand, Julian, and Bill New. 2015. *Government Paternalism: Nanny State or Helpful Friend?* Princeton: Princeton University Press.

Lee, Dorothy. 2015. "'Signs and Works': The Miracles in the Gospels of Mark and John." *Colloquium* 47 (1): 89–101.

Leech, Ashley A., David D. Kim, Joshua T. Cohen, and Peter J. Neumann. 2018. "Use and Misuse of Cost-Effectiveness Analysis Thresholds in Low- and Middle-Income Countries: Trends in Cost-per-DALY Studies." *Value in Health* 21 (7): 759–761.

Leget, Carlo. 2015. "Why Good Quality Care Needs Philosophy More Than Compassion: Comment on 'Why and How Is Compassion Necessary to Provide Good Quality Healthcare?'." *International Journal of Health Policy and Management* 4 (10): 677–679.

Leget, Carlo, and Gert Olthuis. 2007. "Compassion as a Basis for Ethics in Medical Education." *Journal of Medical Ethics* 33: 617–620.

Leland, Brian D., Alexia M. Torke, Lucia D. Wocial, and Paul R. Helft. 2017. "Futility Disputes: A Review of the Literature and Proposed Model for Dispute Navigation through Trust Building." *Journal of Intensive Care Medicine* 32 (9): 523–527.

Leo XIII. 1891. *Rerum Novarum: Encyclical Letter on the Condition of Workers.* Vatican City: The Holy See.

Leshem, Dotan. 2016. "What Did the Ancient Greeks Mean by Oikonomia?" *Journal of Economic Perspectives* 30 (1): 225–38.

Lessard, Chantale, André-Pierre Contandriopoulos, and Marie-Dominique Beaulieu. 2010. "The Role (or not) of Economic Evaluation at the Micro Level: Can Bourdieu's Theory Provide a Way Forward for Clinical Decision-Making?" *Social Science & Medicine* 70 (12): 1948–1956.

Lester, Helen, and Martin Roland. 2009. "Performance Measurement in Primary Care." In *Performance Measurement for Health System Improvement: Experiences, Challenges, and Prospects,* edited by Peter Smith, Elias Mossialos, Irene Papanicolas and S. Leatherman, 371–405. Cambridge; New York: Cambridge University Press.

Levesque, Jean-Frédéric, Mark F. Harris, and Grant Russell. 2013. "Patient-Centred Access to Health Care: Conceptualising Access at the Interface of Health Systems and Populations." *International Journal for Equity in Health* 12 (18): 1–9.

Levine, Amy-Jill. 2006. *The Misunderstood Jew: The Church and the Scandal of the Jewish Jesus.* San Francisco: HarperSanFrancisco.

2015. *Short Stories by Jesus: The Enigmatic Parables of a Controversial Rabbi.* New York: HarperOne.

Levinson, Wendy, Karen Born, and Daniel Wolfson. 2018. "Choosing Wisely Campaigns: A Work in Progress – Evolution in the Ability of Choosing Wisely Campaigns to Reduce Health Care Overuse." *JAMA* 319 (19): 1975–1976.

Levy, Neil. 2019. "Taking Responsibility for Responsibility." *Public Health Ethics* 12 (2): 103–113.

Lewis, Ebony, Magnolia Cardona-Morrell, Kok Y. Ong, Steven A. Trankle, and Ken Hillman. 2016. "Evidence Still Insufficient That Advance Care Documentation Leads to Engagement of Healthcare Professionals in End-of-Life Discussions: A Systematic Review." *Palliative Medicine* 30 (9): 807–824.

Lewis, Maureen. 2007. "Informal Payments and the Financing of Health Care in Developing and Transition Countries." *Health Affairs* 26 (4): 984–997.

Lewison, Grant, Ajay Aggarwal, Philip Roe, Henrik Møller, Charlotte Chamberlain, and Richard Sullivan. 2018. "UK Newspaper Reporting of the NHS Cancer Drugs Fund, 2010 to 2015: A Retrospective Media Analysis." *Journal of the Royal Society of Medicine* 111 (10): 366–373.

Li, Alvin Ho-ting, Karen S. Palmer, Monica Taljaard, J. Michael Paterson, Adalsteinn Brown, Anjie Huang, Husayn Marani, Lauren Lapointe-Shaw, Daniel Pincus, Marian S. Wettstein, Girish S. Kulkarni, David Wasserstein, and Noah Ivers. 2020. "Effects of Quality-Based Procedure Hospital Funding Reform in Ontario, Canada: An Interrupted Time Series Study." *PLOS ONE* 15 (8): e0236480.

Liberatore, Matthew J. 2013. "Six Sigma in Healthcare Delivery." *International Journal of Health Care Quality Assurance* 26 (7): 601–626.

Lightbown, Andrew. 2014. "What's It All About?" In *Theonomics: Reconnecting Economics with Virtue and Integrity*, edited by Andrew Lightbown and Peter Sills, 1–15. Durham: Sacristy Press.

Link, Bruce George and Jo Carol Phelan. 2005. "Fundamental Sources of Health Inequalities." In *Policy Challenges in Modern Health Care*, edited by D. Mechanic, L. B. Rogut, D. C. Colby and J. R. Knickman. New Brunswick, NJ: Rutgers University Press.

Lipsitch, Marc, Nicholas G. Evans, and Owen Cotton-Barratt. 2017. "Underprotection of Unpredictable Statistical Lives Compared to Predictable Ones." *Risk Analysis* 37 (5): 893–904.

Little, Miles, Wendy Lipworth, and Ian Kerridge. 2022. "An Archeology of Corruption in Medicine." *Journal of Bioethical Inquiry* 19 (1): 109–116.

Littlejohns, Peter, Kalipso Chalkidou, Anthony J. Culyer, Albert Weale, Annette Rid, Katharina Kieslich, Clare Coultas, Catherine Max, Jill Manthorpe, Benedict Rumbold, Victoria Charlton, Helen Roberts, Ruth Faden, James Wilson, Carleigh Krubiner, Polly Michell, Gry Wester, Jennifer A. Whitty, and Selena Knight. 2019. "National Institute for Health and Care Excellence, Social Values and Healthcare Priority Setting." *Journal of the Royal Society of Medicine* 112 (5): 173–179.

Lloyd, Peter, and Donald MacLaren. 2019. "Should We Tax Sugar and If So How?" *Australian Economic Review* 52 (1): 19–40.

Löblová, Olga, Marcell Csanádi, Piotr Ozierański, Zoltán Kaló, Lawrence King, and Martin McKee. 2019. "Alternative Access Schemes for Pharmaceuticals in Europe: Towards an Emerging Typology." *Health Policy* 123 (7): 630–634.

Löfmark, Rurik, and Tore Nilstun. 2002. "Conditions and Consequences of Medical Futility – from a Literature Review to a Clinical Model." *Journal of Medical Ethics* 28 (2): 115–119.

Lohfink, Norbert. 1995. *Option for the Poor: The Basic Principle of Liberation Theology in the Light of the Bible.* Berkeley, CA: Bibal Press.

Lomas, James, Karl Claxton, Stephen Martin, and Marta Soares. 2018. "Resolving the "Cost-Effective but Unaffordable" Paradox: Estimating the Health Opportunity Costs of Nonmarginal Budget Impacts." *Value in Health* 21 (3): 266–275.

Longenecker, Bruce W. 2009a. "Afterword." In *Engaging economics: New Testament Scenarios and Early Christian Reception*, edited by Bruce W. Longenecker and Kelly D. Liebengood, 307–311. Grand Rapids, MI: Wm. B. Eerdmans Publishing.

2009b. "The Poor in Galatians 2:10: The Interpretative Paradigm of the First Centuries." In *Engaging Economics: New Testament Scenarios and Early Christian Reception*, edited by Bruce W. Longenecker and Kelly D. Liebengood, 205–221. Grand Rapids, MI: Wm. B. Eerdmans Publishing.

2009c. "The Story of the Samaritan and the Innkeeper (Luke 10:30–35): A Study in Character Rehabilitation." *Biblical Interpretation* 17 (4): 422–447.

2010. *Remember the Poor: Paul, Poverty, and the Greco-Roman World.* Grand Rapids, MI: W.B. Eerdmans Pub.

Longley, Clifford. 2014. *Just Money: How Catholic Social Teaching Can Redeem Capitalism.* London: Theos.

Lopez, Marianne Hamilton, Gregory W. Daniel, Nicholas C. Fiore, Aparna Higgins, and Mark B. McClellan. 2020. "Paying for Value from Costly Medical Technologies: A Framework for Applying Value-Based Payment Reforms." *Health Affairs* 39 (6): 1018–1025.

Love-Koh, James, Richard Cookson, Nils Gutacker, Thomas Patton, and Susan Griffin. 2019. "Aggregate Distributional Cost-Effectiveness Analysis of Health Technologies." *Value in Health* 22 (5): 518–526.

Lukes, Steven. 1974. *Power: A Radical View.* Oxford: Macmillan Press.

2009. *Power: A Radical View.* New York: Palgrave Macmillan.

Lundh, Andreas, Sergio Sismondo, Joel Lexchin, Octavian Busuioc, and Lisa Bero. 2012. *Industry Sponsorship and Research Outcome Cochrane Database of Systematic Reviews* 12 (MR000033): 1–113.

Lustig, Andrew. 2017. "The Image of God and Human Dignity: A Complex Conversation." *Christian Bioethics*: 23 (3): 317–334.

Luyten, Jeroen, and Albert Jan van Hoek. 2021. "Integrating Alternative Social Value Judgments into Cost-Effectiveness Analysis of Vaccines: An Application to Varicella-Zoster Virus Vaccination." *Value in Health* 24 (1): 41–49.

Maani, Nason, Jeff Collin, Sharon Friel, Anna B. Gilmore, Jim McCambridge, Lindsay Robertson, and Mark P. Petticrew. 2020. "Bringing the Commercial Determinants of Health Out of the Shadows: A Review of How the Commercial Determinants Are Represented in Conceptual Frameworks." *European Journal of Public Health* 30 (4): 660–664.

Macdonald, Nathan. 2004. "Listening to Abraham – Listening to Yhwh: Divine Justice and Mercy in Genesis 18:16–33." *The Catholic Biblical Quarterly* 66 (1): 25–43.

MacNamara, Vincent. 1998. "The Distinctiveness of Christian Morality." In *Christian Ethics: An Introduction*, edited by Bernard Hoose, 149–160. London: Continuum.

Macnicol, John. 2006. *Age Discrimination: An Historical and Contemporary Analysis*. Cambridge: Cambridge University Press.

Maddox, Marion. 2013. "Prosper, Consume and Be Saved." *Critical Research on Religion* 1 (1): 108–115.

Magi, Margus, and Erik Allander. 1981. "Towards a Theory of Perceived and Medically Defined Need." *Sociology of Health & Illness* 3 (1): 49–71.

Magnusson, Roger S., and Paul E. Griffiths. 2015. "Who's Afraid of the Nanny State? Introduction to a Symposium." *Public Health* 129 (8): 1017–1020.

Main, Ben, Marcell Csanadi, and Piotr Ozieranski. 2022 (in press). "Pricing Strategies, Executive Committee Power and Negotiation Leverage in New Zealand's Containment of Public Spending on Pharmaceuticals." *Health Economics, Policy and Law*: 1–18.

Malan, Gert J. 2014. "Is Rewritten Bible/Scripture the Solution to the Synoptic Problem?" *HTS Teologiese Studies/Theological Studies* 70 (1): 1–10.

Malchow, Bruce V. 1996. *Social Justice in the Hebrew Bible: What Is New and What Is Old*. Collegeville, MN: Liturgical Press.

Malpani, Rohit, and Alex Maitland. 2021. *Dose of Reality: How Rich Countries and Pharmaceutical Corporations Are Breaking Their Vaccine Promises*. People's Vaccine Alliance. https://webassets.oxfamamerica.org/media/documents/A_Dose_of_Reality-Briefing_Note_kOW1yUs.pdf.

Mannion, Russell. 2014. "Enabling Compassionate Health Care: Perils, Prospects and Perspectives." *International Journal of Health Policy and Management* 2 (3): 115–117.

Mannion, Russell, and Jeffrey Braithwaite. 2012. "Unintended Consequences of Performance Measurement in Healthcare: 20 Salutary Lessons from the English National Health Service." *Internal Medicine Journal* 42 (5): 569–574.

Marchildon, Gregory P., Shuli Brammli-Greenberg, Mark Dayan, Antonio Giulio De Belvis, Coralie Gandré, David Isaksson, Madelon Kroneman, Neuner-Jehle S. Stefan, Ingrid Sperre Saunes, Steven Thomas, Karsten Vrangbæk, and Wilm Quentin. 2021 (in press). "Achieving Higher Performing Primary Care through Patient Registration: A Review of Twelve High-Income Countries." *Health Policy*. 125 (12): 1507–1516.

Margolis, Howard. 1984. *Selfishness, Altruism, and Rationality: A Theory of Social Choice*. Chicago: University of Chicago Press.

Markovitz, Adam A., and Andrew M. Ryan. 2017. "Pay-for-Performance: Disappointing Results or Masked Heterogeneity?" *Medical Care Research and Review* 74 (1): 3–78.

Marmor, Theodore R. 2004. *Fads in Medical Care Management and Policy*. London: The Nuffield Trust.

2007. *Fads, Fallacies and Foolishness in Medical Care Management and Policy*. Singapore: World Scientific Publishing.

Marmot, Michael. 2005a. "Introduction." In *Social Determinants of Health*, edited by Michael Marmot and Richard Wilkinson, 1–16. Oxford: Oxford University Press.

2005b. "Social Determinants of Health Inequalities." *Public Health* 365: 1099–1106.

2018. "Inclusion Health: Addressing the Causes of the Causes." *The Lancet* 391 (10117): 186–188.

2020. "Health Equity in England: The Marmot Review 10 Years On." *British Medical Journal* 368: m693.

Marmot, Michael, and Ruth Bell. 2019. "Social Determinants and Non-communicable Diseases: Time for Integrated Action." *British Medical Journal* 364: l251.

Marshall, Christopher D. 2012. *Compassionate Justice: An Interdisciplinary Dialogue with Two Gospel Parables on Law, Crime, and Restorative Justice.* Eugene, OR: Cascade.

Martin, John, Shannon Mills, and Mary E. Foley. 2018. "Innovative Models of Dental Care Delivery and Coverage: Patient-Centric Dental Benefits Based on Digital Oral Health Risk Assessment." *Dental Clinics of North America* 62 (2): 319–325.

Marx, Karl. 2010. "Critique of the Gotha Programme." In *Marx and Engels Collected works. Volume 24: 1874–188*, edited by Karl Marx and Friedrich Engels. London: Lawrence & Wishart.

Marxsen, Willi. 1993. *New Testament Foundations for Christian Ethics* (translated by O.C. Dean). Edinburgh: T&T Clark.

Mash, Rachel. 2021. "The Green Anglican Movement and Climate Change." In *World Scientific Encyclopedia of Climate Change*, edited by Jan W. Dash, 257–260. Singapore: World Scientific.

Massaro, Thomas J. 2018. "'He Drinks from His Own Wells': The Jesuit Roots of the Ethical Teachings of Pope Francis." *Journal of Catholic Social Thought* 15 (2): 353–373.

Massingale, Bryan N. 2016. "Theology in the Public Sphere in the Twenty-First Century." *Horizons* 43 (2): 351–356. https://doi.org/10.1017/hor.2016.110.

Masters, Rebecca, Elspeth Anwar, Brendan Collins, Richard Cookson, and Simon Capewell. 2017. "Return on Investment of Public Health Interventions: A Systematic Review." *Journal of Epidemiology and Community Health* 71 (8): 827–834.

Matera, Frank J. 1999. *New Testament Ethics: The Legacies of Jesus and Paul.* Louisville, KY: Wetminster John Knox Press.

Mattingly, T Joseph, and Linda Simoni-Wastila. 2017. "Patient-Centered Drug Approval: The Role of Patient Advocacy in the Drug Approval Process." *Journal of Managed Care & Specialty Pharmacy* 23 (10): 1078–1082.

May, Peter, Melissa M. Garrido, J. Brian Cassel, Amy S. Kelley, Diane E. Meier, Charles Normand, Thomas J. Smith, and R. Sean Morrison. 2017. "Cost Analysis of a Prospective Multi-site Cohort Study of Palliative Care

Consultation Teams for Adults with Advanced Cancer: Where Do Cost-Savings Come From?" *Palliative Medicine* 31 (4): 378–386.

Maynard, Alan. 1979. "Pricing, Demanders, and the Supply of Health Care." *International Journal of Health Services* 9 (1): 121–133.

1997. "Evidence-Based Medicine: An Incomplete Method for Informing Treatment Choices." *The Lancet* 349 (9045): 126–128.

Maynard, Alan, and Karen Bloor. 2010. "Patient Reported Outcome Measurement: Learning to Walk before We Run." *J R Soc Med* 103 (4): 129–132.

Mazurenko, Olena, Heather L. Taylor, and Nir Menachemi. 2022 (in press). "The Impact of Narrow and Tiered Networks on Costs, Access, Quality, and Patient Steering: A Systematic Review." *Medical Care Research and Review* 79 (5): 607–617.

McCabe, Christopher, Mike Paulden, James O'Mahony, Richard Edlin, and Anthony Culyer. 2016. "Life at a Premium: Considering an End-of-Life Premium in Value-Based Reimbursement." In *Care at the End of Life: An Economic Perspective*, edited by Jeff Round, 123–139. Cham: Springer International Publishing.

McCartney, James J. 1980. "The Development of the Doctrine of Ordinary and Extraordinary Means of Preserving Life in Catholic Moral Theology before the Karen Quinlan Case." *The Linacre Quarterly* 47 (3): 215–224.

McClain, Zachary, Linda A. Hawkins, and Baligh R. Yehia. 2016. "Creating Welcoming Spaces for Lesbian, Gay, Bisexual, and Transgender (LGBT) Patients: An Evaluation of the Health Care Environment." *Journal of Homosexuality* 63 (3): 387–393.

McCoy, David, Simukai Chigudu, and Taavi Tillmann. 2017. "Framing the Tax and Health Nexus: A Neglected Aspect of Public Health Concern." *Health Economics, Policy and Law* 12 (2): 179–194.

McCoy, Matthew S., Michael Carniol, Katherine Chockley, John W. Urwin, Ezekiel J. Emanuel, and Harald Schmidt. 2017. "Conflicts of Interest for Patient-Advocacy Organizations." *New England Journal of Medicine* 376 (9): 880–885.

McDaid, David, Franco Sassi, and Sherry Merkur. 2015. "Supporting Effective and Efficient Policies: The Role of Economic Analysis." In *Promoting Health, Preventing Disease: The Economic Case*, edited by David McDaid, Franco Sassi and Sherry Merkur, 19–32. Maidenhead: Open University Press.

McDaid, David, and Matthias Wismar. 2015. "Making an Economic Case for Intersectoral Action." In *Promoting Health, Preventing Disease: The Economic Case*, edited by David McDaid, Franco Sassi and Sherry Merkur, 293–312. Maidenhead: Open University Press.

McDonald, J. I. H. 1996. "The View from the Ditch – and Other Angles: Interpreting the Parable of the Good Samaritan." *Scottish Journal of Theology* 49 (1): 21–37.

McDougall, Jean A., Wesley E. Furnback, Bruce C. M. Wang, and Jörg Mahlich. 2020. "Understanding the Global Measurement of Willingness to Pay in Health." *Journal of Market Access & Health Policy* 8 (1): 1717030.

McFarland, Ian A. 2001. "Who Is My Neighbor?: The Good Samaritan as a Source for Theological Anthropology." *Modern Theology* 17 (1): 57–66.

McFarland, Sophie, Anne Coufopolous, and Deborah Lycett. 2021. "The Effect of Telehealth versus Usual Care for Home-Care Patients with Long-Term Conditions: A Systematic Review, Meta-analysis and Qualitative Synthesis." *Journal of Telemedicine and Telecare* 27 (2): 69–87.

McGregor, Sue. 2001. "Neoliberalism and Health Care." *International Journal of Consumer Studies* 25 (2): 82–89.

McGuire, Thomas G. 2000. "Physician Agency." In *Handbook of Health Economics, Volume 1A*, edited by A. J. Culyer and J. P. Newhouse, 461–536. Amsterdam: Elsevier.

McHugh, Neil, Rachel M. Baker, Helen Mason, Laura Williamson, Job van Exel, Rohan Deogaonkar, Marissa Collins, and Cam Donaldson. 2015. "Extending Life for People with a Terminal Illness: A Moral Right and an Expensive Death? Exploring Societal Perspectives." *BMC Medical Ethics* 16 (14).

McHugh, Neil, José Luis Pinto-Prades, Rachel Baker, Helen Mason, and Cam Donaldson. 2020. "Exploring the Relative Value of End of Life QALYs: Are the Comparators Important?" *Social Science & Medicine* 245: 112660.

McHugh, Neil, Job van Exel, Helen Mason, Jon Godwin, Marissa Collins, Cam Donaldson, and Rachel Baker. 2018. "Are Life-Extending Treatments for Terminal Illnesses a Special Case? Exploring Choices and Societal Viewpoints." *Social Science & Medicine* 198: 61–69.

McIntyre, Di. 2007. "Pay the Piper and Call the Tune: Changing Health Care Financing Mechanisms to Address Public-Private Health Sector Mix Inequities." In *The Economics of Health Equity*, edited by Di McIntyre and Gavin Mooney, 174–196. Cambridge: Cambridge University Press.

McIntyre, Di, and Joseph Kutzin. 2016. *Health Financing Country Diagnostic: A Foundation for National Strategy Development*. Geneva: World Health Organization.

McIntyre, Di, Filip Meheus, and John-Arne Røttingen. 2017. "What Level of Domestic Government Health Expenditure Should We Aspire to for Universal Health Coverage?" *Health Economics, Policy and Law* 12 (2): 125–137.

McKee, Martin, and David Stuckler. 2018. "Revisiting the Corporate and Commercial Determinants of Health." *American Journal of Public Health* 108 (9): 1167–1170.

McKie, John, and Jeff Richardson. 2003. "The Rule of Rescue." *Social Science and Medicine* 56 (12): 2407–2419.

McKie, John, Jeff Richardson, Peter Singer, and Helga Kuhse. 1998. *The Allocation of Health Care Resources: An Ethical Evaluation of the 'QALY' Approach*. Aldershot: Ashgate/Dartmouth.

McKnight, D Harrison, and Norman L. Chervany. 2000. "What Is Trust? A Conceptual Analysis and an Interdisciplinary Model." *AMCIS proceedings* (382): 827–832.

Meadors, Gary T. 1985. "The 'Poor' in the Beatitudes of Matthew and Luke." *Grace Theological Journal* 6 (2): 305–314.

Meadow, William, Anne Pohlman, Dan Reynolds, Leah Rand, Camil Correia, Ella Christoph, and Jesse Hall. 2014. "Power and Limitations of Daily Prognostications of Death in the Medical ICU for Outcomes in the Following 6 Months." *Critical Care Medicine* 42 (11): 2387–2392.

Mealand, David L. 1980. *Poverty and Expectation in the Gospels*. London: SPCK.

Meeks, M. Douglas. 1989. *God the Economist: The Doctrine of God and Political Economy*. Minneapolis, MN: Fortress Press.

Meheus, Filip, and Di McIntyre. 2017. "Fiscal Space for Domestic Funding of Health and Other Social Services." *Health Economics, Policy and Law* 12 (2): 159–177.

Meier, Stephan. 2006. *The Economics of Non-selfish Behaviour: Decisions to Contribute Money to Public Goods*. Cheltenham, UK: Edward Elgar.

Mendelson, Aaron, Karli Kondo, Cheryl Damberg, Allison Low, Makalapua Motúapuaka, Michele Freeman, Maya O'Neil, Rose Relevo, and Devan Kansagara. 2017. "The Effects of Pay-for-Performance Programs on Health, Health Care Use, and Processes of Care: A Systematic Review." *Annals of Internal Medicine* 166 (5): 341–353.

Mensch, Barbara S., Erica K. Chuang, Andrea J. Melnikas, and Stephanie R. Psaki. 2019. "Evidence for Causal Links between Education and Maternal and Child Health: Systematic Review." *Tropical Medicine & International Health* 24 (5): 504–522.

Merton, Robert K. 1936. "The Unanticipated Consequences of Purposive Social Action." *American Sociological Review* 1 (6): 894–904.

Metzl, Jonathan M., and Helena Hansen. 2014. "Structural Competency: Theorizing a New Medical Engagement with Stigma and Inequality." *Social Science & Medicine* 103: 126–133.

Mikton, Christopher, Vânia de la Fuente-Núñez, Alana Officer, and Etienne Krug. 2021. "Ageism: A Social Determinant of Health That Has Come of Age." *The Lancet* 397 (10282): 1333–1334.

Mill, John Stuart. 1977. *Essays on Politics and Society* (Edited by J.M. Robson). Toronto, London: University of Toronto Press; Routledge & Kegan Paul.

Miller, David. 2017. "Solidarity and Its Sources." In *The Strains of Commitment: The Political Sources of Solidarity in Diverse Societies*, edited by Keith Banting and Will Kymlicka, 62–79. Oxford: Oxford University Press.

Miller, Harold D. 2009. "From Volume to Value: Better Ways to Pay for Health Care." *Health Affairs* 28 (5): 1418–1428.

Miller, Pavla, and David Hayward. 2016. "Social Policy 'Generosity' at a Time of Fiscal Austerity: The Strange Case of Australia's National Disability Insurance Scheme." *Critical Social Policy* 37 (1): 128–147.

Miller, Susan. 2012. "'I Came That They May Have Life, and Have It Abundantly' (John 10:10): An Ecological Reading of John's Gospel." *The Expository Times* 124 (2): 64–71.

Mills, Mackenzie, and Panos Kanavos. 2020. "Do Pharmaceutical Budgets Deliver Financial Sustainability in Healthcare? Evidence from Europe." *Health Policy* 124 (3): 239–251.

Milstein, Ricarda, and Jonas Schreyoegg. 2016. "Pay for Performance in the Inpatient Sector: A Review of 34 P4P Programs in 14 OECD Countries." *Health Policy* 120 (10): 1125–1140.

Mintrom, Michael. 2019. "New Zealand's Wellbeing Budget Invests in Population Health." *The Milbank Quarterly* 97 (4): 893–896.

Mintzberg, Henry. 1975. *Impediments to the Use of Management Information*. New York: National Association of Accountants, The Society of Industrial Accountants of Canada, Ontario.

2017. *Managing the Myths of Health Care: Bridging the Separations between Care, Cure, Control, and Community*. Oakland, CA: Berrett-Koehler.

Mirelman, Andrew, and Richard Cookson. 2020. "Financial protection." In *Distributional Cost-Effectiveness Analysis Quantifying Health Equity Impacts and Trade-Offs*, edited by Richard Cookson, Susan Griffin, Ole Frithjof Norheim and Anthony J. Culyer. Oxford: Oxford University Press.

Mirowski, Philip. 1991. *More Heat Than Light: Economics as Social Physics, Physics as Nature's Economics*. Cambridge: Cambridge University Press.

1992. "Do Economists Suffer from Physics Envy?" *Finnish Economic Papers* 5 (1): 61–68.

Misak, Cheryl J., Douglas B. White, and Robert D. Truog. 2014. "Medical Futility: A New Look at an Old Problem." *Chest* 146 (6): 1667–1672.

Mitchell, Imogen, Jeanette Lacey, Matthew Anstey, Cathy Corbett, Carol Douglas, Christine Drummond, Michel Hensley, Amber Mills, Caroline Scott, and Jo-Anne Slee. 2021. "Understanding End-of-Life Care in Australian Hospitals." *Australian Health Review* 45 (5): 540–547.

Mitchell, Polly, Alan Cribb, and Vikki Entwistle. 2021. "Made to Measure: The Ethics of Routine Measurement for Healthcare Improvement." *Health Care Analysis* 29 (1): 39–58.

Mitton, Craig, and Cam Donaldson. 2001. "Twenty-Five Years of Programme Budgeting and Marginal Analysis in the Health Sector, 1974–1999." *Journal of Health Services & Research Policy* 6 (4): 239–248.

Moccia, Salvatore. 2017. "Evangelii Gaudium: A European Perspective." *Journal of Vincentian Social Action* 2 (2): 27–34.

Mohammadshahi, Marita, Shahrooz Yazdani, Alireza Olyaeemanesh, Ali Akbari Sari, Mehdi Yaseri, and Sara Emamgholipour Sefiddashti. 2019. "A Scoping Review of Components of Physician-induced Demand for Designing a Conceptual Framework." *Journal of Preventive Medicine & Public Health* 52 (2): 72–81.

Moldovan, Andrada, and Steven Van de Walle. 2013. "Gifts or Bribes? Attitudes on Informal Payments in Romanian Health Care." *Public Integrity* 15 (4): 385–402.

Mont, Daniel. 2007. "Measuring Health and Disability." *The Lancet* 369 (9573): 1658–1663.

Montero, Roman A. 2019. *Jesus's Manifesto: The Sermon on the Plain*. Eugene, OR: Wipf and Stock Publishers.

Mooney, Gavin. 1986. *Economics, Medicine and Health Care*. Hertfordshire: Harvester Wheatsheaf.

2001. "Communitarianism and Health Economics." In *The Social Economics of Health Care*, edited by John Bryan Davis, 40–60. London: Routledge.

Moore, Randall F. 1996. "Caring for Identified versus Statistical Lives: An Evolutionary View of Medical Distributive Justice." *Ethology and Sociobiology* 17 (6): 379–401.

Moore, Sharon. 2017. "From State to Market: Reclaiming a Critical Ethics of Elder Care." In *Critical Ethics of Care in Social Work: Transforming the Politics and Practices of Caring*, edited by Bob Pease, Anthea Vreugdenhil and Sonya Stanford, 84–93. London: Routledge.

Moradpour, Javad, and Aidan Hollis. 2021. "The Economic Theory of Cost-Effectiveness Thresholds in Health: Domestic and International Implications." *Health Economics* 30 (5): 1139–1151.

Morata, Lauren. 2018. "An Evolutionary Concept Analysis of Futility in Health Care." *Journal of Advanced Nursing* 74 (6): 1289–1300.

Morden, Nancy E., Carrie H. Colla, Thomas D. Sequist, and Meredith B. Rosenthal. 2014. "Choosing Wisely – The Politics and Economics of Labeling Low-Value Services." *New England Journal of Medicine* 370 (7): 589–592.

Morris, John, Deborah White, and Gill Bradnock. 2012. "Primary Dental Care: Time to Revise the Definition? Prim Dent Care 2000. 7 (3): 93–96." *Primary Dental Care: Journal of the Faculty of General Dental Practitioners (UK)* 19 (3): 102–110.

Morris, Leon. 2008. *Luke: Tyndale New Testament Commentaries*. Nottingham: Inter-Varsity Press.

Mott, Stephen Charles. 2011. *Biblical Ethics and Social Change*. New York: Oxford University Press.

Mounsey, Sarah, Lennert Veerman, Stephen Jan, and Anne Marie Thow. 2020. "The Macroeconomic Impacts of Diet-Related Fiscal Policy for NCD Prevention: A Systematic Review." *Economics & Human Biology* 37: 100854.

Moynihan, Ray, and L. Bero. 2017. "Toward a Healthier Patient Voice: More Independence, Less Industry Funding." *JAMA Internal Medicine* 177 (3): 350–351.

Moynihan, Ray, Jenny Doust, and David Henry. 2012. "Preventing Overdiagnosis: How to Stop Harming the Healthy." *BMJ* 344.

Muers, Stephen. 2020. *Culture and Values at the Heart of Policy Making: An Insider's Guide*. Bristol: Policy Press.

Mügge, Daniel. 2022. "Economic Statistics as Political Artefacts." *Review of International Political Economy* 29 (1): 1–22.

Mullan, Fitzhugh. 2001. "A Founder of Quality Assessment Encounters A Troubled System Firsthand." *Health Affairs* 20 (1): 137–141.

Munari, Stephanie C., Alyce N. Wilson, Ngaree J. Blow, Caroline S. E. Homer, and Jeanette E. Ward. 2021. "Rethinking the Use of 'Vulnerable'." *Australian and New Zealand Journal of Public Health* 45 (3): 197–199.

Murdoch, Jamie, Charlotte Salter, John Ford, Elizabeth Lenaghan, Alice Shiner, and Nicholas Steel. 2020. "The 'Unknown Territory' of Goal-Setting: Negotiating a Novel Interactional Activity within Primary Care Doctor-Patient Consultations for Patients with Multiple Chronic Conditions." *Social Science & Medicine*: 113040.

Musikanski, Laura. 2014. "Happiness in Public Policy." *Journal of Social Change* 6 (1): 55–85.

Nanavaty, Merena, Mkaya Mwamburi, Anagha Gogate, John Proach, Abner Nyandege, and Zeba M. Khan. 2015. "The Use of Incremental Cost-Effectiveness Ratio Thresholds in Health Technology Assessment Decisions." *Journal of Clinical Pathways* 1 (1): 29–36.

National Academies of Sciences Engineering and Medicine. 2017. *Accounting for Social Risk Factors in Medicare Payment: Identifying Social Risk Factors.* Washington, DC: National Academies Press.

2020. *Framework for Equitable Allocation of COVID-19 Vaccine*. Washington, DC: National Academies Press.

Navarria, Andrea, Valentina Drago, Lucia Gozzo, Laura Longo, Silvana Mansueto, Giacomo Pignataro, and Filippo Drago. 2015. "Do the Current Performance-Based Schemes in Italy Really Work? 'Success Fee': A Novel Measure for Cost-Containment of Drug Expenditure." *Value in Health* 18 (1): 131–136.

Nche, George C. 2020. "The Church Climate Action: Identifying the Barriers and the Bridges." *Transformation* 37 (3): 222–241.

Nelson, Julie A. 2003. "How Did 'the Moral' Get Split from 'the Economic'?" In *Toward a Feminist Philosophy of Economics*, edited by Drucilla K Barker, Edith Kuiper, 134–141. London: Routledge.

Neumann, Peter J. 2005. *Using Cost-Effectiveness Analysis to Improve Health Care: Opportunities and Barriers*. Oxford: Oxford University Press.

Neumann, Peter J., James D. Chambers, Françoise Simon, and Lisa M. Meckley. 2011. "Risk-Sharing Arrangements That Link Payment for Drugs to Health Outcomes Are Proving Hard to Implement." *Health Affairs* 30 (12): 2329–2337.

Neumann, Peter J., Daniel A. Ollendorf, and Joshua T. Cohen. 2021. "Value-Based Drug Pricing in the Biden Era: Opportunities and Prospects." *Health Services Research* 56 (6): 1093–1099.

Neumann, Peter J., Eileen A. Sandberg, Chaim M. Bell, Patricia W. Stone, and Richard H. Chapman. 2000. "Are Pharmaceuticals Cost-Effective? A Review of the Evidence." *Health Affairs* 19 (2): 92–109.

Neumann, Peter J., Gillian D. Sanders, Louise B. Russell, Joanna E. Siegel, and Theodore G. Ganiats. 2017. *Cost-Effectiveness in Health and Medicine* (2nd ed). New York: Oxford University Press.

Newbert, Scott L. 2018. "Achieving Social and Economic Equality by Unifying Business and Ethics: Adam Smith as the Cause of and Cure for the Separation Thesis." *Journal of Management Studies* 55 (3): 517–544.

Newhouse, Joseph P., and Anna D. Sinaiko. 2008. "What We Know and Don't Know about the Effects of Cost Sharing of the Demand for Medical Care – and So What?" In *Incentives and Choice in Health Care*, edited by Frank A Sloan and Hirschel Kasper, 85–102. Cambridge: MIT Press.

Newhouse, Joseph P., and the Health Insurance Experiment Group. 1993. *Free for All? Lessons from the RAND Health Insurance Experiment.* Cambridge, MA: Harvard University Press.

New Zealand Treasury. 2019. *The Wellbeing Budget.* Wellington, NZ: Treasury.

Nguengang-Wakap, Stéphanie, Deborah M. Lambert, Annie Olry, Charlotte Rodwell, Charlotte Gueydan, Valérie Lanneau, Daniel Murphy, Yann Le Cam, and Ana Rath. 2020. "Estimating Cumulative Point Prevalence of Rare Diseases: Analysis of the Orphanet Database." *European Journal of Human Genetics* 28 (2): 165–173.

Nolan, Brian, and Luis Valenzuela. 2019. "Inequality and Its Discontents." *Oxford Review of Economic Policy* 35 (3): 396–430.

Nord, Erik. 1999. *Cost-Value Analysis in Health Care: Making Sense Out of QALYs.* Cambridge: Cambridge University Press.

2005. "Values for Health States in QALYs and DALYs: Desirability versus Well-Being and Worth." In *Quality of Life and Human Difference: Genetic Testing, Health Care, and Disability*, edited by David Wasserman, Robert Wachbroit and Jerome Bickenbach, 125–141. New York: Cambridge University Press.

Norheim, Ole Frithjof. 2015. "Ethical Perspective: Five Unacceptable Trade-Offs on the Path to Universal Health Coverage." *International Journal of Health Policy and Management* 4 (11): 711–714.

Norsigian, Judy. 2019. "Our Bodies Ourselves and the Women's Health Movement in the United States: Some Reflections." *American Journal of Public Health* 109 (6): 844–846.

Noseworthy, Tom W., John J. McGurran, David C. Hadorn, and Steering Committee of the Western Canada Waiting List Project. 2003. "Waiting for Scheduled Services in Canada: Development of Priority-Setting Scoring Systems." *Journal of Evaluation in Clinical Practice* 9 (1): 23–31.

Novak, David. 2019. *Athens and Jerusalem: God, Humans, and Nature (The Gifford Lectures 2017).* Toronto: University of Toronto Press.

Nozick, Robert. 1974. *Anarchy, State, and Utopia.* Oxford: Blackwell.

Nussbaum, Martha C. 1996. "Compassion: The Basic Social Emotion." *Social Philosophy and Policy* 13 (1): 27–58.

2000. "The Costs of Tragedy: Some Moral Limits of Cost-Benefit Analysis." *The Journal of Legal Studies* 29 (S2): 1005–1036.

2013. *Political Emotions: Why Love Matters for Justice.* Cambridge: Harvard University Press.

Nyman, John A. 2004. "Is 'Moral Hazard' Inefficient? The Policy Implications of a New Theory." *Health Affairs* 23 (5): 194–199.

2007. "American Health Policy: Cracks in the Foundation." *Journal of Health Politics, Policy and Law* 32 (5): 759–783.

O' Mahony, Seamus. 2016. *The Way We Die Now*. London: Head of Zeus
O'Neill, Onora. 2000. *Bounds of Justice*. Cambridge: Cambridge University Press.
2002. *Towards Justice and Virtue: A Constructive Account of Practical Reasoning*. Cambridge: Cambridge University Press.
O'Toole, Robert F. 1981. "Activity of the Risen Jesus in Luke-Acts." *Biblica* 62 (4): 471–498.
Oakman, Douglas E. 2008. *Jesus and the Peasants*. Eugene, OR: Wipf and Stock Publishers.
Ochalek, Jessica, and James Lomas. 2020. "Reflecting the Health Opportunity Costs of Funding Decisions within Value Frameworks: Initial Estimates and the Need for Further Research." *Clinical Therapeutics* 42 (1): 44–59.
Ogundeji, Yewande Kofoworola, John Martin Bland, and Trevor Andrew Sheldon. 2016. "The Effectiveness of Payment for Performance in Health Care: A Meta-analysis and Exploration of Variation in Outcomes." *Health Policy* 120 (10): 1141–1150.
Oliver, Adam. 2019. *Reciprocity and the Art of Behavioural Public Policy*. Cambridge: Cambridge University Press.
Olofsson, Sara., Ulf-Göran Gerdtham, Lars Hultkrantz, and Ulf Persson. 2018. "Measuring the End-of-Life Premium in Cancer Using Individual ex ante Willingness to Pay." *The European Journal of Health Economics* 19 (6): 807–820.
Olofsson, Sara, Ulf G. Gerdtham, Lars Hultkrantz, and Ulf Persson. 2019. "Dread and Risk Elimination Premium for the Value of a Statistical Life." *Risk Analysis* 39 (11): 2391–2407.
Olsen, Jan Abel, and RoseAnne Misajon. 2020. "A Conceptual Map of Health-Related Quality of Life Dimensions: Key Lessons for a New Instrument." *Quality of Life Research* 29 (3): 733–743.
Olson, Rebecca E., Alexandra Smith, Phillip Good, Emily Neate, Cody Hughes, and Janet Hardy. 2021. "Emotionally Reflexive Labour in End-of-Life Communication." *Social Science & Medicine* 291: 112928.
Onakpoya, Igho J., Elizabeth A. Spencer, Matthew J. Thompson, and Carl J. Heneghan. 2015. "Effectiveness, Safety and Costs of Orphan Drugs: An Evidence-Based Review." *BMJ Open* 5 (6).
Ong, Wee Loon, Richard Khor, Mathias Bressel, Phillip Tran, Jo Tedesco, Keen Hun Tai, David Ball, Gillian Duchesne, and Farshad Foroudi. 2017. "Patterns of Health Services Utilization in the Last Two Weeks of Life among Cancer Patients: Experience in an Australian Academic Cancer Center." *Asia-Pacific Journal of Clinical Oncology* 13 (6): 400–406.
Oosthuizen, André J., and Laetus O. K. Lategan. 2015. "'Managing the Household of God': The Contribution from Management Sciences to the Sustainability of the Church as an Organization." *Stellenbosch Theological Journal* 1 (2): 551–568.
Oppenheimer, Daniel M, and Christopher Y Olivola, eds. 2011. *The Science of Giving: Experimental Approaches to the Study of Charity*. New York, NY: Psychology Press.

Or, Zeynep, Chantal Cases, Melanie Lisac, Karsten Vrangbæk, Ulrika Winblad, and Gwyn Bevan. 2010. "Are Health Problems Systemic? Politics of Access and Choice under Beveridge and Bismarck Systems." *Health Economics, Policy and Law* 5 (3): 269–293.

Organisation for Economic Cooperation and Development. 2017. *Tackling Wasteful Spending on Health*. Paris: OECD.

2019a. *Health at a Glance 2019: OECD Indicators*. Paris: OECD Publishing.

2019b. *Measuring What Matters: The Patient Reported Indicator Surveys. Patient-Reported Indicators for Assessing Health System Performance*. Paris: OECD.

2021. *How's Life? 2020: Measuring Well-Being*. Paris: OECD Publishing.

Oslington, Paul. 2012. "God and the Market: Adam Smith's Invisible Hand." *Journal of Business Ethics* 108 (4): 429–438.

Ostrom, Elinor. 1990. *Governing the Commons: The Evolution of Institutions for Collective Action*. Cambridge: Cambridge University Press.

2010. "Beyond Markets and States: Polycentric Governance of Complex Economic Systems." *American Economic Review* 100 (3): 641–672.

Ottersen, Trygve, Riku Elovainio, David B. Evans, David McCoy, Di McIntyre, Filip Meheus, Suerie Moon, Gorik Ooms, and John-Arne Røttingen. 2017. "Towards a Coherent Global Framework for Health Financing: Recommendations and Recent Developments." *Health Economics, Policy and Law* 12 (2): 285–296.

Otteson, James. 2015. "Adam Smith." In *The Oxford Handbook of the History of Ethics*, edited by Roger Crisp. Oxford: Oxford University Press.

Ottmann, Goetz, Jacqui Allen, and Peter Feldman. 2013. "A Systematic Narrative Review of Consumer-Directed Care for Older People: Implications for Model Development." *Health & Social Care in the Community* 21 (6): 563–581.

Pace, Jessica, Narcyz Ghinea, Ian Kerridge, and Wendy Lipworth. 2018. "An Ethical Framework for the Creation, Governance and Evaluation of Accelerated Access Programs." *Health Policy* 122 (9): 984–990.

Pace, Jessica, Ian Kerridge, Sallie Pearson, and Wendy Lipworth. 2021. "Physicians' Attitudes towards Accelerated Access to Medicines." *Health Economics, Policy and Law* 16 (2): 154–169.

Padula, William V., and Mark J. Sculpher. 2021. "Ideas about Resourcing Health Care in the United States: Can Economic Evaluation Achieve Meaningful Use?" *Annals of internal medicine* 174 (1): 80–85.

Palmer, Andrew J., Julie A. Campbell, Barbara de Graaff, Nancy Devlin, Hasnat Ahmad, Philip M. Clarke, Mingsheng Chen, and Lei Si. 2021. "Population Norms for Quality Adjusted Life Years for the United States of America, China, the United Kingdom and Australia." *Health Economics* 30 (8): 1950–1977.

Palmer, Karen S., Thomas Agoritsas, Danielle Martin, Taryn Scott, Sohail M Mulla, Ashley P Miller, Arnav Agarwal, Andrew Bresnahan, Afeez Abiola Hazzan, Rebecca A Jeffery, Arnaud Merglen, Ahmed Negm, Reed A.

Siemieniuk, Neera Bhatnagar, Irfan A. Dhalla, John N. Lavis, John J. You, Stephen J. Duckett, and Gordon H. Guyat. 2014. "Activity-Based Funding of Hospitals and Its Impact on Mortality, Readmission, Discharge Destination, Severity of Illness, and Volume of Care: A Systematic Review and Meta-analysis." *PLOS ONE* 9 (10): e109975.

Palmer, Karen S., Adalsteinn D. Brown, Jenna M. Evans, Husayn Marani, Kirstie K. Russell, Danielle Martin, and Noah M. Ivers. 2018a. "Correction: Qualitative Analysis of the Dynamics of Policy Design and Implementation in Hospital Funding Reform." *PLOS ONE* 13 (3): e0194280.

2018b. "Qualitative Analysis of the Dynamics of Policy Design and Implementation in Hospital Funding Reform." *PLOS ONE* 13 (1): e0191996.

2018c. "Standardising Costs or Standardising Care? Qualitative Evaluation of the Implementation and Impact of a Hospital Funding Reform in Ontario, Canada." *Health Research Policy and Systems* 16 (74): 1–15.

Pan, Stephen W., Gabriella Stein, Barry Bayus, Weiming Tang, Allison Mathews, Cheng Wang, Chongyi Wei, and Joseph D. Tucker. 2017. "Systematic Review of Innovation Design Contests for Health: Spurring Innovation and Mass Engagement." *BMJ Innovations* 3 (4): 227–237.

Pant, Sirjana, and Sarah Visintini. 2018. *Drugs for Rare Diseases: A Review of National and International Health Technology Assessment Agencies and Public Payers' Decision-Making Processes*. Ottawa: Canadian Agency for Drugs and Technologies in Health.

Papanicolas, Irene. 2012. "Providing Financial Incentives for Improved Quality and Efficiency: A Literature Review of the Effects of Payment for Performance (P4P) Policies." In *The LSE Companion to Health Policy*, edited by Alistair McGuire and Joan Costa-Font, 144–159. Cheltenham: Edward Elgar Publishing.

Papanicolas, Irene, José F Figueroa, E John Orav, and Ashish K Jha. 2017. "Patient Hospital Experience Improved Modestly, but No Evidence Medicare Incentives Promoted Meaningful Gains." *Health Affairs* 36 (1): 133–140.

Papanicolas, Irene, Liana R. Woskie, and Ashish K. Jha. 2018. "Health Care Spending in the United States and Other High-Income Countries." *JAMA* 319 (10): 1024–1039.

Patel, Kant, and Mark E. Rushefsky. 2015. *Health Care in America: Separate and Unequal*. New York: Routledge.

Paul VI. 1965. *Pastoral Constitution on the Church in the Modern World: Gaudium et spes*. Vatican City: The Holy See.

Pauly, Mark V. 2004. "Medicare Drug Coverage and Moral Hazard." *Health Affairs* 23 (1): 113–122.

Pawson, Ray, Joanne Greenhalgh, and Cathy Brennan. 2016. "Demand Management for Planned Care: A Realist Synthesis." *Health Services and Delivery Research* 4 (2): 1–222.

Peck, M. Scott. 1978. *The Road Less Traveled: A New Psychology of Love, Traditional Values, and Spiritual Growth*. New York: Simon and Schuster.

Pedersen, Kusumita P. 2015. "Religious Ethics and the Environment: A Review Essay." *Journal of Religious Ethics* 43 (3): 558–585.

Pekarsky, Brita A. K. 2015. *The New Drug Reimbursement Game: A Regulator's Guide to Playing and Winning.* Cham: Springer International Publishing: Adis.

Pencheon, David, and Jeremy Wight. 2020. "Making Healthcare and Health Systems Net Zero." *British Medical Journal* 368: m970.

Pennington, Becky, Monica Hernandez-Alava, Stephen Pudney, and Allan Wailoo. 2019. "The Impact of Moving from EQ-5D-3L to -5L in NICE Technology Appraisals." *PharmacoEconomics* 37 (1): 75–84.

Pennington, Mark, Rachel Baker, Werner Brouwer, Helen Mason, Dorte Gyrd Hansen, Angela Robinson, and Cam Donaldson. 2015. "Comparing WTP Values of Different Types of QALY Gain Elicited from the General Public." *Health Economics* 24 (3): 280–293.

Percy, Martyn. 2014. "Foreword: Theonomics?" In *Theonomics: Reconnecting Economics with Virtue and Integrity*, edited by Andrew Lightbown and Peter Sills. Durham: Sacristy Press.

Pescheny, Julia V., Gurch Randhawa, and Yannis Pappas. 2019. "The Impact of Social Prescribing Services on Service Users: A Systematic Review of the Evidence." *European Journal of Public Health* 30 (4): 664–673.

Phelps, Andrea C., Paul K. Maciejewski, Matthew Nilsson, Tracy A. Balboni, Alexi A. Wright, M. Elizabeth Paulk, Elizabeth Trice, Deborah Schrag, John R. Peteet, Susan D. Block, and Holly G. Prigerson. 2009. "Religious Coping and Use of Intensive Life-Prolonging Care Near Death in Patients with Advanced Cancer." *JAMA* 301 (11): 1140–1147.

Phillips, Russell S., Neil S. Wenger, Joan Teno, Robert K. Oye, Stuart Youngner, Robert Califf, Peter Layde, Norman Desbiens, Alfred F. Connors, Joanne Lynn, and Support Investigators For the. 1996. "Choices of Seriously Ill Patients about Cardiopulmonary Resuscitation: Correlates and Outcomes." *The American Journal of Medicine* 100 (2): 128–137.

Pickett, Kate E., and Richard G. Wilkinson. 2015. "Income Inequality and Health: A Causal Review." *Social Science & Medicine* 128: 316–326.

Piketty, Thomas. 2020. *Capital and Ideology.* Cambridge, MA: Harvard University Press.

Pilch, John J. 2000. *Healing in the New Testament: Insights from Medical and Mediterranean Anthropology.* Minneapolis, MN: Fortress Press.

2012. *A Cultural Handbook to the Bible.* Grand Rapids, MI: Wm. B. Eerdmans.

2016. "Sickness and Healing in Luke-Acts." In *The Social World of Luke-Acts Models for Interpretation*, edited by Jerome Henry Neyrey. Peabody, MA: Hendrickson Publishers.

Pilkington, Bryan C. 2017. "Putting Image into Practice: Imago Dei, Dignity, and Their Bioethical Import." *Christian Bioethics* 23 (3): 299–316.

Pius XI. 1937. *Divini Redemptoris: Encyclical of Pope Pius XI on Atheistic Communism.* Vatican City: The Holy See.

Pomey, Marie-Pascale, Pierre-Gerlier Forest, Claudia Sanmartin, Carolyn De Coster, and Madeleine Drew. 2010. "Wait Time Management Strategies for Scheduled Care: What Makes Them Succeed?" *Healthcare Policy* 5 (3): 66–81.

Pontifical Council for Justice and Peace. 2004. *Compendium of the Social Doctrine of the Church.* Cittá del Vaticano: Libreria Editrice Vaticana.

Pope, Gregory C. 2011. "Overview of Pay for Performance Models and Issues." In *Pay for Performance in Health Care: Methods and Approaches,* edited by Jerry Cromwell, Michael G. Trisolini, Gregory C. Pope, Janet B. Mitchell and Leslie M. Greenwald, 33–75. Research Triangle Park, NC: RTI Press.

Pope, Stephen J. 1993. "The 'Preferential Option for the Poor': An Ethic for 'Saints and Heroes'?" *Irish Theological Quarterly* 59 (3): 161–176.

Porter, Elisabeth. 2006. "Can Politics Practice Compassion?" *Hypatia* 21 (4): 97–123.

Porter, Michael E., and Robert S. Kaplan. 2016. "How to Pay for Health Care." *Harvard Business Review* 94 (7): 88–102.

Porter, Michael E., Stefan Larsson, and Thomas H. Lee. 2016. "Standardizing Patient Outcomes Measurement." *New England Journal of Medicine* 374 (6): 504–506.

Porter, Michael E., and Elizabeth Olmsted Teisberg. 2004. "Redefining Competition in Health Care." *Harvard Business Review* 82 (6): 64–77.

2006. *Redefining Health Care: Creating Value-Based Competition on Results.* Boston, MA: Harvard Business School Press.

Posner, Eric A., and Cass R. Sunstein. 2017. "Moral Commitments in Cost-Benefit Analysis." *Virginia Law Review* 103 (8): 1809–1860.

Pourtaleb, Arefeh, Mehdi Jafari, Hesam Seyedin, and Ali Akhavan Behbahani. 2020. "New Insight into the Informal Patients' Payments on the Evidence of Literature: A Systematic Review Study." *BMC Health Services Research* 20 (14): 1–11.

Pressman, Jeffrey, and Aaron Wildavsky. 1973. *Implementation: How Great Expectations in Washington Are Dashed in Oakland or, Why It's Amazing That Federal Programs Work at All, This Being a Saga of the Economic Development Administration as Told by Two Sympathetic Observers Who Seek to Build Morals on a Foundation of Ruined Hopes.* Berkeley: University of California Press.

Proctor, Mark A. 2019. "'Who Is My Neighbor?' Recontextualizing Luke's Good Samaritan (Luke 10:25–37)." *Journal of Biblical Literature* 138 (1): 203–219.

Prodinger, Birgit, and Paul Taylor. 2018. "Improving Quality of Care through Patient-Reported Outcome Measures (PROMs): Expert Interviews Using the NHS PROMs Programme and the Swedish Quality Registers for Knee and Hip Arthroplasty as Examples." *BMC Health Services Research* 18 (87): 1–13.

Prügl, Elisabeth. 2021. "Untenable Dichotomies: De-gendering Political Economy." *Review of International Political Economy* 28 (2): 295–306.

Puyol, Angel. 2018. "The Uncomfortable Truths of Healthcare Prioritisation." In *Prioritising Health Services or Muddling Through,* edited by Juan del Llano Señarís and Salvador Peiró Moreno, 125–143. Madrid: Springer Healthcare.

Quentin, Wilm, Tit Albreht, Alexia Bezzina, Lucie Bryndova, Antoniya Dimova, Sophie Gerkens, Iwona Kowalska-Bobko, Sarah Mantwill, Zeynep Or, and Selina Rajan. 2020. "Adjusting Hospital Inpatient Payment Systems for COVID-19." *Eurohealth* 26 (2): 88–92.

Quinn, Kevin. 2015. "The 8 Basic Payment Methods in Health Care." *Annals of Internal Medicine* 163 (4): 300–306.

Radant, Nancy, Richard Blackford, Tamara Porch, Paul Shahbaz, and Richard E. Butman. 1985. "From Jerusalem to Jericho Revisited: A Study in Helping Behavior." *Journal of Psychology and Christianity* 4: 48–55.

Ragupathy, Rajan, and Michael Jameson. 2016. "Pharmaceutical Funding Decisions Must Balance Therapeutic Innovation, Opportunity Costs and Patient Equity." *New Zealand Medical Journal* 129 (1440): 22–24.

Ragupathy, Rajan, June Tordoff, Pauline Norris, and David Reith. 2012. "Key Informants' Perceptions of How PHARMAC Operates in New Zealand." *International Journal of Technology Assessment in Health Care* 28 (4): 367–373.

Rajan, Dheepa, Eva Brocard, Charlotte Poulussen, Kira Koch, Naomi Limaro Nathan, Katja Rohrer-Herold, and Pascal Melihan-Chenin. 2022. "Beyond Consultations and Surveys: Enhancing Participatory Governance in Health Systems." *Eurohealth* 28 (1): 9–13.

Ramirez, Steven A. 2017. "Social Justice and Capitalism: An Assessment of the Teachings of Pope Francis from a Law and Macroeconomics Perspective." *Seattle University Law Review* 40 (4): 1229–1259.

Ran, Tao, and Sajal K. Chattopadhyay. 2016. "Economic Evaluation of Community Water Fluoridation: A Community Guide Systematic Review." *American Journal of Preventive Medicine* 50 (6): 790–796.

Rand, Leah Z., and Aaron S. Kesselheim. 2021. "Controversy over Using Quality-Adjusted Life-Years in Cost-Effectiveness Analyses: A Systematic Literature Review." *Health Affairs* 40 (9): 1402–1410.

Raphael, Dennis, ed. 2009. *Social Determinants of Health: Canadian Perspectives* (2nd ed). Toronto: Canadaian Scholars' Publishing.

Raven, Sea. 2012. *Theology from Exile – Commentary on the Revised Common Lectionary for an Emerging Christianity. Volume 1: The Year of Luke.* Gerradstown, WV: Raven.

Rawles, John. 1989. "Castigating QALYs." *Journal of Medical Ethics* 15 (3): 143–147.

Rawls, John. 1997. "The Idea of Public Reason Revisited." *The University of Chicago Law Review* 64 (3): 765–807.

1999. *A Theory of Justice* (Revised edition). Boston: Belknap Press.

Rawstorn, Jonathan C., Nicholas Gant, Artur Direito, Christina Beckmann, and Ralph Maddison. 2016. "Telehealth Exercise-Based Cardiac Rehabilitation: A Systematic Review and Meta-analysis." *Heart* 102 (15): 1183–1192.

Reader, Soran. 2003. "Distance, Relationship and Moral Obligation." *The Monist* 86 (3): 367–381.

Reibling, Nadine, and Claus Wendt. 2012. "Gatekeeping and Provider Choice in OECD Healthcare Systems." *Current Sociology* 60 (4): 489–505.

Reilly, Richard. 2008. *Ethics of Compassion: Bridging Ethical Theory and Religious Moral Discourse*. Lanham, MD: Lexington Books.

Reinhardt, Uwe. 2012. "Divide et impera: Protecting the Growth of Health Care Incomes (COSTS)." *Health Economics* 21 (1): 41–54.

Reiser, Stanley J. 1980. "Refusing Treatment for Mental Illness: Historical and Ethical Dimensions." *The American Journal of Psychiatry* 137 (3): 329–331.

Reschovsky, James D., Larisa Converse, and Eugene C. Rich. 2015. "Solving the Sustainable Growth Rate Formula Conundrum Continues Steps toward Cost Savings and Care Improvements." *Health Affairs* 34 (4): 689–696.

Reumann, John Henry Paul. 1957. "The Use of Oikonomia and Related Terms in Greek Sources to about A.D. 100, as a Background for Patristic Applications." PhD, Graduate School, University of Pennsylvania.

Rice, Thomas. 2015. "Reflecting on 'Valuing Lives and Life Years: Anomalies, Implications, and an Alternative'." *Health Economics, Policy and Law* 10 (4): 405–409.

Rice, Thomas, and Jill Bernstein. 1990. "Volume Performance Standards: Can They Control Growth in Medicare Services?" *The Milbank Quarterly* 68 (3): 295–319.

Rich, Eugene C., Timothy K. Lake, Christal Stone Valenzano, and Myles M. Maxfield. 2013. "Paying the Doctor: Evidence-Based Decisions at the Point-of-Care and the Role of Fee-for-Service Incentives." *Journal of Comparative Effectiveness Research* 2 (3): 235–247.

Richardson, Jeff. 1998. "Supplier Induced Demand Reconsidered." In *Economics and Health 1998*, edited by Jonathan C. Baldry, 143–66. Sydney: School of Health Services Management.

Richardson, Jeff, and John McKie. 2005. "Empiricism, Ethics and Orthodox Economic Theory: What Is the Appropriate Basis for Decision-Making in the Health Sector?" *Social Science & Medicine* 60 (2): 265–275.

Ricoeur, Paul. 1965. *History and Truth*. Evanston, IL: Northwestern University Press.

1992. *Oneself as Another (translated by Kathleen Blamey)*. Chicago, IL: University of Chicago Press.

1995. "Love and Justice." *Philosophy & Social Criticism* 21 (5–6): 23–39.

2007. *Reflections on the Just*. Chicago; London: University of Chicago Press.

Robbins, Lionel. 1932. *An Essay on the Nature and Significance of Economic Science*. London: Macmillan.

Robbins, Vernon K. 2004. "The Sensory-Aesthetic Texture of the Compassionate Samaritan Parable in Luke 10." In *Literary Encounters with the Reign of God*, edited by Sharon H. Ringe and Hyun Chul Paul Kim, 247–262. New York: T & T Clark International.

Robinson, James C. 2001. "Theory and Practice in the Design of Physician Payment Incentives." *The Milbank Quarterly* 79 (2): 149–77.

Robson, Alex, and Francesco Paolucci. 2012. "Private Health Insurance Incentives in Australia: The Effects of Recent Changes to Price Carrots and Income Sticks." *The Geneva Papers on Risk and Insurance. Issues and Practice* 37 (4): 725–744.

Rocque, Rhea J., Caroline Beaudoin, Ruth Ndjaboue, Laura Cameron, Louann Poirier-Bergeron, Rose-Alice Poulin-Rheault, Catherine Fallon, Andrea C. Tricco, and Holly O. Witteman. 2021. "Health effects of climate change: an overview of systematic reviews." *BMJ Open* 11 (6): e046333.

Rodriguez-Martin, Ana-Maria, Panagiota Zacharopoulou, A. Bassim Hassan, and Apostolos Tsiachristas. 2018. "Cost-Effectiveness of Healthcare Interventions for Rare Cancers: Evidence from a Systematic Literature Review and Meta-Sanalysis." *Journal of Cancer Policy* 18: 1–10.

Rodriguez Santana, Idaira, Anne Mason, Nils Gutacker, Panagiotis Kasteridis, Rita Santos, and Nigel Rice. 2022 (in press). "Need, Demand, Supply in Health Care: Working Definitions, and Their Implications for Defining Access." *Health Economics, Policy and Law*: 1–13.

Rodwin, Marc A., Julien Mancini, Ségolène Duran, Anne-Céline Jalbert, Patrice Viens, Dominique Maraninchi, Anthony Gonçalves, and Patricia Marino. 2021. "The Use of 'Added Benefit' to Determine the Price of New Anti-cancer Drugs in France, 2004–2017." *European Journal of Cancer* 145: 11–18.

Romeder, Jean-Marie, and John R. McWhinnie. 1977. "Potential Years of Life Lost between Ages 1 and 70: An Indicator of Premature Mortality for Health Planning." *International Journal of Epidemiology* 6 (2): 143–151.

Romer, Paul. 2020. "The Dismal Kingdom: Do Economists Have Too Much Power." *Foreign Affairs* 99 (2): 150–157.

Rosano, Aldo, Christian Abo Loha, Roberto Falvo, Jouke van der Zee, Walter Ricciardi, Gabriella Guasticchi, and Antonio Giulio de Belvis. 2013. "The Relationship between Avoidable Hospitalization and Accessibility to Primary Care: A Systematic Review." *The European Journal of Public Health* 23 (3): 356–360.

Rose, Geoffrey. 1985. "Sick Individuals and Sick Populations." *International Journal of Epidemiology* 14 (1): 32–38.

Rose, Susannah L., Janelle Highland, Matthew T. Karafa, and Steven Joffe. 2017. "Patient Advocacy Organizations, Industry Funding, and Conflicts of Interest." *JAMA Internal Medicine* 177 (3): 344–350.

Rosenbaum, Lisa. 2017. "The Less-Is-More Crusade – Are We Overmedicalizing or Oversimplifying?" *New England Journal of Medicine* 377 (24): 2392–2397.

2022a. "Metric Myopia — Trading Away Our Clinical Judgment." *New England Journal of Medicine* 386 (18): 1759–1763.

2022b. "Peers, Professionalism, and Improvement—Reframing the Quality Question." *New England Journal of Medicine* 386 (19): 1850–1854.

2022c. "Reassessing Quality Assessment — The Flawed System for Fixing a Flawed System." *New England Journal of Medicine* 386 (17): 1663–1667.

Rosenberg, Leah B. 2020. "What Are Two Days Worth? Facing Dilemmas Together at the End of Life." *New England Journal of Medicine* 382 (10): 890–891.

Rosenberg, Marjorie A., Dennis G. Fryback, and David A. Katz. 2000. "A Statistical Model to Detect DRG Upcoding." *Health Services and Outcomes Research Methodology* 1 (3–4): 233–52.

Rosoff, Philip M. 2019. "When Religion and Medicine Clash: Non-beneficial Treatments and Hope for a Miracle." *HEC Forum* 31 (2): 119–139.

Roukema, Riemer. 2004. "The Good Samaritan in Ancient Christianity." *Vigiliae Christianae* 58 (1): 56–74.

Rowlands, Anna. 2014. "Fraternal Traditions: Anglican Social Theology and Catholic Social Teaching in a British Context." In *Anglican Social Theology: Renewing the Vision Today*, edited by Malcolm Brown, 133–174. London: Church House.

Ruden, Sarah. 2021. *The Gospels*. New York, NY: Modern Library.

Rumbold, Benedict, Victoria Charlton, Annette Rid, Polly Mitchell, James Wilson, Peter Littlejohns, Catherine Max, and Albert Weale. 2019. "Affordability and Non-Perfectionism in Moral Action." *Ethical Theory and Moral Practice.*

Russell, Louise B. 1986. *Is Prevention Better than Cure? Studies in Social Economics.* Washington, D.C.: Brookings Institution.

1989a. *Medicare's New Hospital Payment System: Is It Working?* Washington: The Brookings Institution.

1989b. *Medicare's New Hospital Payment System: Is It Working?* Washington, D.C.: The Brookings Institution.

1994. *Educated Guesses: Making Policy about Medical Screening Tests.* Berkeley, CA: University of California Press.

2007. *Prevention's Potential for Slowing the Growth of Medical Spending.* Washington: D.C.: National Coalition on Health Care.

Ryan, Maurice. 2021. "Revisiting the Parable of the Good Samaritan." *Studies in Christian-Jewish Relations* 16 (1).

Ryan, Patrick, and Anne Preisz. 2022. "Towards a Broader Concept of Wellbeing in Evaluating Paediatric Quality of Life." *Journal of Paediatrics and Child Health* 58 (1): 24–29.

Sacks, Jonathan. 2020. *Morality: Restoring the Common Good in Divided Times.* London: Hodder Stoughton.

Sagovsky, Nicholas. 2008. *Christian Tradition and the Practice of Justice.* London: Society for Promoting Christian Knowledge.

2017. "Public Theology, the Public Sphere and the Struggle for Social Justice." In *A Companion to Public Theology*, edited by Sebastian Kim and Katie Day, 251–270. Leiden: Brill.

Saiman, Chaim. 2007. "Jesus' Legal Theory – A Rabbinic Reading." *Journal of Law and Religion* 23 (1): 97–130.

Saing, Sopany, Naomi van der Linden, Christopher Hayward, and Stephen Goodall. 2019. "Why Is There Discordance between the Reimbursement of High-Cost 'Life-Extending' Pharmaceuticals and Medical Devices? The Funding of Ventricular Assist Devices in Australia." *Applied Health Economics and Health Policy* 17 (4): 421–431.

Sakowsky, Ruben Andreas. 2021. "Disentangling the Welfarism/Extra-Welfarism Distinction: Towards a More Fine-Grained Categorization." *Health Economics* 30 (9): 2307–2311.

Salas-Vega, Sebastian, Emily Shearer, and Elias Mossialos. 2020. "Relationship between Costs and Clinical Benefits of New Cancer Medicines in Australia, France, the UK, and the US." *Social Science & Medicine* 258: 113042.

Salcher-Konrad, Maximilian, Arnoupe Jhass, Huseyin Naci, Marselia Tan, Yousef El-Tawil, and Adelina Comas-Herrera. 2020. "COVID-19 Related Mortality and Spread of Disease in Long-Term Care: A Living Systematic Review of Emerging Evidence." *medRxiv*: 2020.06.09.20125237.

Salomon, Joshua A., Theo Vos, Daniel R Hogan, Michael Gagnon, Mohsen Naghavi, Ali Mokdad, Nazma Begum, Razibuzzaman Shah, Muhammad Karyana, and Soewarta Kosen. 2012. "Common Values in Assessing Health Outcomes from Disease and Injury: Disability Weights Measurement Study for the Global Burden of Disease Study 2010." *The Lancet* 380 (9859): 2129–2143.

Sample, Tex. 2016. *A Christian Justice for the Common Good*. Nashville: Abingdon Press.

Sampson, Chris, David Parkin, and Nancy Devlin. 2020. *Drop Dead: Is Anchoring at 'Dead' a Theoretical Requirement in Health State Valuation?* London: Office of Health Economics. www.ohe.org/publications/drop-dead-anchoring-%E2%80%98dead%E2%80%99-theoretical-requirement-health-state-valuation#.

Sampson, Christopher J. 2016. "Identifying Objects of Value at the End of Life." In *Care at the End of Life: An Economic Perspective*, edited by Jeff Round. Cham: Adis.

Sandel, Michael J. 2012. *What Money Can't Buy: The Moral Limits of Markets*. New York: Farrar, Straus and Giroux.

Sanders, William. 2021. *Big Picture Essays on Australian Indigenous Policy: Deep Structures and Decolonising*. Canberra: Australian National University, Centre for Aboriginal Economic Policy Research (CAEPR).

Sanderson, Marie, Pauline Allen, Valerie Moran, Imelda McDermott, and Dorota Osipovic. 2020. "Agreeing the Allocation of Scarce Resources in the English NHS: Ostrom, Common Pool Resources and the Role of the State." *Social Science & Medicine* 250: 112888.

Sandhu, Sahil, Hugh Alderwick, and Laura M. Gottlieb. 2022 (in press). "Financing Approaches to Social Prescribing Programs in England and the United States." *The Milbank Quarterly* n/a (n/a).

Sarri, Grammati, Andreas Freitag, Boglarka Szegvari, Irina Mountian, Diana Brixner, Neil Bertelsen, Zoltán Kaló, and Sheela Upadhyaya. 2021. "The Role of Patient Experience in the Value Assessment of Complex Technologies – Do HTA Bodies Need to Reconsider How Value Is Assessed?" *Health Policy* 125 (5): 593–601.

Sasiadek, Adam. 2017. "Varieties of Catholic Social Justice Initiatives since Rerum Novarum and Their Implications for Contemporary Labor and Employment Policy." *Journal of Catholic Legal Studies* 50 (1): 257–278.

Sassi, Franco, Leonard Archard, and Julian Le Grand. 2001. "Equity and the Economic Evaluation of Healthcare." *Health Technology Assessment* 5 (3): 1–138.

Sawyer, John F. A. 1974. "The Meaning of בְּצֶלֶם אֱלֹהִםי ('in the Image of God') in Genesis 1–11." *Journal of Theological Studies* 25 (2): 418–426.

Saxby, Karinna, Sonja C. de New, and Dennis Petrie. 2020. "Structural Stigma and Sexual Orientation Disparities in Healthcare Use: Evidence from Australian Census-Linked-Administrative Data." *Social Science & Medicine* 255: 113027.

Schaffer, Sarah Karlsberg, Donna Messner, Jorge Mestre-Ferrandiz, Ellen Tambor, and Adrian Towse. 2018. "Paying for Cures: Perspectives on Solutions to the 'Affordability Issue'." *Value in Health* 21 (3): 276–279.

Scharf, Kimberly A., and Mirco Tonin, eds. 2018. *The Economics of Philanthropy: Donations and Fundraising*. Cambridge: MIT Press.

Scharper, Stephen Bede. 1998. *Redeeming the Time: A Political Theology of the Environment*. New York: Continuum.

Scheerens, Charlotte, Kristof Faes, Peter Pype, Kim Beernaert, Guy Joos, Eric Derom, Joachim Cohen, Luc Deliens, and Kenneth Chambaere. 2020. "Earlier Palliative Home Care Is Associated with Patient-Centred Medical Resource Utilisation and Lower Costs in the Last 30 Days before Death in COPD: A Population-Level Decedent Cohort Study." *European Respiratory Journal* 55 (5): 1901139.

Schein, Edgar H. 1992. *Organizational Culture and Leadership*. San Francisco: Jossey Bass.

Schellenberg, Ryan S. 2018. "Subsistence, Swapping, and Paul's Rhetoric of Generosity." *Journal of Biblical Literature* 137 (1): 215–234.

Schelling, Thomas C. 1968. "The Life You Save May Be Your Own." In *Problems in Public Expenditure*, edited by Samuel B. Chase, 127–162. Washington, DC: Brookings Institution.

Schilling, Chris, Duncan Mortimer, and Kim Dalziel. 2016. "Using CART to Identify Thresholds and Hierarchies in the Determinants of Funding Decisions." *Medical Decision Making* 37 (2): 173–182.

Schmidt, Volker H. 2004. "Models of Health Care Rationing." *Current Sociology* 52 (6): 969–988.

Schneider, Paul P. 2021. "Social Tariffs and Democratic Choice – Do Population-Based Health State Values Reflect the Will of the People?" *Health Economics* 30 (1): 104–112.

2022. "The QALY Is Ableist: On the Unethical Implications of Health States Worse than Dead." *Quality of Life Research* 31 (5): 1545–1522.

Schneiderman, Lawrence J. 2011. "Defining Medical Futility and Improving Medical Care." *Journal of Bioethical Inquiry* 8 (2): 123–131.

Schoen, Cathy, Robin Osborn, David Squires, and Michelle M. Doty. 2013. "Access, Affordability, and Insurance Complexity Are Often Worse in the United States Compared to Ten Other Countries." *Health Affairs* 32 (12): 2205–2215.

Schoukens, Paul. 2008. "The Right to Access Health Care: Health Care according to International and European Social Security Law Instruments." In *International Health Law: Solidarity and Justice in Health Care*, edited by A. den Exter, 17–48. Antwerpen: Maklu.

Schwarzer, Ruth, Ursula Rochau, Kim Saverno, Beate Jahn, Bernhard Bornschein, Nikolai Muehlberger, Magdalena Flatscher-Thoeni, Petra Schnell-Inderst, Gaby Sroczynski, Martina Lackner, Imke Schall, Ansgar Hebborn, Karl Pugner, Andras Fehervary, Diana Brixner, and Uwe Siebert. 2015. "Systematic Overview of Cost-Effectiveness Thresholds in Ten Countries across Four Continents." *Journal of Comparative Effectiveness Research* 4 (5): 485–504.

Scott, Anthony, Miao Liu, and Jongsay Yong. 2018. "Financial Incentives to Encourage Value-Based Health Care." *Medical Care Research and Review* 75 (1): 3–32.

Scott, Ian A., and Stephen J. Duckett. 2015. "In Search of Professional Consensus in Defining and Reducing Low-Value Care." *The Medical Journal of Australia* 203 (4): 179–81.

Scotton, Richard B., and Christine R. Macdonald. 1993. *The Making of Medibank*. Vol. No. 76. Sydney: School of Health Services Management, University of NSW.

Scovronick, Noah, Maddalena Ferranna, Francis Dennig, and Mark Budolfson. 2020. "Valuing Health Impacts in Climate Policy: Ethical Issues and Economic Challenges: Study Examines the Ethical Issues and Economic Challenges of Valuing Health Impacts in Climate Policy." *Health Affairs* 39 (12): 2105–2112.

Sculpher, Mark, and Stephen Palmer. 2020. "After 20 Years of Using Economic Evaluation, Should NICE Be Considered a Methods Innovator?" *PharmacoEconomics* 38 (3): 247–257.

Sculpher, Mark, Paul Revill, Jessica M. Ochalek, and Karl Claxton. 2017. "How Much Health for the Money? Using Cost-Effectiveness Analysis to Support Benefits Plan Decisions." In *What's In, What's Out: Designing Benefits for Universal Health Coverage*, edited by Amanda Glassman, Ursula Giedion and Peter C Smith, 115–140. Washington, DC: Center for Global Development.

Seaman, Karla L., Max K. Bulsara, Frank M. Sanfilippo, Anna Kemp-Casey, Elizabeth E. Roughead, Caroline Bulsara, Gerald F. Watts, and David B. Preen. 2021. "Exploring the Association between Stroke and Acute Myocardial Infarction and Statins Adherence Following a Medicines Co-payment Increase." *Research in Social and Administrative Pharmacy* 17 (10): 1780–1785.

Segal, Leonie, Kim Dalziel, and Duncan Mortimer. 2010. "Fixing the Game: Are between-Silo Differences in Funding Arrangements Handicapping Some Interventions and Giving Others a Head-Start?" *Health Economics* 19 (4): 449–465.

Seixas, Brayan V., François Dionne, and Craig Mitton. 2021. "Practices of Decision Making in Priority Setting and Resource Allocation: A Scoping Review and Narrative Synthesis of Existing Frameworks." *Health Economics Review* 11 (2): 1–11.

Seixas, Brayan V., Dean A. Regier, Stirling Bryan, and Craig Mitton. 2021. "Describing Practices of Priority Setting and Resource Allocation in Publicly

Funded Health Care Systems of High-Income Countries." *BMC Health Services Research* 21 (90): 1–15.

Selby, Peter. 2014. *An Idol Unmasked: A Faith Perspective on Money*. London: Darton, Longman & Todd.

Self, Peter. 1976. *Econocrats and the Policy Process: The Politics and Philosophy of Cost-Benefit Analysis*. London: Macmillan.

Self, Sharmistha, and Richard Grabowski. 2003. "How Effective Is Public Health Expenditure in Improving Overall Health? A Cross–Country Analysis." *Applied Economics* 35 (7): 835–845.

Sen, Amartya. 1977. "Rational Fools: A Critique of the Behavioral Foundations of Economic Theory." *Philosophy & Public Affairs* 6 (4): 317–344.

1979. "Utilitarianism and Welfarism." *The Journal of Philosophy* 76 (9): 463–489.

1987. *On ethics and economics*. Malden, MA: Blackwell.

1993. "Does Business Ethics Make Economic Sense?" *Business Ethics Quarterly* 3 (1): 45–54.

2000. "The Discipline of Cost-Benefit Analysis." *The Journal of Legal Studies* 29 (S2): 931–952.

2009. *The Idea of Justice*. Cambridge: Harvard University Press.

2017. *Collective Choice and Social Welfare (Expanded edition)*. London: Penguin Books.

Sendi, Pedram. 2021. "Dealing with Bad Risk in Cost-Effectiveness Analysis: The Cost-Effectiveness Risk-Aversion Curve." *PharmacoEconomics* 39 (2): 161–169.

Shadmi, Efrat, Yingyao Chen, Inês Dourado, Inbal Faran-Perach, John Furler, Peter Hangoma, Piya Hanvoravongchai, Claudia Obando, Varduhi Petrosyan, Krishna D. Rao, Ana Lorena Ruano, Leiyu Shi, Luis Eugenio de Souza, Sivan Spitzer-Shohat, Elizabeth Sturgiss, Rapeepong Suphanchaimat, Manuela Villar Uribe, and Sara Willems. 2020. "Health Equity and COVID-19: Global Perspectives." *International Journal for Equity in Health* 19 (104): 1–16.

Shaffer, Victoria A., and Laura D. Scherer. 2018. "Too Much Medicine: Behavioral Science Insights on Overutilization, Overdiagnosis, and Overtreatment in Health Care." *Policy Insights from the Behavioral and Brain Sciences* 5 (2): 155–162.

Shafrin, Jason, Syvart Dennen, Priti Pednekar, Kelly Birch, Menaka Bhor, Julie Kanter, and Peter Neumann. 2021. "For Which Diseases Do Broader Value Elements Matter Most? An Evaluation across 20 ICER Evidence Reports." *Journal of Managed Care & Specialty Pharmacy* 27 (5): 650–659.

Shah, Koonal. 2016. "Does Society Place Special Value on End of Life Treatments?" In *Care at the End of Life: An Economic Perspective*, edited by Jeff Round, 155–166. Cham: Springer International Publishing.

Shah, Koonal K., Richard Cookson, Anthony J. Culyer, and Peter Littlejohns. 2012. "NICE's Social Value Judgements about Equity in Health and Health Care." *Health Economics, Policy and Law* 8 (2): 145–165.

Shah, Koonal K., Aki Tsuchiya, and Allan J. Wailoo. 2018. "Valuing Health at the End of Life: A Review of Stated Preference Studies in the Social Sciences Literature." *Social Science & Medicine* 204: 39–50.

Sharma, Eesha, and Vicki G Morwitz. 2016. "Saving the Asses: The Impact of Perceived Efficacy on Charitable Giving to Single vs. Multiple Beneficiaries." *Organizational Behavior and Human Decision Processes* 135: 45–54.

Sharma, Umesh. 2021. "Managing Well-Being Outcomes-Based Approach to Public Sector Accountability in New Zealand." In *Public Sector Reform and Performance Management in Developed Economies*, edited by Zahirul Hoque. New York, NY: Taylor and Francis.

Shea, Sue, and Christos Lionis. 2017. "The Call for Compassion in Health Care." In *The Oxford Handbook of Compassion Science*, edited by Emma M Seppälä, Emiliana Simon-Thomas, Stephanie L Brown, Monica C Worline, C Daryl Cameron and James R Doty, 457–474. Oxford: Oxford University Press.

Sheppard, David. 1983. *Bias to the Poor*. London: Hodder & Stoughton.

Sherman, Jodi D., Andrea MacNeill, and Cassandra Thiel. 2019. "Reducing Pollution from the Health Care Industry." *JAMA* 322 (11): 1043–1044.

Sherman, Jodi D., Cassandra Thiel, Andrea MacNeill, Matthew J. Eckelman, Robert Dubrow, Harriet Hopf, Robert Lagasse, Joseph Bialowitz, Anthony Costello, McGain Forbes, Rachel Stancliffe, Paul Anastas, Laura Anderko, Mark Baratz, Stefi Barna, Urvashi Bhatnagar, Jason Burnham, Yizhen Cai, Andy Cassels-Brown, Alexander F. P. Cimprich, Heidi Cole, Lorea Coronado-Garcia, Brett Duane, Gabriella Grisotti, Arthy Hartwell, Varshini Kumar, Ann Kurth, Michael Leapman, Daniel S. Morris, Michael Overcash, Abhijeet G. Parvatker, David Pencheon, Adam Pollard, Bernard Robaire, Karl Rockne, Blair L. Sadler, Beth Schenk, Tushar Sethi, L. Scott Sussman, Jeff Thompson, Janet M. Twomey, Sten H. Vermund, Daniel Vukelich, Natasha Wasim, Debbie Wilson, Steven B. Young, Julie Zimmerman, and Melissa M. Bilec. 2020. "The Green Print: Advancement of Environmental Sustainability in Healthcare." *Resources, Conservation and Recycling* 161: 104882.

Shiell, Alan, and Penelope Hawe. 1996. "Health Promotion Community Development and the Tyranny of Individualism." *Health Economics* 5 (3): 241–247.

Shiell, Alan, Penelope Hawe, and Janelle Seymour. 1997. "Values and Preferences Are Not Necessarily the Same." *Health Economics* 6 (5): 515–518.

Shriver, Donald W., and E. Richard Knox. 1985. "Taxation in the History of Protestant Ethics." *The Journal of Religious Ethics* 13 (1): 134–160.

Shuster, Sam. 2019. "The Life Improvement Value: A New Measure of Cost-Efficiency." *The Lancet* 394 (10212): 1903–1904.

Shuttleworth, Russell. 2017. "Critical Engagements with the Politics of Care and Disability." In *Critical Ethics of Care in Social Work: Transforming the Politics and Practices of Caring*, edited by Bob Pease, Anthea Vreugdenhil and Sonya Stanford, 161–171. London: Routledge.

Siciliani, Luigi, James Michael Gaughan, Nils Gutacker, Hugh Stanley Emrys Gravelle, and Martin John Chalkley. 2021. *Paying for Health Gains*. York: Centre for Health Economics, University of York.

Simon, Herbert A. 1993. "Altruism and Economics." *The American Economic Review* 83 (2): 156–161.

Simons, Robert G. 1995. *Competing Gospels: Public Theology and Economic Theory*. Alexandria, NSW: E.J. Dwyer.

Sinclair, Shane, Neil A. Hagen, Carole Chambers, Braden Manns, Anita Simon, and George P Browman. 2008. "Accounting for Reasonableness: Exploring the Personal Internal Framework Affecting Decisions about Cancer Drug Funding." *Health Policy* 86 (2–3): 381–390.

Singer, Kurt. 1958. "Oikonomia: An Inquiry into Beginnings of Economic Thought and Language." *Kyklos* 11 (1): 29–57.

Singh, Ankur, Diana Contreras Suarez, Emily You, Ludmila Fleitas Alfonzo, and Tania King. 2021. "Role of Social Support in the Relationship between Financial Hardship and Multimorbidity – a Causal Mediation Analysis." *European Journal of Public Health* 31 (3): 482–487.

Singh, Neha S., Roxanne J. Kovacs, Rachel Cassidy, Søren R. Kristensen, Josephine Borghi, and Garrett W. Brown. 2021. "A Realist Review to Assess for Whom, under What Conditions and How Pay for Performance Programmes Work in Low- and Middle-Income Countries." *Social Science & Medicine* 270: 113624.

Siverskog, Jonathan, and Martin Henriksson. 2019. "Estimating the Marginal Cost of a Life Year in Sweden's Public Healthcare Sector." *The European Journal of Health Economics* 20 (5): 751–762.

Slovic, Paul. 2010. *The Feeling of Risk: New Perspectives on Risk Perception*. London: Routledge.

Small, Deborah A. 2011. "Sympathy Biases and Sympathy Appeals: Reducing Social Distance to Boost Charitable Contributions." In *The Science of Giving: Experimental Approaches to the Study of Charity*, edited by Daniel M Oppenheimer and Christopher Y Olivola. New York, NY: Psychology Press.

Smee, Clive. 2005. *Speaking Truth to Power: Two Decades of Analysis in the Department of Health*. Oxford: Radcliffe Publishing.

Smith, Adam. 1759/1979. *The Theory of Moral Sentiments*. Oxford: Clarendon Press.

1775/1979. *An Inquiry into the Nature and Causes of the Wealth of Nations*. Oxford: Clarendon Press.

Smith, George Patrick. 2010. *Distributive Justice and the New Medicine*. Cheltenham, UK: Edward Elgar.

Smith, Peter C. 2005. "User Charges and Priority Setting in Health Care: Balancing Equity and Efficiency." *Journal of Health Economics* 24 (5): 1018–1029.

Smith, Peter, Elias Mossialos, Irene Papanicolas, and S. Leatherman, eds. 2009. *Performance Measurement for Health System Improvement: Experiences, Challenges, and Prospects*. Cambridge, NY: Cambridge University Press.

Smith, Sarah, Mark Ottoni-Wilhelm, and Kimberley Scharf. 2018. "The Donation Response to Natural Disasters." In *The Economics of Philanthropy: Donations and Fundraising*, edited by Kimberly A. Scharf and Mirco Tonin, 239–261. Cambridge: MIT Press.

Snodgrass, Klyne. 2008. *Stories with Intent: A Comprehensive Guide to the Parables of Jesus*. Grand Rapids, MI: William B. Eerdmans.

Soards, Marion L. 2010. "Luke." In *The New Oxford Annotated Bible: The New Revised Standard Version with Apocrypha,* edited by Michael David Coogan, Marc Zvi Brettler, Carol A. Newsom and Pheme Perkins. Oxford: Oxford University Press.

Soares, Marta O., Mark J. Sculpher, and Karl Claxton. 2020. "Health Opportunity Costs: Assessing the Implications of Uncertainty Using Elicitation Methods with Experts." *Medical Decision Making* 40 (4): 448–459.

Soekhai, Vikas, Esther W. de Bekker-Grob, Alan R. Ellis, and Caroline M. Vass. 2019. "Discrete Choice Experiments in Health Economics: Past, Present and Future." *PharmacoEconomics* 37 (2): 201–226.

Sölle, Dorothee. 1990. *Thinking about God: An Introduction to Theology*. London, Philadelphia: SCM Press; Trinity Press International.

Sommers, Benjamin D., Kathryn L. Clark, and Arnold M. Epstein. 2018. "Early Changes in Health Insurance Coverage under the Trump Administration." *New England Journal of Medicine* 378 (11): 1061–1063.

Sommet, Nicolas, and Dario Spini. 2022. "Financial Scarcity Undermines Health across the Globe and the Life Course." *Social Science & Medicine* 292: 114607.

Song, Zirui. 2021. "Taking Account of Accountable Care." *Health Services Research* 56 (4): 573–577.

Spencer, A. John, Loc G. Do, and Diep H. Ha. 2018. "Contemporary Evidence on the Effectiveness of Water Fluoridation in the Prevention of Childhood Caries." *Community Dentistry and Oral Epidemiology* 46 (4): 407–415.

Spencer, Anne, Oliver. Rivero-Arias, Ruth Wong, Aki Tsuchiya, Han Bleichrodt, Rhiannon Tudor Edward, Richard Norman, Andrew Lloyd, and Phillip Clarke. 2022. "The QALY at 50: One Story Many Voices." *Social Science & Medicine* 296: 114653.

Spencer, Nick. 2017. *The Political Samaritan: How Power Hijacked a Parable.* London: Bloomsbury Publishing.

Spohn, William C. 2005. "Scripture." In *The Oxford Handbook of Theological Ethics*, edited by Gilbert Meilaender and William Werpehowski, 93–111. Oxford: Oxford University Press.

Sripa, Poompong, Benedict Hayhoe, Priya Garg, Azeem Majeed, and Geva Greenfield. 2019. "Impact of GP Gatekeeping on Quality of Care, and Health Outcomes, Use, and Expenditure: A Systematic Review." *British Journal of General Practice* 69 (682): e294–e303.

Stabile, Mark. 2015. "Determining What Should Be Included in a Publicly Funded Health Care System: Reflecting on 'Individual Responsibility for What? A

Conceptual Framework for Exploring the Suitability of Private Financing in a Publicly Funded Health-Care System'." *Health Economics, Policy and Law* 10 (4): 425–430.

Stantcheva, Stefanie. 2022. "Inequalities in the Times of a Pandemic." *Economic Policy* 37 (109): 5–41.

Starfield, Barbara. 1992. *Primary Care: Concept, Evaluation and Policy*. New York: Oxford University Press.

Starfield, Barbara, Leiyu Shi, and James Macinko. 2005. "Contribution of Primary Care to Health Systems and Health." *The Milbank Quarterly* 83 (3): 457–502.

Stark, Oded. 2000. "On the Evolution of Altruism." In *The Economics of Reciprocity, Giving, and Altruism*, edited by Louis-André Gérard-Varet, Serge-Christophe Kolm and Jean Mercier Ythier, 352–358. Basingstoke, Hampshire: Macmillan.

Stavrianos, Kyriakos. 2012. "The Parable of the Good Samaritan in Patristic Thought." *Greek Orthodox Theological Review* 57 (1–4): 29–48.

Stavropoulou, Charitini. 2012. "The Doctor-Patient Relationship: A Review of the Theory and Policy." In *The LSE Companion to Health Policy*, edited by Alistair McGuire and Joan Costa-Font, 314–326. Cheltenham: Edward Elgar Publishing.

Stein, Janice Gross 2001. *The Cult of Efficiency*. Toronto: Anansi.

Steinbrook, Robert. 2015. "The Repeal of Medicare's Sustainable Growth Rate for Physician Payment." *JAMA* 313 (20): 2025–2026.

Steinbusch, Paul J. M., Jan B. Oostenbrink, Joost J. Zuurbier, and Frans J. M. Schaepkens. 2007. "The Risk of Upcoding in Casemix Systems: A Comparative Study." *Health Policy* 81 (2–3): 289–299.

Steinmann, Gijs, Hester van de Bovenkamp, Antoinette de Bont, and Diana Delnoij. 2020. "Redefining Value: A Discourse Analysis on Value-Based Health Care." *BMC Health Services Research* 20 (862): 1–13.

Stenhouse, Paul. 2013. "The Good Samaritan: The Unidentified Man Who Fell among Robbers on the Jericho Road." *Compass* 47 (2): 35–41.

Stepurko, Tetiana, Milena Pavlova, and Wim Groot. 2017. "Informal Payments in Health Care." In *The Handbook of Business and Corruption: Cross-sectoral Experiences*, edited by Michael S Assländer and Sarah Hudson, 305–327. Bingley: Emerald Group Publishing.

Stevenson, Fiona A., Geraldine Leydon-Hudson, Elizabeth Murray, Maureen Seguin, and Rebecca Barnes. 2021. "Patients' Use of the Internet to Negotiate about Treatment." *Social Science & Medicine*: 114262.

Stibbe, Mark W. G. 1994. "A Tomb with a View: John 11.1–44 in Narrative-Critical Perspective." *New Testament Studies* 40 (1): 38–54.

Stiglitz, Joseph E., Jean-Paul Fitoussi, and Martine Durand. 2018. *Beyond GDP: Measuring What Counts for Economic and Social Performance*. Paris: OECD Publishing.

Stivers, Laura A. 2011. *Disrupting Homelessness: Alternative Christian Approaches*. Minneapolis, MN: Fortress Press.

Stone, Deborah. 2008. *The Samaritan's Dilemma: Should Government Help Your Neighbor?* New York, NY: Nation Books.

Story, Cullen I. K. 1976. "The Nature of Paul's Stewardship with Special Reference to I and II Corinthians " *The Evangelical Quarterly.* 48 (4): 212–229.

Strahan, Joshua Marshall. 2016. "Jesus Teaches Theological Interpretation of the Law: Reading the Good Samaritan in Its Literary Context." *Journal of Theological Interpretation* 10 (1): 71–86.

Strategic Review of Health and Medical Research (Chair: Simon McKeon). 2013. *Final Report: Better Health through Research.* Canberra, ACT: Dept. of Health and Ageing.

Strathern, Marilyn. 1997. "'Improving Ratings': Audit in the British University system." *European Review* 5 (3): 305–321.

Street, Andrew, and Stephen Duckett. 1996. "Are Waiting Lists Inevitable?" *Health Policy* 36 (1): 1–15.

Suggate, Alan M. 2014. "The Temple Tradition." In *Anglican Social Theology: Renewing the Vision Today*, edited by Malcolm Brown, 28–73. London: Church House.

Sundmacher, Leonie, Diana Fischbach, Wiebke Schuettig, Christoph Naumann, Uta Augustin, and Cristina Faisst. 2015. "Which Hospitalisations Are Ambulatory Care-Sensitive, to What Degree, and How Could the Rates Be Reduced? Results of a Group Consensus Study in Germany." *Health Policy* 119 (11): 1415–1423.

Sunstein, Cass R. 2004. "Valuing Life: A Plea for Disaggregation." *Duke Law Journal* 54 (2): 385–445.

2010. "Moral Heuristics and Risk." In *Emotions and Risky Technologies*, edited by Sabine Roeser, 3–16. Dordrecht: Springer.

2013. "The Value of a Statistical Life: Some Clarifications and Puzzles." *Journal of Benefit-Cost Analysis* 4 (2): 237–261.

2014. *Valuing life: Humanizing the Regulatory State.* Chicago and London: University of Chicago Press.

Swerissen, Hal, and Beth R. Crisp. 2004. "The Sustainability of Health Promotion Interventions for Different Levels of Social Organization." *Health Promotion International* 19 (1): 123–130.

Szende, Agota, Mark Oppe, and Nancy J Devlin. 2007. *EQ-5D Value Sets: Inventory, Comparative Review and User Guide.* Dordrecht: Springer.

Taboada, Paulina. 2002. "What Is Appropriate Intensive Care? A Roman Catholic Perspective." In *Allocating Scarce Medical Resources: Roman Catholic Perspectives*, edited by H Tristram Engelhardt Jr and Mark J Cherry, 53–73. Washington, DC: Georgetown University Press.

Taksler, Glen B., and Michael B. Rothberg. 2017. "Assessing Years of Life Lost Versus Number of Deaths in the United States, 1995–2015." *American Journal of Public Health* 107 (10): 1653–1659.

Tamez, Elsa. 1982. *Bible of the Oppressed* (Translated from the Spanish by Matthew J. O'Connell). Maryknoll, NY: Orbis.

1990. *The Scandalous Message of James: Faith without Works Is Dead.* New York: Crossroad.

Tanenbaum, Sandra J. 2009. "Pay for Performance in Medicare: Evidentiary Irony and the Politics of Value." *Journal of Health Politics Policy and Law* 34 (5): 717–746.

2016. "What Is the Value of Value-Based Purchasing?" *Journal of Health Politics, Policy and Law* 41 (5): 1033–1045.

Tanner, Denise. 2020. "'The Love That Dare Not Speak Its Name': The Role of Compassion in Social Work Practice." *The British Journal of Social Work* 50 (6): 1688–1705.

Tay-Teo, Kiu, André Ilbawi, and Suzanne R. Hill. 2019. "Comparison of Sales Income and Research and Development Costs for FDA-Approved Cancer Drugs Sold by Originator Drug Companies." *JAMA Network Open* 2 (1): e186875–e186875.

Tello, Juan E., Erica Barbazza, and Kerry Waddell. 2020. "Review of 128 Quality of Care Mechanisms: A Framework and Mapping for Health System Stewards." *Health Policy* 124 (1): 12–24.

Temel, Jennifer S., Joseph A. Greer, Alona Muzikansky, Emily R. Gallagher, Sonal Admane, Vicki A. Jackson, Constance M. Dahlin, Craig D. Blinderman, Juliet Jacobsen, William F. Pirl, J. Andrew Billings, and Thomas J. Lynch. 2010. "Early Palliative Care for Patients with Metastatic Non-Small-Cell Lung Cancer." *New England Journal of Medicine* 363 (8): 733–742.

Temple, William. 1950/1976. *Christianity and social order.* London: Shepheard-Walwyn.

Tenbensel, Tim, Samantha Eagle, and Toni Ashton. 2012. "Comparing Health Policy Agendas across Eleven High Income Countries: Islands of Difference in a Sea of Similarity." *Health Policy* 106 (1): 29–36.

Teng, Andrea M., Amanda C. Jones, Anja Mizdrak, Louise Signal, Murat Genç, and Nick Wilson. 2019. "Impact of sugar-sweetened beverage taxes on purchases and dietary intake: Systematic review and meta-analysis." *Obesity Reviews* 20 (9).

Terris, Milton. 1999. "The Neoliberal Triad of Anti-health Reforms: Government Budget Cutting, Deregulation, and Privatization." *Journal of Public Health Policy* 20 (2): 149–167.

Tetlock, Philip E. 2000. "Coping with Trade-Offs: Psychological Constraints and Political Implications." In *Elements of Reason: Cognition, Choice, and the Bounds of Rationality*, edited by Arthur Lupia, Mathew D McCubbins and Samuel L Popkin, 239–263. Cambridge: Cambridge University Press.

Thaler, Richard H. 2000. "From Homo Economicus to Homo Sapiens." *Journal of Economic Perspectives* 14 (1): 133–141.

Thomas, Hayley R., Laura Deckx, Nicolas A. Sieben, Michele M. Foster, and Geoffrey K. Mitchell. 2020. "General Practitioners' Considerations When Deciding Whether to Initiate End-of-Life Conversations: A Qualitative Study." *Family Practice* 37 (4): 554–560.

Thomas, Hedley. 2007. *Sick to Death: A Manipulative Surgeon and a Health System in Crisis – a Disaster Waiting to Happen.* Crows Nest, NSW: Allen & Unwin.

Thomas, Robyn L., Mohamed Y. Zubair, Barbara Hayes, and Michael A. Ashby. 2014. "Goals of Care: A Clinical Framework for Limitation of Medical Treatment." *Medical Journal of Australia* 201 (8): 452–455.

Thompson, James. D. 1967. *Organizations in Action: Social Science Bases of Administrative Theory* New York: McGraw Hill.

Thow, Anne Marie, Holly L. Rippin, Georgina Mulcahy, Keeva Duffey, and Kremlin Wickramasinghe. 2022. "*Sugar-Sweetened Beverage Taxes in Europe: Learning for the Future.*" *European Journal of Public Health* 32 (2): 273–280.

Tinbergen, Jan. 1952. *On the Theory of Economic Policy.* Amsterdam: North-Holland Publishing Company.

Tinghőg, Gustav, Per Carlsson, and Carl H. Lyttkens. 2010. "Individual Responsibility for What? A Conceptual Framework for Exploring the Suitability of "Private Financing in a Publicly Funded Health-Care System." *Health Economics, Policy and Law* 5 (2): 201–223.

Titmuss, Richard M. 1974. *Social Policy: An Introduction.* London: George Allen and Unwin.

Toffoli, Luisa, Trudy Rudge, and Lynne Barnes. 2011. "The Work of Nurses in Private Health: Accounting for the Intangibles in Care Delivery." *Health Sociology Review* 20 (3): 338–351.

Torbica, Aleksandra, Rosanna Tarricone, and Michael Drummond. 2018. "Does the Approach to Economic Evaluation in Health Care Depend on Culture, Values, and Institutional Context?" *The European Journal of Health Economics* 19 (6): 769–774.

Torke, Alexia M., George Fitchett, Saneta Maiko, Emily S. Burke, James E. Slaven, Beth Newton Watson, Steven Ivy, and Patrick O. Monahan. 2020. "The Association of Surrogate Decision Makers' Religious and Spiritual Beliefs with End-of-Life Decisions." *Journal of Pain and Symptom Management* 59 (2): 261–269.

Totten, Annette M., Dana M. Womack, Karen B. Eden, Marian S. McDonagh, Jessica C. Griffin, Sara Grusing, and William R. Hersh. 2016. *Telehealth: Mapping the Evidence for Patient Outcomes from Systematic Reviews.* Rockville, MD: Agency for Healthcare Research and Quality.

Townes, Emilie M. 1998. *Breaking the Fine Rain of Death: African American Health Issues and a Womanist Ethic of Care.* New York: Continuum.

Tracy, David. 1981. "Defending the Public Character of Theology." *The Christian Century* 98 (April): 350–356.

Tran, Linda Diem, Frederick J. Zimmerman, and Jonathan E. Fielding. 2017. "Public Health and the Economy Could Be Served by Reallocating Medical Expenditures to Social Programs." *SSM – Population Health* 3: 185–191.

Tran, Nam, Jeffrey W. Poss, Christopher Perlman, and John P. Hirdes. 2019. "Case-Mix Classification for Mental Health Care in Community Settings: A Scoping Review." *Health Services Insights* 12: 1–12.

Trujillo, Antonio J., Taruja Karmarkar, Caleb Alexander, William Padula, Jeremy Greene, and Gerard Anderson. 2020. "Fairness in Drug Prices: Do Economists Think Differently from the Public?" *Health Economics, Policy and Law* 15 (1): 18–29.

Trzeciak, Stephen, and Anthony Mazzarelli. 2019. *Compassionomics: The Revolutionary Scientific Evidence That Caring Makes a Difference*. Pensacola, FL: Studer.

Trzeciak, Stephen, Brian W. Roberts, and Anthony J. Mazzarelli. 2017. "Compassionomics: Hypothesis and Experimental Approach." *Medical Hypotheses* 107: 92–97.

Tsourapas, Angelos, and Emma Frew. 2011. "Evaluating 'Success' in Programme Budgeting and Marginal Analysis: A Literature Review." *Journal of Health Services Research & Policy* 16 (3): 177–183.

Tuller, David. 2020. "For LGBTQ Patients, High-Quality Care in a Welcoming Environment." *Health Affairs* 39 (5): 736–739.

Tuohy, Carolyn H., Colleen M. Flood, and Mark Stabile. 2004. "How Does Private Finance Affect Public Health Care Systems? Marshaling the Evidence from OECD Nations." *J Health Politics, Policy and Law* 29 (3): 359–396.

Turnbull, Alison E., Gabriel T. Bosslet, and Erin K. Kross. 2019. "Aligning Use of Intensive Care with Patient Values in the USA: Past, Present, and Future." *The Lancet Respiratory Medicine* 7 (7): 626–638.

Tutu, Desmond. 1999. *No Future without Forgiveness*. London: Rider.

Tuzzio, Leah, Andrew L. Berry, Kathy Gleason, Jennifer Barrow, Elizabeth A. Bayliss, Marlaine Figueroa Gray, Thomas Delate, Zoe Bermet, Connie S. Uratsu, Richard W. Grant, and James D. Ralston. 2022. "Aligning Care with the Personal Values of Patients with Complex Care Needs." *Health Services Research* 56 (S1): 1037–1044.

Twomey, Gerald Sean. 2005. *The "Preferential Option for the Poor" in Catholic Social Thought from John XXIII to John Paul II*. Lewiston, NY: Edwin Mellen Press.

2006. "Pope John Paul II and the "Preferential Option for the Poor"." *Journal of Catholic Legal Studies* 45 (2): 321–368.

Ubel, Peter A. 2000. "Are Preferences for Equity over Efficiency in Health Care Allocation 'All or Nothing'?" *Medical Care* 38 (4): 366–73.

Ubel, Peter A., George Loewenstein, Dennis Scanlon, and Mark Kamlet. 1996. "Individual Utilities Are Inconsistent with Rationing Choices: A Partial Explanation of Why Oregon's Cost-Effectiveness List Failed." *Medical Decision Making* 16 (2): 108–115.

Ubel, Peter A., George Loewenstein, Norbert Schwarz, and Dylan Smith. 2005. "Misimagining the Unimaginable: The Disability Paradox and Health Care Decision Making." *Health Psychology* 24 (4S): S57–S62.

Ulrich, Peter. 2000. "Integrative Economic Ethics – Towards a Conception of Socio-Economic Rationality." In *Contemporary Economic Ethics and Business Ethics*, edited by Peter Koslowski, 37–54. Berlin, Heidelberg: Springer Berlin Heidelberg.

United Kingdom. Her Majesty's Treasury. 2018. *The Green Book. Central Government Guidance on Appraisal and Evaluation*. London: HM Treasury. www.gov.uk/government/publications/the-green-book-appraisal-and-evaluation-in-central-governent.

United Nations. 2016. *Transforming Our World: The 2030 Agenda for Sustainable Development*. UN (New York). https://sustainabledevelopment.un.org/content/documents/21252030%20Agenda%20for%20Sustainable%20Development%20web.pdf.

Unwin, Julia. 2018. *Kindness, Emotions and Human Relationships: The Blind Spot in Public Policy*. Dunfermline, Scotland: Carnegie UK Trust.

Valentelyte, Gintare, Conor Keegan, and Jan Sørensen. 2021. "Analytical Methods to Assess the Impacts of Activity-Based Funding (ABF): A Scoping Review." *Health Economics Review* 11 (17): 1–16.

Valizadeh-Haghi, Saeideh, Shahabedin Rahmatizadeh, Ali Soleimaninejad, Seyedeh Fatemeh Mousavi Shirazi, and Parisa Mollaei. 2021. "Are Health Websites Credible Enough for Elderly Self-Education in the Most Prevalent Elderly Diseases?" *BMC Medical Informatics and Decision Making* 21 (31): 1–9

van Baal, Pieter, Meg Perry-Duxbury, Pieter Bakx, Matthijs Versteegh, Eddy van Doorslaer, and Werner Brouwer. 2019. "A Cost-Effectiveness Threshold Based on the Marginal Returns of Cardiovascular Hospital Spending." *Health Economics* 28 (1): 87–100.

Van de Ven, Wynand P. M. M. 2011. "Risk Adjustment and Risk Equalization: What Needs to Be Done?" *Health Economics, Policy and Law* 6 (1): 147–156.

Van de Ven, Wynand P. M. M., Konstantin Beck, Carine Van de Voorde, Jürgen Wasem, and Irit Zmora. 2007. "Risk Adjustment and Risk Selection in Europe: 6 Years Later." *Health Policy* 83 (2–3): 162–179.

van der Zee, Jouke, and Madelon Kroneman. 2007. "Bismarck or Beveridge: A Beauty Contest between Dinosaurs." *BMC Health Services Research* 7: 94.

van Doorslaer, Eddy, Adam Wagstaff, Hattem van der Burg, Terkel Christiansen, Guido Citoni, Rita Di Biase, Ulf- G. Gerdtham, Mike Gerfin, Lorna Gross, Unto Häkinnen, Jürgen John, Paul Johnson, Jan Klavus, Claire Lachaud, Jørgen Lauritsen, Robert Leu, Brian Nolan, João Pereira, Carol Propper, Frank Puffer, Lise Rochaix, Martin Schellhorn, Gun Sundberg, and Olaf Winkelhake. 1999. "The Redistributive Effect of Health Care Finance in Twelve OECD Countries." *Journal of Health Economics* 18 (3): 291–313.

Van Eck, Ernest, and Robert J Van Niekerk. 2018. "The Samaritan 'brought him to an inn': Revisiting πανδοχεῖον in Luke 10: 34." *HTS Teologiese Studies/Theological Studies* 74 (4): 1–11.

Van Elderen, Bastiaan. 1978. "Another Look at the Parable of the Good Samaritan." In *Saved by Hope: Essays in Honor of Richard C. Oudersluys*, edited by James I. Cook, 109–119. Grand Rapids, MI: Eerdmans.

Van Staveren, Irene. 2007. "Beyond Utilitarianism and Deontology: Ethics in Economics." *Review of Political Economy* 19 (1): 21–35.

Varela, Jordi 2018. "Priorities of Modern Clinical Management." In *Prioritising Health Services or Muddling Through*, edited by Juan del Llano Señarís and Salvador Peiró Moreno, 77–91. Madrid: Springer Healthcare.

Vaux, Kenneth L. 2010. *Journey into an Interfaith World: Jews, Christians, and Muslims in a World Come of Age*. Eugene, OR: Wipf and Stock.

Vecchio, Riccardo, and Carla Cavallo. 2019. "Increasing Healthy Food Choices through Nudges: A Systematic Review." *Food Quality and Preference* 78: 103714.

Verkerk, Eva W., Marit A. C. Tanke, Rudolf B. Kool, Simone A. van Dulmen, and Gert P. Westert. 2018. "Limit, Lean or Listen? A Typology of Low-Value Care That Gives Direction in De-implementation." *International Journal for Quality in Health Care.*

Viljoen, Francois P. 2013. "Righteousness and Identity Formation in the Sermon on the Mount." *HTS Teologiese Studies/Theological Studies* 69 (1): a1300.

Viney, Rosalie, Richard Norman, Madeleine T. King, Paula Cronin, Deborah J. Street, Stephanie Knox, and Julie Ratcliffe. 2011. "Time Trade-Off Derived EQ-5D Weights for Australia." *Value in Health* 14 (6): 928–936.

Viscusi, W. Kip, and Clayton J. Masterman. 2017. "Income Elasticities and Global Values of a Statistical Life." *Journal of Benefit-Cost Analysis* 8 (2): 226–250.

Viscusi, W. Kip, Joel Huber, and Jason Bell. 2014. "Assessing Whether There Is a Cancer Premium for the Value of a Statistical Life." *Health Economics* 23 (4): 384–396.

Visvanathan, Renuka, Azmeraw T. Amare, Steve Wesselingh, Richard Hearn, Sue McKechnie, Jane Mussared, and Maria C. Inacio. 2019. "Prolonged Wait Time Prior to Entry to Home Care Packages Increases the Risk of Mortality and Transition to Permanent Residential Aged Care Services: Findings from the Registry of Older South Australians (ROSA)." *The Journal of Nutrition, Health & Aging* 23 (3): 271–280.

Vivot, Alexandre, Justine Jacot, Jean David Zeitoun, Philippe H. Ravaud, Perrine Créquit, and Raphaël Porcher. 2017. "Clinical Benefit, Price and Approval Characteristics of FDA-Approved New Drugs for Treating Advanced Solid Cancer, 2000–2015." *Annals of Oncology* 28 (5): 1111–1116.

Vlaanderen, Floris P., Marit A. Tanke, Bastiaan R. Bloem, Marjan J. Faber, Frank Eijkenaar, Erik F. T. Schut, and Patrick P. T. Jeurissen. 2019. "Design and Effects of Outcome-Based Payment Models in Healthcare: A Systematic Review." *European Journal of Health Economics* 20 (2): 217–232.

Vokinger, Kerstin N., Thomas J. Hwang, Thomas Grischott, Sophie Reichert, Ariadna Tibau, Thomas Rosemann, and Aaron S. Kesselheim. 2020. "Prices and Clinical Benefit of Cancer Drugs in the USA and Europe: A Cost–Benefit Analysis." *The Lancet Oncology* 21 (5): 664–670.

Volf, Miroslav. 2011. *A Public Faith: How Followers of Christ Should Serve the Common Good.* Grand Rapids, MI: Brazos.

Vollset, Stein Emil, Emily Goren, Chun-Wei Yuan, Jackie Cao, Amanda E. Smith, Thomas Hsiao, Catherine Bisignano, Gulrez S. Azhar, Emma Castro, Julian Chalek, Andrew J. Dolgert, Tahvi Frank, Kai Fukutaki, Simon I. Hay, Rafael Lozano, Ali H. Mokdad, Vishnu Nandakumar, Maxwell Pierce, Martin Pletcher, Toshana Robalik, Krista M. Steuben, Han Yong Wunrow, Bianca S. Zlavog, and Christopher J. L. Murray. 2020. "Fertility, Mortality, Migration, and Population Scenarios for 195 Countries and Territories from 2017 to 2100: A Forecasting Analysis for the Global Burden of Disease Study." *The Lancet* 396 (10258): 1285–1306.

Volmink, Heinrich C., Melanie Y. Bertram, Ruxana Jina, Alisha N. Wade, and Karen J. Hofman. 2014. "Applying a Private Sector Capitation Model to the Management of Type 2 Diabetes in the South African Public Sector: A Cost-Effectiveness Analysis." *BMC Health Services Research* 14 (444): 1–9.

Vos, Theo, Rob Carter, Jan Barendregt, Cathrine Mihalopoulos, Lennert Veerman, Anne Magnus, Linda Cobiac, Melanie Bertram, Angela Wallace, and ACE–Prevention Team. 2010. *Assessing Cost-Effectiveness in Prevention (ACE–Prevention): Final Report.* Brisbane and Melbourne: University of Queensland and Deakin University.

Vreman, Rick A., Inkatuuli Heikkinen, Ad Schuurman, Claudine Sapede, Jordi Llinares Garcia, Niklas Hedberg, Dimitrios Athanasiou, Jens Grueger, Hubert G. M. Leufkens, and Wim G. Goettsch. 2019. "Unmet Medical Need: An Introduction to Definitions and Stakeholder Perceptions." *Value in Health* 22 (11): 1275–1282.

Wagstaff, Adam. 2009. "Measuring Financial Protection in Health." In *Performance Measurement for Health System Improvement: Experiences, Challenges, and Prospects*, edited by Peter Smith, Elias Mossialos, Irene Papanicolas and S. Leatherman, 114–137. Cambridge, NY: Cambridge University Press.

Wagstaff, Adam, and Eddy van Doorslaer. 2000. "Equity in Health Care Finance and Delivery." In *Handbook of Health Economics*, edited by Anthony J. Culyer and Joseph P. Newhouse. Amsterdam: Elsevier Science BV.

Wagstaff, Adam, Eddy van Doorslaer, Hattem van der Burg, Samuel Calonge, Terkel Christiansen, Guido Citoni, Ulf- G. Gerdtham, Mike Gerfin, Lorna Gross, Unto Häkinnen, Paul Johnson, Jürgen John, Jan Klavus, Claire Lachaud, Jørgen Lauritsen, Robert Leu, Brian Nolan, Encarna Perán, João Pereira, Carol Propper, Frank Puffer, Lise Rochaix, Marisol Rodríguez, Martin Schellhorn, Gun Sundberg, and Olaf Winkelhake. 1999. "Equity in the Finance of Health Care: Some Further International Comparisons." *Journal of Health Economics* 18 (3): 263–290.

Waitzkin, Howard. 1991. *The Politics of Medical Encounters: How Patients and Doctors Deal with Social Problems.* New Haven: Yale University Press.

2000. *The Second Sickness: Contradictions of Capitalist Health Care.* Lanham, MD: Rowman & Littlefield Publishers.

Waldron, Jeremy. 2003. "Who Is My Neighbor?: Humanity and Proximity." *The Monist* 86: 333–354.

Walsh, Michael J. 1991. "Introduction." In *Proclaiming Justice & Peace: Papal Documents from Rerum Novarum through Centesimus Annus*, edited by Michael J. Walsh and Brian Davies. Mystic, CT: Twenty-Third Publications.

Walton, Ronald. 1969. "Need: A Central Concept." *Social Service Quarterly* 43 (1): 13–17.

Walzer, Michael. 1983. *Spheres of Justice: A Defense of Pluralism and Equality*. New York: Basic books.

Wammes, Joost Johan Godert, Geert Frederix, Paulien Govaert, Domino Determann, Silvia Evers, Aggie Paulus, Niek Stadhouders, Patrick Jeurissen, Wija Oortwijn, and Eddy M. M. Adang. 2020. "Case-Studies of Displacement Effects in Dutch Hospital Care." *BMC Health Services Research* 20 (263): 1–12.

Wammes, Joost Johan Godert, Philip J. van der Wees, Marit A. C. Tanke, Gert P. Westert, and Patrick P. T. Jeurissen. 2018. "Systematic Review of High-Cost Patients' Characteristics and Healthcare Utilisation." *BMJ Open* 8 (9): e023113.

Wang, Shuhong, Debra Gum, and Tracy Merlin. 2018. "Comparing the ICERs in Medicine Reimbursement Submissions to NICE and PBAC – Does the Presence of an Explicit Threshold Affect the ICER Proposed?" *Value in Health* 21 (8): 938–943.

Ward, Thomas, Ruben E. Mujica-Mota, Anne E. Spencer, and Antonieta Medina-Lara. 2022 (in press). "Incorporating Equity Concerns in Cost-Effectiveness Analyses: A Systematic Literature Review." *PharmacoEconomics*.

Warf, Barney. 2021. "The Coronavirus Pandemic and American Neoliberalism." *Geographical Review* 111 (4): 496–509.

Waring, Marilyn. 1988. *If Women Counted: A New Feminist Economics*. San Francisco: Harper & Row.

1999. *Counting for Nothing: What Men Value and What Women Are Worth*. Wellington, NZ: Allen & Unwin.

2003. "Counting for Something! Recognising Women's Contribution to the Global Economy through Alternative Accounting Systems." *Gender & Development* 11 (1): 35–43.

2018. *Still Counting: Wellbeing, Women's Work and Policy-Making*. Wellington, NZ: Bridget Williams Books.

Warren, Emma, Bradley H. Curtis, Nan Jia, and R. Wendell Evans. 2016. "The Caries Management System: Updating Cost-effectiveness with 4-Year Posttrial Data." *International Journal of Technology Assessment in Health Care* 32 (3): 107–115.

Warren, Emma, Christine Pollicino, Bradley Curtis, Wendell Evans, Alexandra Sbaraini, and Eli Schwarz. 2010. "Modeling the Long-Term Cost-Effectiveness of the Caries Management System in an Australian Population." *JVAL Value in Health* 13 (6): 750–760.

Warrington, Keith. 2006. "Acts and the Healing Narratives: Why?" *Journal of Pentecostal Theology* 14 (2): 189–217.

Waszek, Norbert. 1984. "Two Concepts of Morality: A Distinction of Adam Smith's Ethics and Its Stoic Origin." *Journal of the History of Ideas* 45 (4): 591–606. https://doi.org/10.2307/2709375. www.jstor.org/stable/2709375.

Waterman, Anthony Michael Charles. 2002. "Economics as Theology: Adam Smith's Wealth of Nations." *Southern Economic Journal* 68 (4): 907–921.

2004. *Political Economy and Christian Theology since the Enlightenment: Essays in Intellectual History*. Basingstoke: Palgrave Macmillan.

Weale, Albert. 2015. "Reflecting on 'Are Health Problems Systemic? Politics of Access and Choice under Beveridge and Bismarck Systems'." *Health Economics, Policy and Law* 10 (4): 431–435.

Weale, Albert, and Sarah Clark. 2010. "Co-payments in the NHS: An Analysis of the Normative Arguments." *Health Economics, Policy and Law* 5 (2): 225–246.

Weeks, Jane C., E. Francis Cook, Steven J. O'Day, Lynn M. Peterson, Neil Wenger, Douglas Reding, Frank E. Harrell, Peter Kussin, Neil V. Dawson, Jr Alfred F. Connors, Joanne Lynn, and Russell S. Phillips. 1998. "Relationship between Cancer Patients' Predictions of Prognosis and Their Treatment Preferences." *JAMA* 279 (21): 1709–1714.

Weil, Max Harry. 1989. "Alternatives to Rationing." In *Rationing of Medical Care for the Critically Ill*, edited by Martin A Strosberg, I Alan Fein and James D Carroll. Washington, DC: Brookings Institution.

Weinfeld, Moshe. 1990. "The Charge of Hypocrisy in Matthew 23 and in Jewish Sources." *Immanuel* 24/25: 52–58.

1995. *Social Justice in Ancient Israel and in the Ancient Near East*. Jerusalem; Minneapolis: The Magnes Press/The Hebrew Univ Fortress Press.

Welby, Justin. 2016. "National Life: Shared Values and Public Policy Priorities." *Hansard – House of Lords* 777 (2 December): 415–421.

2017. *Dethroning Mammon: Making Money Serve Grace (the Archbishop of Canterbury's Lent book 2017)*. London: Bloomsbury.

2018. "Archbishop of Canterbury's Speech at the Trades Union Congress – 12 September, 2018." www.archbishopofcanterbury.org/speaking-and-writing/speeches/archbishop-canterburys-speech-tuc.

Welch, H. Gilbert, Lisa Schwartz, and Steve Woloshin. 2011. *Overdiagnosed: Making People Sick in the Pursuit of Health*. Boston, MA: Beacon Press.

Wendt, Claus, and Jürgen Kohl. 2010. "Translating Monetary Inputs into Health Care Provision: A Comparative Analysis of the Impact of Different Modes of Public Policy." *Journal of Comparative Policy Analysis: Research and Practice* 12 (1): 11–31.

Wenell, Karen J. 2017. "Kingdom, Not Kingly Rule: Assessing the Kingdom of God as Sacred Space." *Biblical Interpretation* 25 (2): 206–233.

Wenham, Gordon J. 2000. *Story as Torah: Reading Old Testament Ethically*. Edinburgh: T & T Clark.

Wennberg, John E., Benjamin A. Barnes, and Michael Zubkoff. 1982. "Professional Uncertainty and the Problem of Supplier-Induced Demand." *Social Science & Medicine* 16 (7): 811–824.

Wennberg, John E., and Megan M. Cooper. 1996. *The Dartmouth Atlas of Health Care*. Hanover, NH: The Center for the Evaluative Clinical Sciences, Dartmouth Medical School.

Wennberg, John E., Jean L. Freeman, and William J. Culp. 1987. "Are Hospital Services Rationed in New Haven or Over-Utilised in Boston?" *The Lancet* 8543 (May 23): 1185–1188.

West, Michael A. 2021. *Compassionate Leadership: Sustaining Wisdom, Humanity and Presence in Health and Social Care*. Sidcup: Swirling Leaf Press.

West, Traci C. 2006. *Disruptive Christian Ethics: When Racism and Women's Lives Matter*. Louisville, KY: Westminster John Knox Press.

Whaley, Christopher. 2018. "The Association between Provider Price and Complication Rates for Outpatient Surgical Services." *Journal of General Internal Medicine* 33 (8): 1352–1358.

White, Ben, Lindy Willmott, and Eliana Close. 2020. "Futile, Non-beneficial, Potentially Inappropriate or 'Disputed' Treatment." In *Contemporary European Perspectives on the Ethics of End of Life Care*, edited by Nathan Emmerich, Pierre Mallia, Bert Gordijn and Francesca Pistoia, 181–198. Cham, Switzerland: Springer.

White, Ben, Lindy Willmott, Eliana Close, and Jocelyn Downie. 2017. "Withholding and Withdrawing Potentially Life-Sustaining Treatment: Who Should Decide?" In *Tensions and Traumas in Health Law*, edited by Ian Freckelton and Kerry Petersen. Annandale: Federation Press.

White, Ben, Lindy Willmott, Eliana Close, Nicole Shepherd, Cindy Gallois, Malcolm H. Parker, Sarah Winch, Nicholas Graves, and Leonie K. Callaway. 2016. "What Does Futility Mean? An Empirical Study of Doctors Perceptions." *Medical Journal of Australia* 204 (8): 318.e1–318.e5.

White, William D., ed. 2003. *Compelled by Data – John D Thompson: Nurse, Health Services Researcher, and Health Administration Educator*. New Haven: Department of Epidemiology and Public Health, Yale University.

Whitehead, Sarah J., and Shehzad Ali. 2010. "Health Outcomes in Economic Evaluation: the QALY and Utilities." *British Medical Bulletin* 96 (1): 5–21.

Whitford, Andrew B. 2008. "The Policy Implications of Economic Reasoning: What We Do Not Know about Moral Hazard in Health Policy." *Evidence & Policy* 4 (1): 69–73.

Whittaker, Brooke A., Deborah R. Gillum, and Judith M. Kelly. 2018. "Burnout, Moral Distress, and Job Turnover in Critical Care Nurses." *International Journal of Studies in Nursing* 3 (3): 108–121.

Wieseler, Beate, Natalie McGauran, and Thomas Kaiser. 2019. "New Drugs: Where Did We Go Wrong and What Can We Do Better?" *BMJ* 366: l4340.

Wight, Jonathan B. 2005. "Adam Smith and Greed." *Journal of Private Enterprise* 21 (1): 46–58.

Wildavsky, Aaron. 1961. "Political Implications of Budgetary Reform." *Public Administration Review* 21 (4): 183–190.

1966. "The Political Economy of Efficiency: Cost-Benefit Analysis, Systems Analysis, and Program Budgeting." *Public Administration Review* 26 (4): 292–310.

1979. *Speaking Truth to Power: The Art and Craft of Policy Analysis*. Boston, MA: Little Brown and Co.

1988. *The New Politics of the Budgetary Process*. Glenview, IL: Scott Foresman.

Wiley, Lindsay F., Micah L. Berman, and Doug Blanke. 2013. "Who's Your Nanny? Choice, Paternalism and Public Health in the Age of Personal Responsibility." *Journal of Law, Medicine & Ethics* 41 (S1): 88–91.

Wilkinson, Iain. 2005. *Suffering: A Sociological Introduction*. Cambridge: Polity.

Wilkinson, Richard G., and Kate Pickett. 2010. *The Spirit Level: Why Equality Is Better for Everyone*. London: Penguin.

Williams, Alan. 1974. "Need as a Demand Concept (with Special Reference to Health)." In *Economic Problems and Social Goals: Aspects of Public Choice*, edited by A. J. Culyer, 60–76. London: Martin Robertson.

1992. "Cost-Effectiveness Analysis: Is It Ethical?" *Journal of Medical Ethics* 18 (1): 7–11.

1993. "Some Methodological Issues in the Use of Cost-Benefit Analysis in Health Care." In *Public and International Economics: Essays in Honour of Professor Hirofumi Shibata*, edited by Ali M. El-Agraa, 42–58. Basingstoke: St. Martin's Press.

1995. *The Measurement and Valuation of Health: A Chronicle*. University of York (York): Centre for Health Economics. https://core.ac.uk/download/pdf/6406540.pdf.

1997a. "Health Economics: The Cheerful Face of the Dismal Science." In *Being Reasonable about the Economics of Health: Selected Essays by Alan Williams*, edited by A. J. Culyer and A. Maynard, 371. London: Edward Elgar.

1997b. "Intergenerational Equity: An Exploration of the 'Fair Innings' Argument." *Health Economics* 6 (2): 117–132.

2001. "How Economics Could Extend the Scope of Ethical Discourse." *Journal of Medical Ethics* 27 (4): 251–255.

Williams, Bernard. 1973. "A Critique of Utilitarianism." In *Utilitarianism: For and Against*, edited by John Jamieson Carswell Smart and Bernard Williams, 77–150. Cambridge: Cambridge University Press.

Williams, Colin C., and Adrian V. Horodnic. 2017. "Rethinking Informal Payments by Patients in Europe: An Institutional Approach." *Health Policy* 121 (10): 1053–1062.

Williams, Rowan. 2012. "Making Moral Decisions." In *The Cambridge Companion to Christian Ethics*, edited by Robin Gill, 3–15. Cambridge: Cambridge University Press.

2015. *Faith in the Public Square*. London: Bloomsbury Continuum.

Williamson, Oliver Eaton. 1975. *Markets and Hierarchies: Analysis and Antitrust Implications*. New York: The Free Press.

1986. *Economic Organization: Firms, Markets and Policy Control*. Hemel Hempstead, England: Wheatsheaf Books Ltd.

2002. "The Theory of the Firm as Governance Structure: From Choice to Contract." *Journal of Economic Perspectives* 16 (3): 171–195.

Willing, Esther, Sarah-Jane Paine, Emma Wyeth, Braden Te Ao, Rhema Vaithianathan, and Papaarangi Reid. 2020. "Indigenous Voices on

Measuring and Valuing Health States." *AlterNative: An International Journal of Indigenous Peoples* 16 (1): 3–9.

Willis, Evan. 1983. *Medical Dominance: The Division of Labour in Australian Health care*. Sydney: Allen & Unwin.

Wilson, James Maxwell Glover, Gunnar Jungner, and World Health Organization. 1968. *Principles and Practice of Screening for Disease. Public Health Papers*. Geneva: World Health Organization.

Wilson, Matt. 2012. *Concrete Faith: The Inside Story of the Eden Network*. Manchester: Message Trust Publications.

Wilson, Michael, Adrian Guta, Kerry Waddell, John Lavis, Robert Reid, and Cara Evans. 2020. "The Impacts of Accountable Care Organizations on Patient Experience, Health Outcomes and Costs: A Rapid Review." *Journal of Health Services Research & Policy* 25 (2): 130–138.

Wilson, Nathan, Ian Couper, Elma de Vries, Steve Reid, Therese J. Fish, and Ben Marais. 2009. "A Critical Review of Interventions to Redress the Inequitable Distribution Of." *Rural and Remote Health* 9 (2): 1060.

Wilson, Rodney. 1997. *Economics, Ethics, and Religion: Jewish, Christian, and Muslim Economic Thought*. New York: New York University Press.

Wilson, Tom, Yuejen Zhao, and John Condon. 2019. "Limited Progress in Closing the Mortality Gap for Aboriginal and Torres Strait Islander Australians of the Northern Territory." *Australian and New Zealand Journal of Public Health* 43 (4): 340–345.

Winant, Gabriel. 2021. *The Next Shift: The Fall of Industry and the Rise of Health Care in Rust Belt America*. Cambridge, MA: Harvard University Press.

Wink, Walter. 1979. "The Parable of the Compassionate Samaritan: A Communal Exegesis Approach." *Review & Expositor* 76 (2): 199–217.

Wiseman, Virginia, Craig Mitton, Mary M. Doyle-Waters, Tom Drake, Lesong Conteh, Anthony T. Newall, Obinna Onwujekwe, and Stephen Jan. 2016. "Using Economic Evidence to Set Healthcare Priorities in Low-Income and Lower-Middle-Income Countries: A Systematic Review of Methodological Frameworks." 25 (S1): 140–161.

Witte, John, and Justin J. Latterell. 2015. "Christianity and Human Rights: Past Contributions and Future Challenges." *Journal of Law and Religion* 30 (3): 353–385.

Wolfe, Alan. 1998. *One Nation, after All: What Middle-Class Americans Really Think About: God, Country, Family, Racism, Welfare, Immigration, Homosexuality, Work, the Right, the Left, and Each Other*. New York: Viking.

Wolfe, Barbara, William Evans, and Teresa E. Seeman, eds. 2012. *The Biological Consequences of Socioeconomic Inequalities*. New York: Russell Sage Foundation.

Wolterstorff, Nicholas. 2008. *Justice: Rights and Wrongs*. Princeton: Princeton University Press.

Woods, Beth, Aimée Fox, Mark Sculpher, and Karl Claxton. 2021. "Estimating the Shares of the Value of Branded Pharmaceuticals Accruing to Manufacturers and to Patients Served by Health Systems." *Health Economics* 30 (11): 2649–2666.

Woods, Beth, Paul Revill, Mark Sculpher, and Karl Claxton. 2016. "Country-Level Cost-Effectiveness Thresholds: Initial Estimates and the Need for Further Research." *Value in Health* 19 (8): 929–935.

Workman, Stephen, Patricia McKeever, William Harvey, and Peter A. Singer. 2003. "Intensive Care Nurses' and Physicians' Experiences with Demands for Treatment: Some Implications for Clinical Practice." *Journal of Critical Care* 18 (1): 17–21.

Worland, Stephen T. 1991. "The Preferential Option, Pope Pius XI, and the Foundations of Social Economics." *Review of Social Economy* 49 (4): 611–627.

World Health Organization. 2001. *International Classification of Functioning, Disability and Health*. Geneva: WHO.

2010. *The World Health Report 2010: Health Systems Financing: The Path to Universal Coverage*. Geneva: WHO.

2014. *Making Fair Choices on the Path to Universal Health Coverage: Final Report of the WHO Consultative Group on Equity and Universal Health Coverage*. Geneva: WHO.

2019. *Health Taxes: A Primer*. Geneva: WHO.

Worline, Monica C., and Jane E. Dutton. 2017. "How Leaders Shape Compassion Processes in Organizations." In *The Oxford Handbook of Compassion Science*, edited by Emma M Seppälä, Emiliana Simon-Thomas, Stephanie L Brown, Monica C Worline, C Daryl Cameron and James R Doty, 435–456. Oxford: Oxford University Press.

Wouters, Sofie, Job van Exel, Rachel Baker, and Werner B. F. Brouwer. 2017. "Priority to End of Life Treatments? Views of the Public in the Netherlands." *Value in Health* 20 (1): 107–117.

Wright, Tom. 2014. *Luke for Everyone*. London: SPCK.

Yeung, C. Albert. 2008. "A Systematic Review of the Efficacy and Safety of Fluoridation." *Evidence-Based Dentistry* 9 (2): 39–43.

Young, Gary J., and Douglas A. Conrad. 2007. "Practical Issues in the Design and Implementation of Pay-for-Quality Programs." *Journal of Healthcare Management* 52 (1): 10–18.

Yuan, Beibei, Li He, Qingyue Meng, and Liying Jia. 2017. "Payment Methods for Outpatient Care Facilities." *Cochrane Database of Systematic Reviews* 3 (CD011153): 1–86.

Yuan, Yaqi. 2021. "Public Satisfaction with Health Care System in 30 Countries: The Effects of Individual Characteristics and Social Contexts." *Health Policy* 125 (10): 1359–1366.

Yuengert, Andrew M. 1999. "The Uses of Economics in Papal Encyclicals." In *Religion and Economics: Normative Social Theory*, edited by James M. Dean and Andrew Michael Charles Waterman, 33–50. Dordrecht: Kluwer Academic.

Yunus, Muhammad, Cam Donaldson, and Jean-Luc Perron. 2020. "COVID-19 Vaccines a Global Common Good." *The Lancet Healthy Longevity* 1 (1): e6–e8.

Zaerpour, Farzad, Diane P. Bischak, Mozart B. C. Menezes, Andrew McRae, and Eddy S. Lang. 2020. "Patient Classification Based on Volume and Case-Mix in the Emergency Department and Their Association with Performance." *Health Care Management Science* 23 (3): 387–400

Zajac, Edward E. 2001. *Political Economy of Fairness*. Cambridge: MIT Press.

Zaresani, Arezou, and Anthony Scott. 2021. "Is the Evidence on the Effectiveness of Pay for Performance Schemes in Healthcare Changing? Evidence from a Meta-Regression Analysis." *BMC Health Services Research* 21 (175): 1–10.

Zeitoun, Mark. 2008. *Power and Water in the Middle East: The Hidden Politics of the Palestinian-Israeli Water Conflict*. London: IB Tauris.

Zink, Jesse. 2017. "Five Marks of Mission: History, Theology, Critique." *Journal of Anglican Studies* 15 (2): 144–166.

Zohar, Danah. 2005. "Spiritually Intelligent Leadership." *Leader to Leader* 2005 (38): 45–51.

Zohar, Danah, and Ian Marshall. 2000. *Spiritual Intelligence: The Ultimate Intelligence*. London: Bloomsbury.

Zuvekas, Samuel H., and Joel W. Cohen. 2016. "Fee-for-Service, While Much Maligned, Remains the Dominant Payment Method for Physician Visits." *Health Affairs* 35 (3): 411–414.

Zvi, Ehud Ben. 1992. "The Dialogue between Abraham and Yhwh in Gen. 18.23–32: A Historical-Critical Analysis." *Journal for the Study of the Old Testament* 17 (53): 27–46.

Zweifel, Peter. 2019. "Do Health System Reforms Stand a Chance?" *Economic Affairs* 39 (2): 232–242.

Zweig, Stefan. 1939. *Beware of Pity*. London: Cassell.

Index

TITLES PUBLISHED IN THE SERIES (*continued from page iii*)

14. *The Market Economy and Christian Ethics*, Peter Sedgwick
15. *Churchgoing and Christian Ethics*, Robin Gill
16. *Inequality and Christian Ethics*, Douglas Hicks
17. *Biology and Christian Ethics*, Stephen Clark
18. *Altruism and Christian Ethics*, Colin Grant
19. *The Public Forum and Christian Ethics*, Robert Gascoigne
20. *Evil and Christian Ethics*, Gordon Graham
21. *Living Together and Christian Ethics*, Adrian Thatcher
22. *The Common Good and Christian Ethics*, David Hollenbach
23. *Self-Love and Christian Ethics*, Darlene Fozard Weaver
24. *Economic Compulsion and Christian Ethics*, Albino Barrera
25. *Genetics and Christian Ethics*, Celia Deane-Drummond
26. *Health Care and Christian Ethics*, Robin Gill
27. *Alcohol, Addiction and Christian Ethics*, Christopher C. H. Cook
28. *Human Evolution and Christian Ethics*, Stephen J. Pope
29. *Media Violence and Christian Ethics*, Jolyon Mitchell
30. *Forgiveness and Christian Ethics*, Anthony Bash
31. *Market Complicity and Christian Ethics*, Albino Barrera
32. *Global Justice, Christology and Christian Ethics*, Lisa Sowle Cahill
33. *Moral Passion and Christian Ethics*, Robin Gill
34. *Hope and Christian Ethics*, David Elliot
35. *Human Dependency and Christian Ethics*, Sandra Sullivan-Dunbar
36. *Biotechnology, Human Nature, and Christian Ethics*, Gerald McKenny
37. *Lying and Christian Ethics*, Christopher O. Tollefsen
38. *Science and Christian Ethics*, Paul Scherz
39. *Gender and Christian Ethics*, Adrian Thatcher